Pediatric Patient Safety
and Quality Improvement

Pediatric Patient Safety and Quality Improvement

Karen S. Frush, MD

Professor of Pediatrics
Division of Pediatric Hospital and Emergency Medicine
Duke Children's Hospital
Durham, North Carolina

Steven E. Krug, MD

Professor of Pediatrics
Head, Division of Emergency Medicine
Ann & Robert H. Lurie Children's Hospital of Chicago
Northwestern University Feinberg School of Medicine
Chicago, Illinois

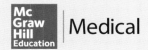 Medical

New York   Chicago   San Francisco   Athens   London   Madrid   Mexico City
Milan   New Delhi   Singapore   Sydney   Toronto

Pediatric Patient Safety and Quality Improvement

1 2 3 4 5 6 7 8 9 0 CTP/CTP 19 18 17 16 15 14

ISBN 978-0-07-182736-2
MHID 0-07-182736-6

This book was set in Minion Pro by Thomson Digital.
The editors were Alyssa K. Fried and Peter J. Boyle.
The production supervisor was Catherine H. Saggese.
Project management was provided by Ritu Joon, Thomson Digtal.
China Translation & Printing Services, Ltd. was printer and binder.

This book was printed on acid-free paper.

Library of Congress Cataloging-in-Publication Data

Pediatric patient safety and quality improvement / editors, Karen Frush, Steven E. Krug.
   p. ; cm.
  Includes bibliographical references and index.
  ISBN 978-0-07-182736-2 (alk. paper)—ISBN 0-07-182736-6 (alk. paper)
  I. Frush, Karen, editor. II. Krug, Steven E., editor.
  [DNLM: 1. Patient Safety. 2. Medical Errors—prevention & control. 3. Pediatrics.
4. Quality Improvement. WX 185]
  R729.8
  363.15--dc23
                                                                    2014027057

McGraw-Hill Education books are available at special quantity discounts to use as premiums and sales promotions, or for use in corporate training programs. To contact a representative please visit the Contact Us pages at www.mhprofessional.com.

Contents

Contributors vii

Preface ix

Chapter 1
Quality Improvement Methods and Improvement Science 1
Binita Patel and Joan Shook

Chapter 2
Applying Quality Improvement in Practice 27
David B. Cooperberg and Alex R. Kemper

Chapter 3
Medical Errors, Adverse Events, and Human Factors 49
John M. Brookey and Doug Bonacum

Chapter 4
Pediatric Medication Safety 73
Lori Kotsonis-Chiampas, Janice Nuuhiwa, and Steven E. Krug

Chapter 5
The Role of Leadership in Safe and Reliable Pediatric Care 103
Allan Frankel and Michael Leonard

Chapter 6
Teamwork and Communication 129
Kyle J. Rehder, Susan M. Hohenhaus, and Heidi B. King

Chapter 7
The Importance of Information Technology in Pediatric patient Safety 157
Eric Tham

Chapter 8
Engaging Patients and Families 181
Leigh Ann Simmons, Sorrel King, and Karen S. Frush

Chapter 9
Special Perspectives for Neonates 205
Chris DeRienzo

Chapter 10
**Professional Accountability and
Pursuit of a Culture of Safety** 239
Gerald B. Hickson and Ilene N. Moore

Index *291*

Contributors

Doug Bonacum, MBA
Vice President
Quality, Patient Safety, and
 Resource Management
Kaiser Permanente
Oakland, California
Chapter 3

John M. Brookey, MD
Assistant Medical Director
Quality, Risk Management, Patient
 Safety
Southern California Permanente
 Medical Group
Pasadena, California
Chapter 3

David B. Cooperberg, MD
Department of Pediatrics
St. Christopher's Hospital for Children
Drexel University College of Medicine
Section of Hospital Medicine
Philadelphia, Pennsylvania
Chapter 2

Chris DeRienzo, MD, MPP
Fellow
Neonatal-Perinatal Medicine
Duke University Health System
Durham, North Carolina
Chapter 9

Allan Frankel, MD
Co-Chief Medical Officer
Pascal Metrics
Washington, DC
Chapter 5

Karen S. Frush, MD
Professor of Pediatrics
Division of Pediatric Hospital and
Emergency Medicine
Duke Children's Hospital
Durham, North Carolina
Chapter 8

Gerald B. Hickson, MD
The Center for Patient and
 Professional Advocacy
Vanderbilt University Medical Center
Nashville, Tennessee
Chapter 10

Susan M. Hohenhaus, LPD, RN, CEN
Executive Director
Emergency Nurses Association
Des Plaines, Illinois
Chapter 6

Alex R. Kemper, MD, MPH, MS
Department of Pediatrics
Duke University School of Medicine
Durham, North Carolina
Chapter 2

Heidi B. King, MS
Director
Department of Defense Patient
 Safety Program
Defense Health Agency
Clinical Support Division
Falls Church, Virginia
Chapter 6

Sorrel King
Josie King Foundation
Baltimore, Maryland
Chapter 8

Lori Kotsonis-Chiampas, PharmD
Medication Safety Coordinator
Department of Pharmacy
Ann & Robert H. Lurie Children's
  Hospital of Chicago
Chicago, Illinois
Chapter 4

Steven E. Krug, MD
Professor of Pediatrics
Head, Division of Emergency
  Medicine
Ann & Robert H. Lurie Children's
  Hospital of Chicago
Northwestern University
  Feinberg School of Medicine
Chicago, Illinois
Chapter 4

Michael Leonard, MD
Co-Chief Medical Officer
Pascal Metrics
Adjunct Professor of Medicine
Duke University
Washington, DC
Chapter 5

Ilene N. Moore, MD, JD
The Center for Patient and
  Professional Advocacy
Vanderbilt University Medical Center
Nashville, Tennessee
Chapter 10

**Janice Nuuhiwa, RN, MSN,
APN/CNS, CPHON®**
Staff Development Specialist
Hematology/Oncology/Stem Cell
  Transplant Division
Ann & Robert H. Lurie Children's
  Hospital of Chicago
Chicago, Illinois
Chapter 4

Binita Patel, MD
Assistant Professor
Pediatrics
Baylor College of Medicine
Texas Children's Hospital
Houston, Texas
Chapter 1

Kyle J. Rehder, MD
Assistant Professor
Division of Pediatric Critical Care
Duke Children's Hospital
Durham, North Carolina
Chapter 6

Joan Shook, MD, MBA
Professor
Pediatrics
Baylor College of Medicine
Texas Children's Hospital
Houston, Texas
Chapter 1

Leigh Ann Simmons, PhD
Duke University School of Nursing
Durham, North Carolina
Chapter 8

Eric Tham, MD, MS
Associate Professor of Pediatrics
Section of Pediatric Emergency
  Medicine
Department of Pediatrics
University of Colorado School of
  Medicine
Director of Research Informatics
The Research Institute
Children's Hospital Colorado
Denver, Colorado
Chapter 7

Preface

Over the past decade, our understanding of patient safety and quality improvement in healthcare has matured, and we have come a long way since the publication of the sentinel Institute of Medicine reports *To Err is Human* and *Crossing the Quality Chasm* at the turn of the millennium. The body of literature has grown, books have been published, and careers launched, as numerous healthcare professionals and leaders, researchers and patient advocates have sought to contribute to the quality improvement and patient safety movement.

We are pleased to offer this book, which is one of the first to provide a view of patient safety and quality improvement with a specific focus on the pediatric population. The book addresses important topics in pediatric patient safety and quality improvement from the perspective of scholars, from clinicians who provide front-line care to children, and from the broad, systems-based perspective of national patient safety leaders and leaders in pediatric care.

Included in these pages are examples of scientifically driven principles, best practices and lessons learned from individual providers, and healthcare systems and communities that have researched and applied improvement methods in the setting of pediatric care. We hope this book is helpful to students and educators in the healthcare professions, to pediatric training programs and practicing clinicians, and to leaders of patient safety programs and pediatric care delivery systems. We believe that, by adopting and implementing these best practices, hospitals and healthcare professionals can achieve safer care and make meaningful changes that will support long-lasting improvements in care delivery to the children and families they are privileged to serve.

QUALITY IMPROVEMENT METHODS AND IMPROVEMENT SCIENCE

1

INTRODUCTION

Science of Improvement

W. Edwards Deming, a statistics professor and physicist, is often considered the father of quality improvement. In the 1950s, Deming helped the Japanese manufacturing industry redefine quality control. His beliefs of cooperation, mistakes as opportunities for improvement, and striving for continual improvement helped the Japanese improve their production process and product quality while reducing costs. Recognizing the success of the Japanese manufacturing industry, in the 1970s, American industries began adopting his theories of management and quality. Finally, during the 1990s, his theories trickled into healthcare improvement efforts. Utilizing these quality improvement methods, healthcare industry leaders, such as Intermountain Healthcare and Geisinger Health System, have now demonstrated improved efficiencies and effectiveness of healthcare processes and outcomes.

Poor outcomes or poor quality are often not the result of bad people. Instead, as Paul Batalden notes, "every system is perfectly designed to achieve exactly the results that it achieves." Critical to improvement is introducing change to a process or system. Often, subject matter knowledge gathered through training and experience will help develop the ideas for change that can then be tested and implemented. For example, to improve care, a team may develop disease-based care guidelines to be instituted on the basis of literature and practical experience. However, for successful adoption, a broader understanding of knowledge and change is required.

Deming described another form of knowledge, called a "system of profound knowledge," that is instrumental in developing effective change and thereby improvement. His theory is composed of four components. The first is an appreciation of a system. The healthcare industry is a complex system of interactions. To accurately assess the impact of changes on the system, an understanding is needed of the interdependencies and relationships among all of the components of the system—doctors, nurses, ancillary staff, patients, treatments, diagnostic tests, and location of care, to name a few. The second component is an understanding of variation. Variation is inherent in every system. A lack of appreciation of variation and its causes will lead to mistakes in dealing with the variation. Individuals may see trends where there are no trends or may try to explain natural or random variation as special events. A fundamental understanding of variation is needed to develop appropriate actions for processes. Building knowledge is the third component to Deming's theory of profound knowledge. In quality improvement, a change represents a prediction. It is predicted that if the change is made, an improvement will result. The more knowledge one has about the current system, the more "accurate" the prediction will be and result in improvement. If the changes do not lead to improvement, the process can be reviewed and the theory modified with new ideas for changes. These iterative cycles of learning by making changes and observing or measuring the results form the foundation of improvement. The final component of profound knowledge is the understanding of the human side of change, how people interact with each other and with the system. Change invariably is difficult and the resistance to change is often encountered in improvement projects. Effective improvement efforts plan for this change resistance by involving affected individuals in the improvement process itself, by communicating rationales for changes, and by using intrinsic motivation factors for reward and recognition. The four components of Deming's theory of profound knowledge do not exist in isolation. Understanding and appreciating their interactions with each other enables true improvement.[1]

QUALITY IMPROVEMENT METHODS

Many quality improvement methods were adapted from continuous quality improvement theories developed by the manufacturing industry. They allow for testing, implementing, and disseminating change through methodical evaluation of the workings of a system. There are numerous approaches or frameworks that improvement teams may employ. Fundamentally, each methodology asks improvement teams to identify a problem, measure the problem, develop interventions to fix the problems, and finally test the created interventions for success. This chapter introduces three common methodologies used for improvement: the Model for Improvement, Lean, and Six Sigma.

MODEL FOR IMPROVEMENT

The Model for Improvement is a simple, yet powerful method for rapid quality improvement introduced by Tom Nolan and Lloyd Provost. It provides a framework for developing, testing, implementing, and spreading changes that can lead to operational efficiencies, revenue enhancement, and improvement in patient care. Improvement efforts can be directed toward processes, products, and services and even one's own personal endeavors (eg, New Year's resolutions). The model begins with three essential questions and then utilizes "plan, do, study, act" (PDSA) cycles to incorporate and study changes (Figure 1-1).[2]

What Are We Trying To Accomplish?

The first step in the improvement journey is to identify what is to be accomplished. This involves creating an aim statement. Aim statements help anchor efforts to a common purpose. In addition, they refocus and redirect efforts when teams stray due to distractions and unwanted variations. Aim statements can be placed into project charters (formal documents) or placed into informal team tools (eg, whiteboard).

Some keys to success when using this methodology include the following:

1. Creating an effective aim statement using the SMART mnemonic.

   Specific: Aims should be written simply and clearly define the system to be improved, the affected patient population, and the approaches to improvement. It defines the what, why, and how of the project.

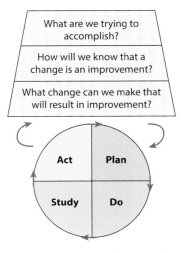

Figure 1-1 ▪ Model for improvement. (Reproduced, with permission, from Langley G, Moen RD, Nolan KM, et al. *The Improvement Guide*. San Francisco, CA: Jossey-Bass; 2009.)

Measurable: Aims should be measurable with detailed numerical goals for improvement. This specificity will aid in creating urgency for change and help focus measurements used in the improvement effort.

Attainable: Aims should be attainable and realistic. They should stretch the team's efforts but should not be so extreme that they cannot be achieved.

Relevant: Choose aims that matter and will garner support due to their relevance. Choose conditions that frequently occur and have great impact on patients. Relevant aims will help teams gather resources that will be required to achieve the goals.

Time bound: Aims should be linked to a time frame with a target date.

EXAMPLES

"During the year (*time bound*), to provide effective care (*specific, relevant*), using an asthma visit checklist (*specific*), at least 90% of patients (*measurable, attainable*) with persistent asthma (*specific*) will be treated with preventative medicines."

"By redesigning the medication administration process (*specific*), we will decrease medication administration errors (*relevant*) by 25% (*measurable, attainable*) by August 2009 (*time bound*)."

2. Once aim statements have been created, teams should avoid "aim drift," where teams retreat deliberately or unconsciously from set goals. It is important to reiterate the aim statement and progress toward that aim throughout the improvement process.
3. Teams may need to refocus the aim during the course of the project. To achieve a system-level goal, initial aims can first target a smaller part of the system with a more focused goal. Once that is achieved, a broader aim can be set.

EXAMPLE

1. "To improve timeliness of care, with the implementation of the new triage process, we will decrease the door to doctor time for all patients presenting to the emergency department by 50% within 6 months of implementation."

   Aim drift: "To improve timeliness of care, with the implementation of the new triage process, we will decrease the door to doctor time for all patients presenting to the emergency department by 30% within 6 months of implementation."

   Refocused aim: "We will decrease the door to doctor time for *level II acuity patients* presenting to the emergency department by 25% within 3 months of implementation."

Table 1-1 **MEASURES: RESEARCH VERSUS PROCESS IMPROVEMENT**		
	Measurement for Research	Measurement for Learning and Process Improvement
Purpose	To discover new knowledge	To bring new knowledge into daily practice
Tests	One large "blind" test	Many sequential, observable tests
Biases	Control for as many biases as possible	Stabilize the biases from test to test
Data	Gather as much data as possible, "just in case"	Gather "just enough" data to learn and complete another cycle
Duration	Can take long periods of time to obtain results	"Small tests of significant changes" accelerate the rate of improvement

Source: Reproduced with permission of the Institute for Healthcare Improvement.[11]

How Will We Know That a Change Is an Improvement?

The second focus of the Model for Improvement involves the creation of measures. Clearly defined measures allow teams to determine the impact of their efforts on testing and implementing change. It is important to remember that the purpose of measuring is to learn and not to judge or draw comparisons, unlike in traditional research (Table 1-1).

There are three major types of quality improvement measures— outcome, process, and balance measures. Every project should include all three types to create a balanced set for monitoring the progress of improvement.[2,3]

1. Outcome measures: Outcome measures define the performance of the system and relate directly to the aim of the project. They encompass the values of the patients.
2. Process measures: Process measures help determine whether an activity has been accomplished—these are the steps in a process working in the intended manner. These measures often help track the progress of the project.
3. Balance measures: Balance measures follow unintended consequences of changes being tested. They also represent other factors that may influence outcome measures, also known as confounders in traditional research methodologies.

EXAMPLE

1. Improving patient handoff of care using a standardized approach and checklist.

   Outcome measure: safety events from a poor handoff
   Process measure: percentage of handoffs that used a standardized approach
   Balance measure: time required to complete handoff process using a new checklist, staff satisfaction with a new process

2. Improving same-day sick visit clinic appointments.

   Outcome measure: percentage of patients receiving same-day sick visit appointments
   Process measure: number of hours available for sick visit appointments per provider
   Balance measure: number of denied well-child visits

When creating measures, teams should define both project-level (global measures) and cycle-level measures. Global measures should be followed throughout the project, whereas cycle-level measures can be used to monitor progress of specific PDSA cycles. For example, for the above-mentioned aim statement regarding improving door to doctor times for the emergency department, the global measure would be time from arrival to time seen by a physician. One specific PDSA cycle could focus on improving the triage process and use the time from arrival to triage completion as a cycle measure.

What Changes Can We Make That Will Result in Improvement?

Change concepts in quality improvement represent general notions or ideas for change that are believed to result in improvement. These concepts can stem from critical appraisal of the current system to evidence-based practices to a patient suggestion. With the aim defined, the improvement team can use change concepts to develop, test, and implement ideas. While "all improvements will require change, not all change will result in improvement".[2] Langley and colleagues identified more than 70 change concepts, which can be grouped into several key categories (Table 1-2).[2]

1. Eliminate waste: Waste represents any activity or resource that does not add value to the "customer" (ie, the patient). Lean methodology, a quality improvement strategy often used for process improvement, seeks to eliminate seven key wastes, known by the Japanese word "muda" (Table 1-3).

Table 1-2 **CHANGE CONCEPTS**	
Change Concept	Examples
Eliminate waste	• Eliminate things that are not used • Eliminate multiple entry • Reduce or eliminate overkill • Reduce controls on the system • Recycle or reuse • Use substitution • Reduce classifications • Remove intermediaries • Match the amount to the need • Use sampling • Change targets or set points
Improve work flow	• Synchronize • Schedule into multiple processes • Minimize handoffs • Move steps in the process close together • Find and remove bottlenecks • Use automation • Smooth workflow • Do tasks in parallel • Consider people as in the same system • Use multiple processing units • Adjust to peak demand
Optimize inventory	• Match inventory to predicted demand • Use pull systems • Reduce choice of features • Reduce multiple brands of same item
Change the work environment	• Give people access to information • Use proper measurements • Take care of basics • Reduce demotivating aspects of pay system • Conduct training • Implement cross-training • Invest more resources in improvement • Focus on core processes and purpose • Share risks • Emphasize natural and logical consequences • Develop alliance/cooperative relationships

(Continued)

Table 1-2 **CHANGE CONCEPTS** *(Continued)*	
Change Concept	**Examples**
Enhance the provider/ customer relationship	• Listen to customers • Coach customers to use product/service • Focus on the outcome to a customer • Use a coordinator • Reach agreement on expectations • Outsource for "free" • Optimize level of inspection • Work with suppliers
Manage time	• Reduce setup or startup time • Set up timing to use discounts • Optimize maintenance • Extend specialist's time • Reduce wait time
Manage variation	• Standardization (create a formal process) • Stop tampering • Develop operational definitions • Improve predictions • Develop contingency plans • Sort product into grades • Desensitize • Exploit variation
Design systems to avoid mistakes	• Use reminders • Use differentiation • Use constraints • Use affordances
Focus on product or service	• Mass customize • Offer product/service anytime • Offer product/service anyplace • Emphasize intangibles • Influence of take advantage of fashion trends • Reduce the number of components • Disguise defects of problems • Differentiate product using quality dimensions

Source: Reproduced, with permission, from Langley G, Moen RD, Nolan KM, et al. *The Improvement Guide*. San Francisco, CA: Jossey-Bass; 2009.

2. Improve workflow: A process is the series of steps that produce a product or service. Teams can work toward eliminating unnecessary or redundant steps. The process can also be reorganized or prioritized to maximize workflow. For example, in a clinic, having the doctor and the nurse take the history at the same time eliminates duplicate questioning of patients, thereby enhancing flow and improving the patient experience.

3. Optimize inventory: Inventory represents waste in organizations. It often represents stockpiled goods, materials, or underutilized workers. In healthcare, patients can also be considered "inventory," patients waiting for beds, waiting to be seen, waiting to be discharged. Efforts at eliminating or minimizing inventory can improve efficiency and costs for organizations.

4. Change the work environment: Changing the work environment can lead to improvements in processes and performance in a system. 5S was developed by the Japanese manufacturing industry. It is an organizing methodology used to enhance workspace efficiency, effectiveness, and safety. Translated into English, 5S encompasses sorting (seiri), straightening (seiton), shining (seiso), standardizing (seiketsu), and sustaining (shitsuke). The 5S system helps create an organized, standardized workspace, enabling individuals to distinguish between normal and abnormal conditions at a glance. Teams can begin by first *sorting*. Clearly distinguish needed equipment, parts, and materials in a work area from unnecessary items and eliminate the latter, leaving only essential items in easily accessible places. Next, *straighten* or organize the workplace such that most frequently utilized items can be easily and quickly located. To improve efficiency, *shine* the workplace by keeping the area clean and in order. The workspace should be *standardized* to ensure consistency for conducting tasks and procedures. Finally, *sustain* accomplishments of reorganization by clearly establishing rules and standard operating procedures.[4]

5. Enhance the provider/customer relationship: Improvement efforts can be directed toward enhancing the patient experience in the healthcare setting. Feedback on needs and expectations of patients can be elicited and utilized to change processes toward a more patient-centered model.

6. Manage time: Change ideas can revolve around improving efficiency by optimizing cycle times and eliminating wait times of processes.

7. Manage variation: Variation in processes and patient care is inherent. Change ideas aimed at reducing unnecessary variation can lead to improvement not only in processes but also in patient outcomes.

8. Design systems to avoid mistakes: Errors are often the result of both human factors and system-related issues. Error proofing involves

designing or redesigning the system to make it less likely for people to make errors. Efforts should be directed toward changing systems rather than changing people's behavior to make the most significant improvements. When error proofing, consider the following techniques:

Make it *impossible* to create the error.
Make it *harder* to create the error.
Make it *obvious* the error has occurred.
Make the system robust to *tolerate* an error.

9. Focus on the product or service: Change can be directed toward improving the product or service itself rather than focusing on the process.

Plan, Do, Study, Act Cycle

The final components of the Model for Improvement are plan, do, study, act (PDSA) cycles. PDSA cycles facilitate the testing and implementation of change using trial and learning methodology. Through an iterative process of repeat PDSA cycles, knowledge is built and changes are implemented that result in improvement.[2]

Plan: Teams begin the plan stage by stating the specific objective for the cycle and developing the questions to be answered during the cycle. Predictions should be made for the test/implementation of change. Detailed plans, including data collection process, should be clearly outlined. When planning, teams should envision subsequent tests that may be needed in future cycles. Teams can scale down scope of cycles by considering limiting tests to a smaller sample of patients, testing only in certain care areas, or involving a small group of physicians. In the initial smaller-scale cycles, testing should not be hindered by attempts at gathering full buy-in or consensus. As the scope of the change expands and efforts are aimed toward implementation rather than testing, garnering wider support becomes vital.

Do: In the do stage, the test of change is conducted and data is collected. In addition, problems and unanticipated results should be noted so that they can be analyzed in the next stage.

Study: In the study phase, the data is analyzed and the results are compared to the predictions made in the plan stage. Teams should consider possible reasons for unsuccessful tests of change. Was the change not properly executed? Were support processes inadequate to allow for the change? Or were the changes implemented successfully; however, the results were not toward desired direction? Lessons learned should be reviewed and summarized to facilitate the next stage and future cycles.

Act: Finally, in the act stage, based on the results of the previous plan, do, study stages, modifications are considered and a plan for new actions is set forth for the upcoming PDSA cycle.

Designs for Testing Changes

One of the most common tests of change is the "before and after test." A change is made and the results are analyzed before and after the intervention using graphical display of data over time, known as run charts (described below in quality improvement tools section). Although simple to perform, the results could represent impact of confounders rather than the intervention itself. To help clarify, other testing designs can be trialed. First, the introduced change can be removed for a period of time and then re-introduced (time series with replication). If the process returns to preimplementation levels with removal but shows improvement after re-introduction, then there can be more belief that the intervention itself caused the results. Another test design could be the addition of a control group (time series with a control group). Comparisons can then be made between the intervention group and the control group. Finally, Deming introduced planned experimentation methodology to testing changes. These statistical approaches can be used to elicit the causes of variation in a process and evaluate the impact of multiple changes to a process. For test cycles incorporating multiple changes at once, planned experimentation allows the distinguishing of individual effects of changes from combined effects of the changes.[3,5]

EXAMPLE

Aim: improving assessment and counseling for childhood obesity

Initial process measures: percentage of patients with a documented body mass index (BMI) and the percentage receiving a handout on healthy weight

Change: standardized vital sign intake including BMI and creation of parental handouts on healthy weight

Before and after trial: process measures would be collected before and after change

Time series with replication: process measures are collected before and after change. The change is removed for a period of time and then re-introduced. Process measures are again measured after re-introduction of change ideas

Time series with control: if two similar practices exist, the changes can be implemented in one group and not the other.

Rapid Cycle Testing and Implementing Changes

Hypotheses are tested through multiple PDSA test cycles from small scale to wider scope of change. One large PDSA cycle with all proposed changes in general should be avoided. It should be considered only when the team has a high degree of belief that the improvement will result in success, the risk of failure is small, and small tests of changes are not possible. With repetitive small cycles of change, teams learn and refine changes with each cycle until they are ready for broader implementation.

PDSA cycles can then be used to implement changes rather than test changes. To successfully implement a permanent change, process support infrastructure may need to be revised or developed. Training programs, technology support, and standardized operating procedures can aid the implementation process. As more people or areas are affected, resistance to change may be encountered; this will need to be addressed to allow successful implementation. Given the larger scale and greater impact of implementation PDSA cycles, in general, they take longer than test cycles. Finally, if adequate testing has been done in testing cycles, failure is not expected when change is implemented. Learning from testing cycles is crucial to successful implementation.[3]

▍LEAN

Lean principles are derived from the Japanese manufacturing industry and the Toyota Production System (TPS), although the term "Lean" was developed in the late 1980s by the Massachusetts Institute of Technology.[6] Traditionally, mass production processes focused on making more products at lower costs and relied on inspection to gauge quality after production. In contrast, Lean production methods centered on customer value and built-in quality by design and methods, creating more products with fewer defects in a shorter amount of time. At the heart of Lean, thinking is the core idea of process improvement by maximizing value and eliminating waste in processes. There are five key principles to Lean thinking.[7,8]

1. **Identify customers and specify value.** Patients represent the core customer for healthcare. However, specific healthcare providers such as nurses, physicians, ancillary staff, subspecialty service consultants, or primary-care physicians can all be considered customers. Identifying the customers allows for defining value from their perspective. This value will then guide improvement efforts. Different improvement efforts have different customers.
2. **Identify the value stream.** All processes are composed of multiple steps. In an ideal process, all steps would have value from the customer's

view. Each step in a process can be grouped into one of three categories: process steps that definitely create value; process steps that create no value but are necessary or required in a system; and process steps that create no value. For example, look at a clinic visit from the patient's perspective. Evaluation by the physician would be a value-added step. However, filling out admission or insurance paperwork is not value-added for the patient but necessary for each visit. Finally, time spent waiting to be seen by the physician represents a purely nonvalue-added step for the patient.

3. **Create flow by eliminating waste.** Lean methodology focuses on maximizing the value-added steps of the value stream and eliminating waste and nonvalue-added steps. This allows for efficient flow of product or service without interruption, detour, or waiting. Table 1-3

Table 1-3 **WASTES IN HEALTHCARE ("MUDA")**		
Waste	Definition	Examples
Delay	Time spent waiting	Waiting to be seen by doctor or nurse, waiting for treatments, waiting for supplies, waiting for paging call back
Overprocessing	Doing more work than is needed by the customer	Duplicate history and physicals (triage nurse, learner, attending), excessive paperwork, unnecessary tests or treatments, placing patient in monitored bed when not needed
Inventory	Producing more than needed. In healthcare, can represent supplies and patients	Specimens waiting for analysis, patients waiting to be seen, extra supplies kept on hand "just in case," drawing "extra" tubes of blood
Transport	Unnecessary transportation of material and people between work areas	Lab specimens through pneumatic tubes, obtaining medications from off floor pharmacies, supplies from central supply
Motion	Excessive movement within a work area	Searching for materials or supplies, traveling distances between floors to care for patients, too many clicks for function in electronic medical record
Overproduction	Producing more than is needed by the customer at the right time	Peripheral intravenous line kept in place longer than needed, delayed discharge, meals for patients who are on nothing by mouth status
Defects	Time and material spent conducting error and fixing error, costs of inspection	Medication errors, mislabeled specimens, illegible handwriting, misdiagnoses, hospital-acquired infections, patient dissatisfaction

lists seven nonvalue-added wastes ("muda") commonly encountered in healthcare.

4. **Let the customer pull value.** In a push system, work is sent to the next step downstream regardless of whether the downstream processes are ready to produce or process the product. If the downstream processes are not ready, capacity is exceeded and bottlenecks result. Excess "inventory" is created. In healthcare, this inventory often represents patients waiting for the next step in their visit. In pull systems, work is done in the process only when the downstream process is demanding the work. Consider scheduling of preoperative patients. In a push system, all patients set for surgery that day would be asked to come in at one time (batching), regardless of consideration of time needed to complete preoperation assessment or scheduled operation time. Bottlenecks would occur and patients would be pushed through the system. In a pull system, patients would be asked to come in throughout the day closer to set surgery time for necessary preoperative procedures (registration, exam, etc). They could be then "pulled" to the operating room once preoperative assessment is completed, minimizing wasted time waiting.

5. **Pursue perfection.** The final principle of Lean highlights the need for continuous improvement of processes in an attempt to create the perfect system where every step adds value for the customer.

SIX SIGMA

Six Sigma is a process improvement methodology focused on reducing defects created by variability in processes. A defect represents any missed target or nonconformance to a standard. At its core, Six Sigma is a quality metric, specifically 3.4 defects per million opportunities for defects. In a Six Sigma process, 99.9997% of products would be defect free! Through the use of data and statistical methods, Six Sigma focuses on the causes of variability and seeks to eliminate or reduce them. Organizations designate trained individuals ("champions," "master black belts," "greenbelts," etc) to lead and implement Six Sigma projects. Similar to PDSA cycles, the define, measure, analyze, improve, control (DMAIC) framework encompasses the five-step Six Sigma process.[9,10]

Define: The first step is to define the problem to be addressed by the team. The customer and their values should be identified. As in the Model for Improvement, the team's primary focus should be to produce a problem or aim statement.

Measure: The current state of process should be outlined. Qualitatively, the current process should be mapped, delineating all the steps involved. Quantitatively, the outcome, process, and balance measures should be outlined and data collected to establish a baseline for improvement efforts.

Analyze: In this step, the data collected is used to identify and prioritize potential root causes. These potential root causes need to be verified by data analysis, often both graphically (eg, scatterplots, boxplots, histograms, etc) and statistically.

Improve: Based on the prioritized root causes in the analyze step, potential solutions are then piloted and process changes are measured. Further changes may need to be tested to achieve the desired goal prior to full-scale implementation.

Control: Once the new process is performing at the desired level, a control plan will help sustain gains. This may involve creating documentation of new process steps and establishing auditing procedures.

QUALITY IMPROVEMENT TOOLS

There are many tools that can be used in improvement efforts. These tools can serve to help define, gather, measure, and analyze a system, process, or problem. Guided by the purpose of the project, teams can utilize the tools as needed. Some projects may need many tools while others may not need any at all. It is important to remember that all key stakeholders should participate to garner a more robust tool as they see issues from different perspectives. Listed below are just a few of the common tools available to gather and organize information and to understand variation.[2,9]

Tools to Gather Information

Process mapping: A process is a series of steps or actions performed to achieve a specific purpose. Process mapping is a method of understanding how the current process or system works. Flow diagrams, value stream mapping, and spaghetti diagrams are different pictorial representations of the actions that comprise a process. Flow diagrams can outline the steps in the current and future process. Value streaming mapping shows process steps and delineates value- from nonvalue-added steps. Spaghetti diagrams depict the actual physical flow of work or material in a process and can be used to optimize the workspace layout. Improvement teams can utilize process mapping methods to first describe and understand work being done. They can then use them to analyze and improve on processes by identifying areas of complexity (unnecessary or redundant work), generating ideas for improvement, and illustrating process improvements. It is important to construct process maps in a room with all stakeholders to accurately describe all steps involved.

Brainstorming: Groups can utilize brainstorming to gather a wide range of ideas around any topic. It can be done in a short period of time, stimulates the creative thinking process, and helps ensure input from all team members. Group members should be given self-stick notes or cards to write down ideas. Encourage members to be creative. Ideas on the notes/cards should then be read out loud. Continue until everyone is out of ideas. The ideas generated are consolidated and grouped using other quality improvement tools such as affinity diagrams or cause and effect diagrams.

Tools for Organizing Information

Innovative information may need arranging in order for it to be used. Many tools are available to accomplish this. Among the most useful are the following.

Key driver diagrams: A key driver diagram allows teams to analyze, organize, and communicate information to help guide improvement efforts by helping to answer the question, "What change can we make that will result in an improvement." To create the diagram, teams must first identify factors, "key drivers," that affect the project and contribute to the results. Once the drivers are outlined, teams can then address each one systematically. These diagrams also provide a measurement framework for monitoring progress (Figure 1-2).

Affinity diagrams: Affinity diagrams are used to organize facts, ideas, and issues into natural groups to identify themes. Ideas or comments garnered during information gathering stages (brainstorming, information from surveys, etc) should be clustered into big groups. Each group should then be given a "header" label that identifies a common theme. Teams can analyze the patterns created on affinity diagrams to establish cause and effect relationships or determine target areas for improvement.

Cause and effect diagrams (Ishikawa or fishbone diagrams): Cause and effect diagrams organize causes contributing to an effect (problem or variation). The effect (problem) is written at the head of a fishbone skeleton and likely causes are arranged along the bones under major headings. The diagrams can help determine root causes of problems using a structured approach.

Failure mode and effects analysis (FMEA): FMEA is a structured approach to identifying the ways in which a product, service, or process can fail to perform its intended function and estimate the risk associated with specific failure causes. Teams can begin by first identifying possible

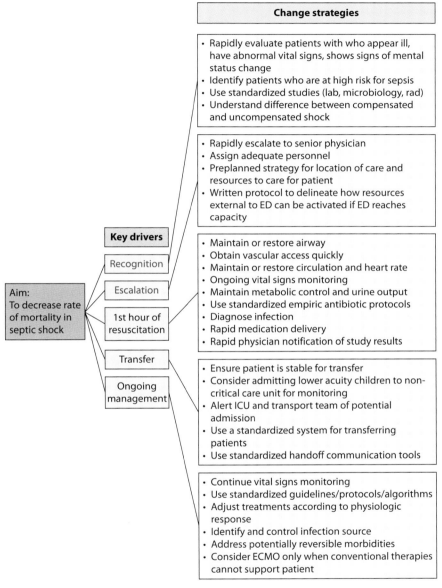

Change strategies

- Rapidly evaluate patients with who appear ill, have abnormal vital signs, shows signs of mental status change
- Identify patients who are at high risk for sepsis
- Use standardized studies (lab, microbiology, rad)
- Understand difference between compensated and uncompensated shock

- Rapidly escalate to senior physician
- Assign adequate personnel
- Preplanned strategy for location of care and resources to care for patient
- Written protocol to delineate how resources external to ED can be activated if ED reaches capacity

- Maintain or restore airway
- Obtain vascular access quickly
- Maintain or restore circulation and heart rate
- Ongoing vital signs monitoring
- Maintain metabolic control and urine output
- Use standardized empiric antibiotic protocols
- Diagnose infection
- Rapid medication delivery
- Rapid physician notification of study results

- Ensure patient is stable for transfer
- Consider admitting lower acuity children to non-critical care unit for monitoring
- Alert ICU and transport team of potential admission
- Use a standardized system for transferring patients
- Use standardized handoff communication tools

- Continue vital signs monitoring
- Use standardized guidelines/protocols/algorithms
- Adjust treatments according to physiologic response
- Identify and control infection source
- Address potentially reversible morbidities
- Consider ECMO only when conventional therapies cannot support patient

Key drivers

Recognition

Escalation

1st hour of resuscitation

Transfer

Ongoing management

Aim:
To decrease rate of mortality in septic shock

Figure 1-2 ■ Sepsis key driver diagram for interventions. Developed by Committee for Quality Transformation, Section of Emergency Medicine, American Academy of Pediatrics, Septic Shock Quality Collaborative, 2013. (Courtesy of Charles G. Macias, MD.)

failure modes and potential effects of each failure. Ratings of the severity of failure (impact on the customer/patient), likelihood of failure, and detectability of failure should be assigned for each failure mode. Risk can then be calculated by multiplying these three ratings. This analysis can guide teams to concentrate efforts on high-priority failure modes and develop both strategies to prevent failure from happening and contingency plans for when failure does occur.

Pareto charts: Pareto charts are based on the "Pareto principle" or "80/20 rule" (named after Italian economist Vilfredo Pareto). The principle states that the majority (80%) of variation of any characteristic is caused by a small number of possible variables (20%). Pareto charts are a type of bar chart in which the horizontal axis represents categories (defects, errors, causes) while the vertical axis represents a count or percent of errors/defects or their impact/outcome. These charts help identify which categories may yield the biggest gains if addressed. It should be noted, though, that the most frequent problems may not have the biggest impact in terms of quality, time, or costs. Therefore, when possible, two Pareto charts should be constructed to identify improvement target areas—one with counts or frequency of data and another that looks at impact (time or effort required to fix problem, dollar impact, etc).

Run charts: Run charts graphically evaluate the impact of changes on a process. Traditionally, results are presented as static points in time, preintervention result and postintervention result. For example, consider the data presented in Figure 1-3. The static bar graph would suggest that the improvement was the result of the intervention performed. However, a single snapshot fails to capture the performance of a healthcare system. If the data is presented over time, one can see that perhaps the intervention had no true effect on the results seen and

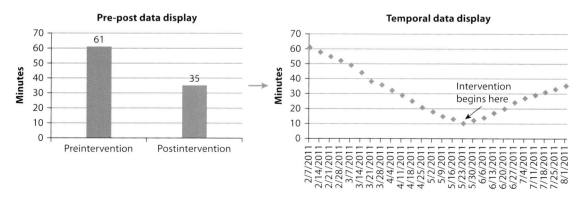

Figure 1-3 ■ Pre- and post data display versus run chart.

may have actually exacerbated the problem. Run charts display data in a temporal manner and visually demonstrate the behavior of a process without statistical calculation. Time is plotted on the x-axis and the observed measure on the y-axis. The center line represents the measure of central tendency (mean or median). Run charts make process improvement visible, allow determination of whether a change is an improvement, and help signal sustainability of the improvement. By adding a median line to a run chart, one can also use probability-based rules to determine whether processes are exhibiting true improvement, nonrandom evidence of change.[3]

Statistical process control charts (Shewhart charts): Statistical process control charts are attributed to the work of Walter A. Shewhart. He believed that every process displays unintended variation, changes that are not purposeful, planned, or guided. These variations lead to inefficiencies, waste, ineffectiveness of care, and medical errors in healthcare. Shewhart believed that by reducing or eliminating unintended variation in processes, one could improve outcomes and lower costs.

There are two types of unintended variation—common cause variation and special cause variation. Common cause variation, also known as random variation, is inherent to the system or process. The root of common cause variation cannot be traced back to a cause since it is the result of random shifts in factors of a system. Special cause variation, also known as assignable variation, is the result of a signal in the process, factors that are not always present in the process. Variation from special cause is not random, can be traced back to its cause, and is potentially modifiable. All processes have common cause variation. Processes that also have special cause variation are said to be "out of control" ("out of statistical control"). Processes that have only common cause variation are said to be "in control" ("in statistical control"). It is vital to identify whether a process is in control as there are different improvement strategies for the two types of variation. To reduce common cause variation, new methods or processes must be developed. In contrast, to reduce special cause variation, the root cause must be found, studied, and action taken based on the special cause.

Statistical process control charts help distinguish special cause from common cause variation in a system or process. It is similar to a run chart but includes two additional lines: an upper and lower control limit. Control limits generally represent three standard deviations above or below the central tendency. Points within the control limits represent common cause variation, while points outside the control limit represent special cause variation. In addition, specific trends formed by data points within the control limits can signal special cause variation. Examples include eight points in a row above or below central tendency, six points in a row steadily increasing or decreasing,

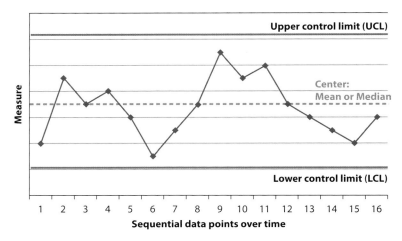

Figure 1-4 ▪ Elements of statistical process control chart.

and fourteen points in a row alternating up and down. Most statistical programs will identify these for you. Finally, there are different types of SPC charts based on the type of data being analyzed—attribute versus continuous data (Figure 1-4; Table 1-4).[3]

Case Study: Improving the Care for Patients Presenting With Suspected Sepsis to an Emergency Department.

Problem: Evidenced-based care guidelines for the management of pediatric sepsis have been established since 2002. Evidence derived from clinical studies has shown that early recognition and initiation of goal-directed therapy via rapid and aggressive fluid resuscitation improves morbidity and mortality. Despite this, in 2009 at the start of the project, it was noted that suspected sepsis care guidelines were not being followed consistently. In addition, system issues were identified at morbidity and mortality conferences leading to poor

Table 1-4	TYPES OF STATISTICAL PROCESS CONTROL CHARTS BASED ON TYPE OF DATA	
Data Type		**SPC Chart**
Attribute	Count (1,2,3,4, etc)	Count or Unit chart
	Classification (yes/no, pass/fail, etc)	Proportion chart
Continuous	Subgroup size of 1 ($n = 1$)	Individual chart (X chart)
	Equal or unequal subgroup size ($n > 1$)	Mean and Sigma bar chart

patient outcomes. A multidisciplinary team consisting of physicians (pediatric emergency medicine, critical care, infectious disease, oncology, bone marrow transplant, organ transplant, and other key subspecialties), nurses, ancillary service members (pharmacy, respiratory therapy, transport team), and information technology personnel was assembled with the mission of improving the care of pediatric patients presenting to the emergency department with concern for septic shock.

What Are We Trying to Accomplish?

Aim statement: By one year, with the implementation of an evidence-based septic shock protocol for patients presenting to the emergency department, we will deliver up to 60 mL/kg of fluids and start appropriate antibiotics within 60 minutes of presentation.

How Will We Know That a Change Is an Improvement?

Outcome measure: Mortality from pediatric septic shock (global measure)
Process measures: Time to initiation of first fluid bolus, time to initiation of third fluid bolus (each bolus constituting 20mL/kg), time to first antibiotic (initial PDSA cycle measures)
Balance measure: Door to doctor time for high-acuity patients

What Changes Can We Make That Will Result in Improvement?

Stakeholder meetings were conducted to identify barriers to recognition and management of septic shock. System changes and process improvement strategies would be used for the improvement effort.

PDSA Cycle 1 Based on evidence of improvements by similar interventions in general emergency department settings for adults, and given the large scope and hospital-wide support of the project, the first cycle was a large-scale test. We anticipated that subsequent cycles would involve fine-tuning initial changes toward full adoption and implementation.

> Plan: Brainstorming sessions were held with key stakeholders. Affinity and fishbone diagrams were used to organize and identify barriers. Using a key driver diagram, the team created change concepts to test (Figure 1-2).
> Do: Direct feedback emails were sent to providers regularly to solicit continued barriers and re-enforce change concepts. Key changes included the following:
>
> > Recognition: Creation of an electronic alert tool from triage to alert ED staff of an at-risk patient.

Recruitment: Members of the hospital transport team recruited to aid bedside nurses in the care of at-risk patients.

Process change: The steps for delivery of antibiotics were modified to expedite care.

Standardization: Standardized evidence-based order sets were implemented to guide care. Standard operating procedures were developed for rapid laboratory test turnaround, nursing administration of fluids and antibiotics, and rapid patient assessment by physicians. A standardized documentation flowsheet was created to facilitate communication of handoffs.

Study: All patients were captured for analysis. Statistical process control charts were created every 2 months and sent to all providers and posted in common areas. Feedback from providers showed that scripting was needed for families and certain supplies were located in an inconvenient location rather than at the bedside.

Act: Initial results showed dramatic improvement in process measures.

Efforts for subsequent PDSA cycles were directed toward creating scripting for families, improving documentation of interventions, improving care area workspace efficiency, developing alternatives for resource recruitment, and introduction of the electronic medical record into the patient care process. The septic shock protocol was integrated into the outpatient oncology urgent

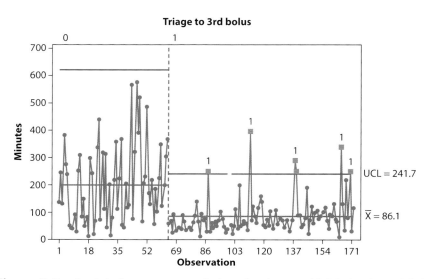

Figure 1-5 ▪ Statistical process control chart for time to third bolus (60 mL/kg). (Courtesy of Binita Patel, MD, Baylor College of Medicine.)

care clinic and our community hospital emergency department. Finally, plans are underway to incorporate into inpatient units.

At the end of the first year, 80% of patients received the third bolus within 60 minutes, and 100% of patients received antibiotics within 60 minutes. For our balance measure, there was no difference in the time to evaluation for other high acuity patients. Finally, preliminary results showed a trend in decreasing mortality; however, data will need to be collected over the next few years to reach statistical significance (Figure 1-5).

IN PRACTICE

- Many quality improvement methodologies exist. Fundamentally, each methodology asks improvement teams to identify a problem, measure the problem, develop interventions to fix the problems, and finally test the created interventions for success.
- Successful quality improvement integrates systems thinking, management of variation, iterative knowledge building, and understanding of human factors.
- Well-constructed aim statements will anchor the team to the overarching improvement goal. They should be specific, measurable, attainable, relevant, and time bound.
- A balanced set of measures – outcome, process, and balance measures – is needed to evaluate the impact of changes.
- Testing small changes via repetitive PDSA cycles allows for successful implementation.
- The patient defines value. Optimizing value-added steps and eliminating waste can improve efficiency, reduce costs, and improve flow.
- Variation is inherent in all systems. Correctly identifying the type of variation (common cause vs. special cause) determines improvement strategies.
- Quality improvement tools can aid gathering information, organizing information, and understanding variation.

FAQs

1. How do I determine which quality improvement method I should use?

   The frameworks for the different methods are similar. Each involves systematically defining a problem, creating measures, implementing change, and studying the effects. Techniques from each framework are often used together in improvement efforts. For example, while the Model for Improvement may form the foundation of your project, Lean techniques for improving flow and eliminating waste can encompass change concepts while Six Sigma techniques can be used to evaluate variation.

2. How do I determine which tools to use?

There are many tools, each with a different purpose. For beginners of quality improvement, quality improvement champions and coaches can help guide selection of tools that may be needed. As individuals gain expertise, the identification and selection of tools will come more naturally. Numerous books and web-based tools exist to help facilitate this determination.

3. What are common causes of failure?
   - Scope of project too large
   - Necessary key stakeholders not involved
   - Lack of leadership support
   - Poorly defined aims
   - Poorly constructed measurement systems
   - Quitting rather than utilizing lessons learned in future cycles

4. How do I get started?

First, find a problem in your own work setting that needs improvement. Make a case for improvement and get buy-in from leadership. Assemble the improvement team and solicit help from quality improvement champions if new to the process. Then, dive in head first! Remember, quality improvement is best learned by doing and often requires multiple PDSA cycles whether within one project or multiple projects over time. Along with quality improvement books, courses (online and in class) are offered throughout the country.

REFERENCES

1. Deming WE. *The New Economics for Industry, Government, Education.* Cambridge, MA: The MIT Press; 2000.
2. Langley G, Moen RD, Nolan KM, et al. *The Improvement Guide.* San Francisco, CA: Jossey-Bass; 2009.
3. Provost LP, Murray SK. *The Health Care Data Guide: Learning from Data for Improvement.* San Francisco, CA: Jossey-Bass; 2011.
4. Hirano H. *5 Pillars of the Visual Workplace.* Cambridge, MA: Productivity Press; 1995.
5. Moen RD, Nolan TW, Provost LP. *Quality Improvement through Planned Experimentation.* New York, NY: McGraw-Hill; 1999.

6. Womack JP, Jones DT, Roos D. *The Machine that Changed the World.* New York, NY: Rawson Associates; 1990.
7. Womack JP, Jones DT. *Lean Thinking.* New York, NY: Free Press, Simon & Schuster; 2003.
8. Zidel TG. *Lean Done Right.* Chicago, IL: Health Administration Press; 2012.
9. George ML, Rowlands D, Price M, et al. *The Lean Six Sigma Pocket Toolbook.* New York, NY: McGraw-Hill; 2005.
10. Arthur J. *Lean Six Sigma for Hospitals.* New York, NY: McGraw-Hill; 2011.
11. Institute for Healthcare Improvement. Science of Improvement: Establishing Measures. Available at: http://www.ihi.org/knowledge/Pages/HowtoImprove/ScienceofImprovementEstablishingMeasures.aspx; Accessed July 16, 2013.

APPLYING QUALITY IMPROVEMENT IN PRACTICE

2

The gaps in care delivery are well recognized by policy makers, patients, and healthcare providers. In the seminal Institute of Medicine (IOM) Report, *Crossing the Quality Chasm*, six specific aims for quality improvement were identified: healthcare should be safe, effective, patient-centered, timely, efficient, and equitable.[1] Rapid-cycle quality improvement methods, which have been effective in diverse fields, including business, engineering, and agriculture, are now being used in healthcare with great success. This chapter will provide an overview of an approach for quality improvement based on the Model for Improvement (see Figure 2-1).[2] The key elements will be:

- Using the Model for Improvement as a framework for improvement
- Selecting an important domain for improvement
- Forming the quality improvement team
- Identifying metrics to track improvement
- Developing interventions to improve quality
- Conducting small Plan-Do-Study-Act cycle tests
- Wide-scale testing
- Implementation for sustainability

USING THE MODEL FOR IMPROVEMENT AS A FRAMEWORK FOR IMPROVEMENT

The answers to the three questions of the Model for Improvement help frame the improvement project. The first section of this chapter will address each of the following essential components in planning the improvement project: selecting the domain for improvement, forming the quality improvement team,

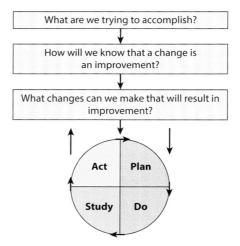

Figure 2-1 ■ Model for improvement. (Adapted, with permission, from Langley GL, Men R, Nolan KM, Nolan TW, Norman CL, Provost LP. The Improvement Guide: A Practical Approach to Enhancing Organizational Performance. Second Edition. San Francisco, CA: Jossey-Bass Publishers; 2009.)

identifying key stakeholders, establishing a shared goal—both with a global aim and specific aims, developing metrics, understanding the existing process by creating a process map, identifying barriers, constructing a key driver diagram to frame a specific aim with complex processes into manageable drivers, and designing focused interventions to actualize these drivers.

SELECTING THE DOMAIN FOR IMPROVEMENT

There is no process that with attention cannot be improved. However, not all processes are equally important and some processes cannot be readily improved. For novice quality improvement teams, we recommend focusing on problems that can be readily modified in order to achieve some preliminary successes. Over time, as the team matures, more challenging topics can be addressed. Ultimately, the goal of quality improvement is to achieve the "triple aim": improving the health of populations, improving patient experiences, and decreasing per capita costs. However, it is unlikely that any one particular project will achieve all the three aims. Over time, as more healthcare providers engage in quality improvement, this overarching goal will be met.[3]

The pediatric quality indicators developed by the US Agency for Healthcare Research and Quality (AHRQ)[4] can provide a good starting point for selecting a domain for quality improvement. Improvement on these indicators can reduce morbidity and mortality. These quality indicators are relevant to both inpatient and outpatient care, and healthcare providers will be increasingly evaluated by their performance in these domains.

When seeking local administrative support and resources, recognize the benefit of choosing a project that aligns with organizational priorities. For some projects, there is an opportunity to improve care both at the local and at the national level. When choosing a project, consider the following questions:

- Will the project address an issue considered to be high-risk?
- Is the healthcare issue common or uncommon?
- Is the process problem-prone?
- Is the problem of national importance, local importance, or both?
- Is there a gap between national standards and local care?

Locally, is there an opportunity to make care safer, more effective, efficient, timely, equitable, and patient-centered? In healthcare, it is common to focus on a problem area or on a particular measure (access, compliance, reliability, flow, readmissions, etc).

For example, when considering the issue of inpatient-to-outpatient medical handover at hospital discharge, colleagues may focus on communication of lab results pending at the time of discharge. A literature review reveals scant data about how to address this issue. However, a policy statement by the National Transitions of Care Collaborative, backed by over 40 physician organizations, lists timely communication of pending lab results as a priority in the safe transition of patients from the inpatient to outpatient environment. After selecting a domain for improvement that addresses the IOM aims for improvement and components of the triple aim, the quality improvement team leader is ready to build the improvement team.

FORMING THE QUALITY IMPROVEMENT TEAM

Successful quality improvement projects are a team effort. The composition of the team will depend on the particular focus. For example, efforts to improve inpatient asthma care could include a physician, nurse, respiratory therapist, hospital administrator, and electronic medical record (EMR) programmer. In contrast, a project to improve outpatient asthma care in a small practice might include only a physician and a nurse. Having a family representative on the quality improvement team can be quite helpful and should be strongly considered, when feasible, for pediatric-focused quality improvement activities. Parents can identify barriers to care and might have insight into care delivery that the healthcare team otherwise lacks. Identifying highly engaged family members and working with these family members to set mutual expectations is critical.

The team should have a leader who is responsible for overseeing all activities of the project. This "champion" should be selected based on interest, experience, and knowledge regarding the topic, as well as leadership skills. If possible, resources, including work time, should be made available to the champion to learn more about the topic to be addressed.

For the project aimed to improve inpatient-to-outpatient medical provider handover focused on pending lab results, the team leader may be a hospitalist who had previously worked as a primary care provider—someone who is knowledgeable and passionate about the issue. In addition, this leader should be connected with a senior leader or a system leader with authority to test changes to the system of interest.

IDENTIFYING KEY STAKEHOLDERS

Stakeholders are anyone who can affect change or who may be affected by the proposed change. Stakeholders may help remove barriers, facilitate the testing of the intervention, assist or implement the change, or may benefit or be harmed by changes in care delivery. In the above example, stakeholders would include hospitalists, nurses, residents, the hospital lab including the microbiology, chemistry, hematology, pathology, and "send-out" areas, admissions department, medical records, hospital administration, hospital-community physician liaisons, primary care providers, primary care provider nursing staff, front office staff, and, of course, patients and their families.

When assembling an improvement team, one should consider each stakeholder's influence and interest. Influence can be categorized as high-level influence (eg, individuals who could change policy or purchase new equipment) and front-line influence (eg, individuals who get things done or perform the tasks that will lead to improvement). Those with both high levels of influence and interest will be most helpful.

When seeking commitment from others, one should demonstrate the extent of this problem locally by describing one or more real-life patient stories that illustrate systems failures that led to patient harm. Utilizing an example through a patient story can help others see, feel, then help change the system to improve patient care. Quality improvement uses a data-driven approach to demonstrate improvement over time. However, supplementing data with real patient stories can be an effective means to gain the support of influential stakeholders.

Perhaps the most important theme in team building is to invite each stakeholder to provide their input and expertise early in the process. Failure to build a collaborative interprofessional team may minimize the impact of a project before it gets started.

A hospitalist leader designs a project to improve the communication of pending lab results to the primary care provider and wonders why the project failed to accomplish its goal. The project details including timeline of interventions, roles and responsibilities, and data collection were meticulously planned. Despite clear communication of expectations, the process did not improve. Residents, hospitalist colleagues, and the medical-surgical unit clerks responsible for faxing communication to the primary care providers were not involved in the planning of the intervention. When interviewed later, the hospitalist realized by neither seeking nor acknowledging the input of key stakeholders early in the planning stage, the leader sabotaged the effort. Quality improvement is a team sport.

ESTABLISH A SHARED GOAL

The quality improvement team needs to establish a shared purpose. As the first question in the IHI Improvement Model asks, "What are we trying to accomplish?" The global aim provides a high-level answer to this question. It is the bumper stick or the slogan. It is what a team member could describe to someone on an elevator ride. It is also a statement of the goal shared by all stakeholders. The improvement team leader needs to establish consensus that this goal is important to everyone and, most of all, important to patients.

For the above example, the global aim is to improve inpatient-to-outpatient medical care provider handover during the transition between inpatient and outpatient care. In early conversations with other stakeholders, primary care providers express their concerns that other essential information about their patients is not being relayed in a timely manner. A survey is performed and "pending results" are one of the seven elements selected to be included in the "essential contents" of discharge communication.

METRICS

A hallmark of successful quality improvement is the use of clearly defined metrics to assess changes over time. There are two general classes of measures: process measures and patient outcome measures. Process measures evaluate healthcare delivery, and patient outcome measures reflect patient-relevant outcomes.[5] Quality improvement activities should include both types of measures. However, some patient-relevant outcomes are too rare to be responsive to a change in care delivery. Therefore, significant effort should be placed on developing process measures that are linked tightly to patient outcome measures.

In addition to selecting outcomes to measure changes in the delivery of care related to the selected domain, we also recommend choosing balancing measures. Balancing measures are used to ensure that improvement in one domain does not lead to worsening care in another domain.[5] This can happen as attention moves from one clinical domain to another.

Developing quality improvement metrics is challenging. There must be a clear way to count events (ie, the numerator), to determine the appropriate population (ie, the denominator), and the metric must be expected to vary over the periods used in the rapid-cycle quality improvement. Whenever possible, we recommend using established quality improvement metrics. This will avoid the challenge of having to develop new metrics and will allow you to benchmark to others. However, choice of metric should reflect the feasibility of measurement using the available resources. The metrics are not useful if it takes a long period of time to obtain the data necessary to assess the impact of interventions.

For each quality improvement project, the team must identify an outcome—ideally a patient outcome—that the team wishes to improve. In the above example, the outcome would be patient harm related to pending lab results. In order to improve the outcome, the team will need to improve one or more related processes. There are two processes that may be linked to improving the outcome in our example. First, improving the process of timely and reliable communication to the primary care provider that there are pending lab results. Secondly, improving the tracking of pending lab results until they are finalized and communicating these results to the patient.

Each outcome measure and process measure should have an accompanying specific aim statement, also called a "SMART" aim statement. The SMART aim should be:

> **S**pecific—answers the question, "Who?" or "what patient population?" In the above example, the Hospital A team might start with the patients on the hospitalist service on the medical–surgical unit. The primary care provider might focus on their patients who are discharged from Hospital A.
> **M**easurable—answers the question, "What?" as in "what will the team improve?"—either to a certain goal or to improve by a certain amount; if it is a rate, then the team must define both the numerator and denominator. For the first process measure, it may be to improve the rate of communication that there are pending lab results at the time of hospital discharge to 95%.
> **A**ction-oriented or Achievable—answers the question, "Where?" By narrowing the scope to a certain clinical area, you may realize improvement sooner (can test a change on a small scale with less risk than full-scale implementation). In this example, starting with the patients on the hospitalist service on the medical–surgical units is a good

starting point. The team could decide to test change on an even smaller scale by testing on one specific nursing unit—4 North.

Realistic—has two contextual considerations:

1. Degree of belief that aim can be reached—this may be based on the best available evidence, experience of others, or simply the degree of belief of the improvement team in the local setting.

2. Quality improvement capacity—this depends on the improvement team's capacity to perform the intended intervention reliably and gather data to track the success process and outcome improvement.

Time-bound—answers the question, "By when?" Setting a time-bound goal drives accountability. In the above example, adding the clause, "within 6 months" or "by January 2015" will help keep the team focused on a concrete goal.

Consider Another Example

In all premature infants born < 32 weeks gestation who are < 2 years of age in the Good Health Center Clinic System, we will increase the rate of bimonthly retinopathy of prematurity ophthalmologic exams to 95% within 12 months.

This aim statement is specific (who = patient population: premature infants born <32 weeks gestation who are < 2 years of age); measurable (what = rate of retinopathy of prematurity ophthalmologic exams); action-oriented/achievable (where = in the Good Health Center Clinic System); realistic (both in terms of degree of belief—others have accomplished rates of 95% and the initial planned interventions and data collection will not overwhelm the system); and time-bound (within 12 months). Note: there is no mention of "how"—that is the intervention. Nor is there an explanation of "why"—that is described in the background/relevance and local context of the problem to be improved.

By building a shared SMART aim through the collaborative input of key stakeholders, the improvement team will increase the likelihood of successful stakeholder engagement and accountability in subsequent steps of the project. For each measure: outcome, process, and/or balancing measure, a team may develop a SMART aim statement. These aim statements serve as the measuring stick for progress throughout the quality improvement project.

UNDERSTANDING THE EXISTING PROCESS

A process map or flow diagram can be used to help an improvement team's understanding of the existing process. Together with representative stakeholders that comprise the improvement team, the group can create a flow chart starting at the beginning and listing chronologically each step in the process until the process is completed. Certain symbols are useful to standardize the flow diagram or process map. Ovals mark the beginning and the end. Rectangles denote the sequential steps in the process, while diamonds highlight a decision branch—essentially a "yes/no" question. A process map is particularly useful when there is a linear process. In healthcare, process maps are useful for any process that has a start and a finish, particularly those involving delays, waiting, or movement from one area to another. Creating and displaying a process map can help identify targets for improvement: steps that represent delay, inefficiency, or ineffectiveness—in other words, nonvalue-added steps.

For the example of Figure 2-2, by mapping out the current state of the initial process as it existed, it became clear to the project team that the current system was flawed. Initially, the team leader considered focusing on efforts to get attending hospitalists to sign the discharge progress note prior to discharge, but quickly realized this was an impractical approach for evening discharges. During an early meeting of key stakeholders, the process map (Figure 2-2) was presented to the multidisciplinary Discharge Planning Committee team. One team member suggested that the attending's signature could be bypassed. The risk manager, who was in attendance for this meeting, agreed noting that the attending needed to sign the discharge summary, but not the discharge progress note. This eliminated one barrier. In a subsequent Plan-Do-Study-Act

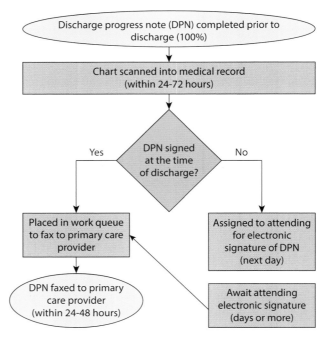

Figure 2-2 ▪ Example of process map: initial handover to primary care provider (faxing the discharge progress note).

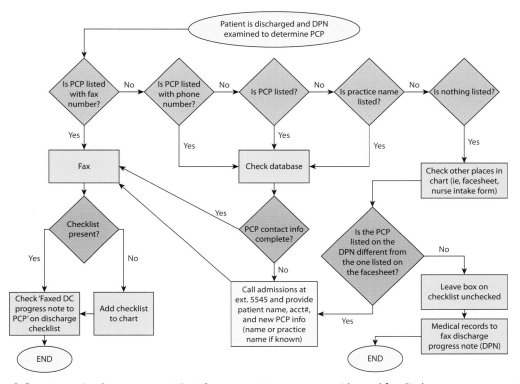

Figure 2-3 ▪ Example of process map: identify correct primary care provider and fax discharge progress note.

cycle, all delays from the above process map were eliminated when the unit clerks began faxing the discharge progress note at the time the chart was dissembled shortly after hospital discharge. A new process map was created for the new process (See Figure 2-3).

IDENTIFY BARRIERS

In quality improvement and in other aspects of life, if one brings a group of individuals together, it is easy for the group to begin a conversation by lamenting a shared obstacle. In fact, identifying barriers can serve as a team building experience. Immediately, diverse team members can find a common connection. Within 5 minutes, a group could fill a flip chart with barriers to accomplishing the shared aim. Common barriers include time, money, apathy, lack of communication, and incoordination. The key to effective teamwork is channeling the frustration into something productive. Ineffective teams focus on insurmountable barriers that require unrealistic amounts of resources or barriers that rarely have impact on the process or actual specific aim.

Focusing on the wrong barriers can waste time and energy and lead to hopelessness and helplessness. Without adequately redirection, an improvement session can fizzle into an unproductive gripe session.

By constructing a process map—listing the sequential steps in the process—a team can identify potential barriers. In the process map below (see Figure 2-3), which was created when the unit clerks began faxing the discharge progress notes, the accurate identification of the primary care provider with accurate contact information represents two barriers readily identified simply by creating a process map.

▌THE KEY DRIVER DIAGRAM[6]

The key driver diagram is a useful tool for breaking down complex issues into smaller, more manageable "drivers."[6] By starting with the SMART aim, the improvement team can list key drivers that are necessary to accomplish the aim. Each of the key drivers are stated in the affirmative. The key drivers answer the question, "What has to go right to accomplish this aim?"

In our example to improve the hospital primary care provider handover of pending lab results, a number of things have to "go right" to accomplish the aim.

First, we need to identify accurately the correct primary care provider with their correct contact information for each patient. Secondly, we need to identify accurately which patients have labs pending at the time of discharge (Figure 2-4).

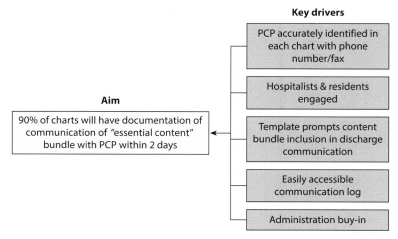

Figure 2-4 ▪ Example of key driver diagram: communication of "essential content" to primary care providers (PCPs).

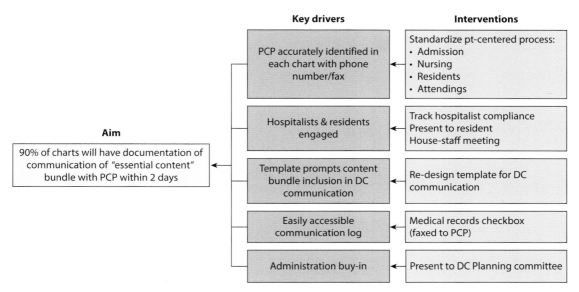

Figure 2-5 ▪ Example of key driver diagram with proposed interventions: communication of "essential contents" to primary care provider.

The key drivers listed can be addressed sequentially or simultaneously in a parallel fashion. Some drivers will require multiple steps—for example, a computer-based decision aid to prompt inclusion of "pending labs" in the "essential content" bundle in discharge communication. Others will require active contribution of front-line staff to refine and improve the process of accurately identifying each patient's primary care provider with their most current contact information. The key driver diagram offers a framework of where to begin in designing interventions to address each key driver (see Figure 2-5).

The key driver diagram allows one to take a complex system and break it down into more manageable drivers. Each key driver, in turn, may lend itself to a key driver diagram with secondary drivers and interventions designed to accomplish a specific aim (Figure 2-6).

COLLECT BASELINE DATA

The first Plan-Do-Study-Act cycle for any project should include each of the above steps to build the team, establish a shared goal, and understand the existing process. The second question from the IHI's Improvement Model asks, "How will we know a change is an improvement?" In measuring success, the team must first collect baseline data. Because data will be plotted over time, the baseline data likewise should be collected over time. Twelve data points is

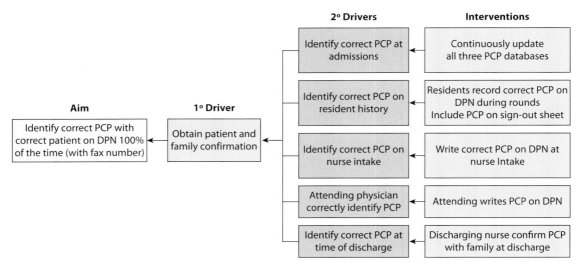

Figure 2-6 ▪ Example of key driver diagram with primary and secondary drivers: identification of correct primary care provider for each patient on the discharge progress note (DPN).

a reasonable number to establish a baseline. In some projects if data is already being collected for another purpose, then it easy to collect a more longitudinal baseline—for example, the past 6 months' worth of data. Otherwise sampling can help establish baseline and can be used to plot data over time to note improvement. If a given outcome is relatively rare—such as a post-discharge serious safety event, then the improvement team will sample all occurrences. Because there are many discharges daily, sampling is an effective means to track improvement in the timeliness of inpatient-to-outpatient medical provider handover.

INITIAL TEST ON A VERY SMALL SCALE

Too often hospitals and healthcare systems implement change throughout their organization without first testing the change on a smaller scale. When change is implemented at scale without initial testing, a team may encounter significant setbacks that may compromise current and future improvement efforts including waste—increased costs, decreased productivity, delays, re-work—each related to inefficiencies and errors magnified on a large scale, and lack of buy-in from front-line staff and administrative stakeholders.

In designing interventions to help accomplish the shared aim, an improvement team can answer the IHI's third question, "What changes can we make that will result in improvement?" Implementing change "at-scale" can magnify the cost and impact of errors. With data collection instruments, an improvement team can design and re-design tools and checklists to meet the team's needs with minimal risk of patient harm. For example, a new process to improve identification and documentation of the accurate primary care provider during rounds (see Figure 2-6) was tested with a single general medicine inpatient team on a single medical–surgical unit. Residents, nurses, and the hospitalist attending the physician provided feedback on the feasibility of the intervention. Updating the discharge progress note during rounds and confirming the primary care provider's name and contact information during rounds saved time and unnecessary steps later in the day. An additional layer of reliability was added by prompting medical students and residents to include the primary care provider's name and contact information on the resident sign-out list. Because this list is used to track follow-up lab results, having the primary care provider's name and contact information increased the feasibility of contacting primary care provider with lab results finalized after hospital discharge.

By testing the new process for accurately identifying the primary care provider on a single pod of a single unit. One 8-bed nursing pod on a single 24-bed medical–surgical unit served as the test unit. On this unit, with two nurses, one unit clerk, and one resident team, the proposed new process was tested. The unit clerk and the nurses encountered specific issues—including inaccurate primary care provider contact information on the admissions paperwork. By detecting this source of misinformation, the team was able to establish a process to provide updated accurate primary care provider contact information to the admissions department. The team traced the process for how one updates the primary care provider contact information in the admissions department. Of significant impact for this project, the team determined that primary care provider database used by the laboratory is the same database used by admissions. During the initial testing phase, the team detected a crucial flaw in the current system—even when inaccurate primary care provider contact information was corrected at the patient level and the unit clerk could fax information that there are pending lab results at the time of discharge to the correct primary care provider, when those results are completed, the lab would not have sent them to the correct primary care provider at the correct facsimile number or address. By linking the update in the primary care provider's contact information at the patient level (by patient/family, nurse, physician, and/or unit clerk) to an update on the admissions/lab primary care provider database, the team helped improve communication and tracking of pending lab results.

Another issue identified and corrected via initial tests of change related directly to communication of pending labs. The current state practice, prior to the intervention, was for residents to complete a template "discharge progress note" to be faxed to the primary care provider. While this form has a prompt to include lab results, there was no prompt to include pending lab results. One member of the team drafted the revised discharge progress note template, and presented this revised template and a brief overview of the project to the hospital Medical Records/Forms Committee. Two months later, the new discharge progress note template was being used throughout the hospital.

PILOT ON A SMALL SCALE

After performing initial tests of change on a very small scale, the changes can be piloted on a small scale. For example, after testing with a single medicine team, the same test could be performed on subspecialty teams, on all teams from a single unit, or on other medicine teams on different medical–surgical units. Additional perspectives can help refine data collection tools and improve processes.

IMPLEMENT ON A LARGER SCALE

Ultimately, successful changes tested and piloted on small scales can be implemented on a larger scale. The habit of identifying the correct primary care provider's name and contact information during rounds and recording this information on the discharge progress note can be spread to all units and services including surgery, medical subspecialties, and the intensive care unit. As these interventions spread, other benefits arose. Teams in the intensive care unit reported improved communication with the primary care provider at other times during the hospitalization including at hospital admission and during times of acute changes in patient status.

Increasingly, there has been an emphasis to accelerate change via the use of multisite quality improvement (QI) learning collaboratives. Via monthly conference calls, participating sites share barriers, keys to success, and lessons learned. Multisite QI learning collaboratives have helped quicken dissemination and spread of innovation—particularly as they relate to patient safety and healthcare quality improvement.

SUBSEQUENT PLAN-DO-STUDY-ACT CYCLES

In the first PDSA cycle, the initial process map was developed (see Figure 2-1). Notably, it was nearly impossible for any fax to reach the primary care provider within 2 days of discharge. The shared goal, including global and specific aim statements, was discussed with the hospitalist attending the physicians. These physicians were asked to "try harder" to sign the discharge progress note prior to discharge. Likewise, the aim statement and process map were discussed in two short meetings with the director of medical records and a single medical records employee responsible for faxing. Once these individuals were informed of the shared goal, the rate of faxing within 2 days of discharge improved from a baseline of 0% to about 25% and reached the goal of 90% for 1 week (see Figure 2-7a). Through a focused effort, hard work, and knowing that this was an organizational priority the goal was achieved in a relatively short timeframe. Unfortunately, success was short-lived. The single employee responsible for faxing went on vacation and was then reassigned to a different role in medical records. The rate of faxing returned to 0% and remained at 0% until a more reliable intervention (faxing by the unit clerk prior to chart arriving to medical records) was implemented (see Figures 2-7b and 2-8). With the new responsibility of the unit clerk faxing the discharge progress note to the correct primary care provider, the improvement team, including the nursing supervisor, unit clerks, admissions staff, and improvement team leader, standardized the process for accurately identifying the correct primary care provider, updating the primary care provider database, and faxing the discharge progress note to the correct primary care provider.

USING RATIONAL SUBGROUPS IN SUBSEQUENT PLAN-DO-STUDY-ACT CYCLES

In the above example, after the unit clerks began faxing the discharge progress note, the faxing rate improved to 74%. While this represented considerable improvement from the previous rate of 0%, it still fell short of the stated goal of 90%. On closer examination, the week-to-week rates ranged from 50 to 100%. By using rational subgroups,[6] in this example stratifying the data based on nursing unit of discharge, the improvement team learned that Unit D had already reached the goal, Units A and B were close, and Unit C's fax rate was less than 50% (see Figure 2-9). The individual unit's success rate was presented to the nursing leaders of each unit. Multiple discussions with the leadership from Unit C led to the hiring of a unit clerk during the nightshift for that unit. Each of the other three units had a nightshift unit clerk who could fax the discharge progress notes for late afternoon and evening discharges. Additional interventions included biweekly performance feedback Unit C leadership and front-line staff along and expanded from sampling to including all discharges from Unit C in data analysis. Finally, the lead unit clerk for Unit D shared with the improvement team her keys to success. The unit clerk from Unit D helped standardize the process for identifying and faxing the discharge progress note to the correct primary care provider (see Figure 2-2).

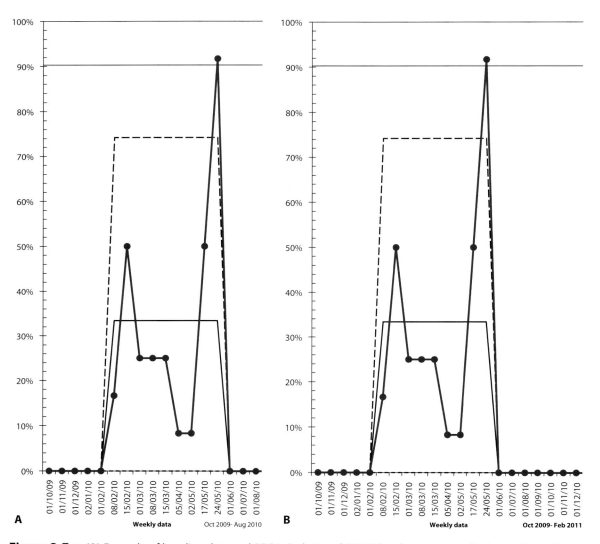

Figure 2-7 ■ (**A**) Example of baseline data and PDSA Cycle 1 and (**B**) With subsequent medical records employee reassignment in January 2010: rate of faxing discharge progress note to primary care providers within 2 days of discharge.

DISPLAYING DATA: RUN CHARTS AND CONTROL CHARTS

Quality improvement is data-driven. Baseline data helps establish a starting point, while a series of sequential interventions and ongoing data collection help determine the temporal, but not causal relationship between interventions

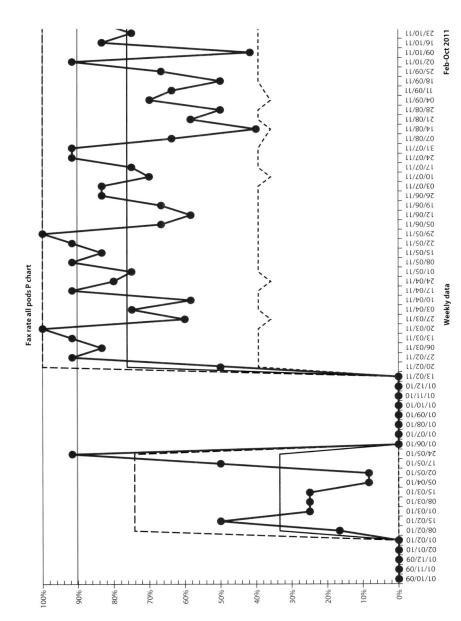

Figure 2-8 ■ Example of baseline data through PDSA Cycle 2 to October 2011: rate of faxing discharge progress note to primary care providers within 2 days of discharge.

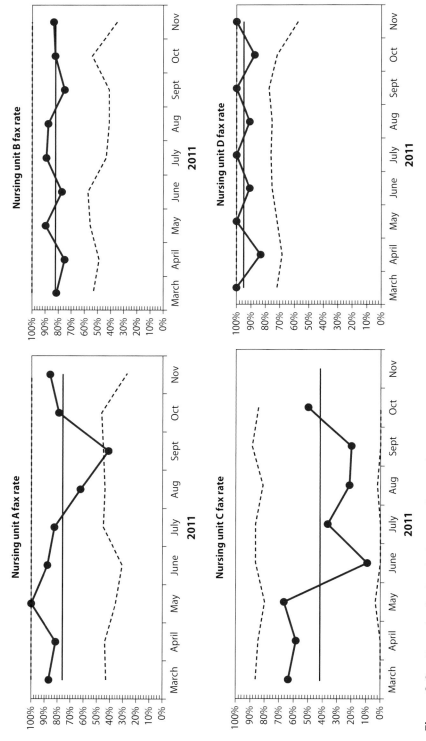

Figure 2-9 ■ Example of rational subgroups: fax rates by nursing unit.

and outcomes. Pre- and post-intervention data that is collected once is limited in its applicability. Performing multiple Plan-Do-Study-Act cycles depends on studying and interpreting data after performing a small test of change or intervention. Each PDSA cycle presents a learning opportunity—both from keys to success as well as lessons learned from failures. In quality improvement, collecting and displaying data over time is essential. Run charts can be used to plot data over time. The x-axis represents time, with each interval of time noted. The y-axis represents the metric studied (which could be a count or a rate). In our example, the rate of faxing the discharge progress note within 2 days of discharge is plotted on the y-axis, where the numerator is the number of times the discharge progress note was faxed to the primary care provider within 2 days of discharge and the denominator is the number of discharges sampled each week.

Statistical process-control charts are a more useful way to demonstrate significant changes over time. The x- and y-axes remain the same. Control charts display the mean or centerline as well as the upper and the lower control limits. The control limits are approximately equal to three standard deviations above and below the mean, respectively.

COMMON CAUSE VERSUS SPECIAL CAUSE VARIATION

Common cause variation is expected variation within a given system. The highest temperature each day in the mid-Atlantic region during the month of October may range from 50 degrees Fahrenheit to 82 degrees. Any number between 50 and 82 degrees is expected or common cause variation. If the temperature reached 98 degrees Fahrenheit or dipped to 20 degrees Fahrenheit, then these changes would be unexpected and outside the norm. They would be the result of special cause variation—a heat wave or a cold front.

With statistical process control charts, there are rules for detecting special cause including a single point outside the upper or lower control limit, eight consecutive points above or below the centerline, six consecutive points increasing or decreasing in value, and two of three points in the outer one-third approaching the upper or lower control limit. When special cause variation is demonstrated, the centerline or mean can be recalculated demonstrating improvement.[7]

Below is an annotated control chart—annotating the sequence of interventions performed over time and demonstrating special cause variation with eight consecutive points above the mean (See Figure 2-10).

GENERALIZABILITY IN QUALITY IMPROVEMENT

Unlike randomized controlled trials, in quality improvement there is no causal link between intervention and improvement. In randomized control trials, similar control groups are formed to minimize confounding variables.

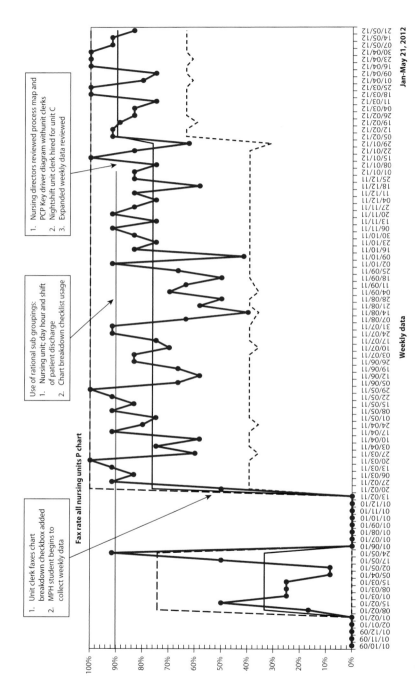

Figure 2-10 ■ Example annotated control chart.

In quality improvement, the aim is real-world improvement. In assessing the relevance of a randomized control trial, one must determine if the controlled study environment is comparable to the uncontrolled clinical environment. Likewise, in quality improvement, the local context of the quality improvement project and the generalizability of the findings to one's own local context are important in seeking to apply lessons learned from others' projects.

CONCLUSION

Quality improvement is a central component of all aspects of healthcare. This is underscored by the expectation that pediatricians participate in meaningful quality improvement activities in order to maintain board certification. In this chapter, we described the most common approach to quality improvement. Ongoing research in quality improvement methods will refine the approach and help identify those strategies that are most likely to lead to success. Regardless, quality improvement will rely on identifying important problems, choosing metrics to assess change, forming a multidisciplinary team, and evaluating tests of change informed by an understanding of the problem and the local resources.

IN PRACTICE

- At the next meeting of your team, discuss areas in need of improvement. What processes could be improved to improve patient experience, reduce costs, and improve quality of care? Are there gaps between evidence-based guidelines and your team's practices?
- Once you have established improvement priorities, define your specific "SMART" aim, collect baseline data, define the current state of your process, and develop a key driver diagram.
- Answer the three questions from the Institute of Healthcare Improvement's Model for Improvement.
  - What are we trying to accomplish? (Aim statement)
  - How will we know a change is an improvement? (Measure)
  - What changes can we make that will result in improvement? (Interventions)
- Perform an initial test of change on a very small scale.
- Perform frequent Plan-Do-Study-Act cycles of change.
- Share data with front-line staff.
- What is the reliability of your intervention(s)?

FAQs

1. Is it okay to jump from aim statement to intervention? My team has several ideas for solutions.

   It is better to define the "Key Drivers" or "what has to go right?" in order for the team to accomplish the aim. Stated in the affirmative, the key drivers can help take a complex issue and break it down into smaller manageable drivers. Each intervention should be directed at helping actualize one or more key drivers.

2. Why not start an intervention at scale? My hospital does it all the time.

   By testing on a very small scale, you can absorb failure in data collection instruments or an intervention's unintended consequences with minimal risk to patients. You also safeguard against losing front-line staff engagement by empowering front-line staff to improve the process and not "handing down" well-intentioned, but ineffective improvement solutions.

The authors would like to thank and acknowledge:

Tess Woerhlen, MPH, Drexel University School for Public Health for her collaboration in developing Figures 2-3, 2-6, and 2-10 and improving hospitalist-to-primary care provider communication.

Lloyd Provost, MS, Associates for Process Improvement, for reviewing and editing this chapter.

REFERENCES

1. Committee on Quality Health Care in America, Institute of Medicine. *Crossing the Quality Chasm: A New Health System for the 21st Century.* Washington, DC: National Academy Press; 2001.
2. Langley GL, Men R, Nolan KM, Nolan TW, Norman CL, Provost LP. *The Improvement Guide: A Practical Approach to Enhancing Organizational Performance.* Second Edition. San Francisco, CA: Jossey-Bass Publishers; 2009.
3. Berwick DB, Nolan TW, Whittington J. The triple aim: care, health, and cost. *Health Affairs.* 2008;27(3):759-769.
4. US Agency for Healthcare Research and Quality (AHRQ) Web site: http://ahrq.gov
5. Provost LP, Murray S. *The Health Care Data Guide: Learning from Data for Improvement.* San Francisco, CA: Jossey-Bass Publishers; 2011.
6. Shewhart WA. *The Economic Control of Quality of Manufactured Product.* New York, NY: D. Van Nostrand; 1931.
7. All figures of control charts including identification of each centerline, upper and lower control limits were created using QI Charts©, Scoville Associates; 2009.

MEDICAL ERRORS, ADVERSE EVENTS, AND HUMAN FACTORS

3

▌ BACKGROUND

Approximately 3.7% of patients hospitalized in New York State in 1984 suffered a disabling adverse event, two-thirds of which were preventable.[1] This data, published by Lucian Leape and colleagues in 1991, was startling to many and initiated widespread discussions about unintended patient harm. Indeed, many experts agree that the modern patient safety movement was conceived with the publication of this research in what became known as the Harvard Medical Practice Study. Leape would later say, "I recognized that my colleagues and I had uncovered a huge problem, but we had no idea what to do about it."

So what Dr Leape did was to study the lessons from human factors engineering and cognitive psychology research regarding human error, culminating in a publication in *JAMA* in 1994 entitled "Error in medicine."[2] If the Harvard study represented the conception of the modern day patient to safety movement, it is fair so say that "Error in Medicine" represents its birth.

In "Error in medicine," Dr Leape reflects, "Can the lessons from cognitive psychology and human factors research that have been successful in accident prevention in aviation and other industries be applied to the practice of medicine? There is every reason to think they could be." Leape concluded that errors must be accepted as evidence of systems' flaws, not character flaws, and until and unless that happens, it is unlikely that any substantial progress will be made in reducing medical errors.[2] While 20 years later, there is still debate about whether or not substantial progress has been made in improving patient safety, one thing is certain: the healthcare industry has significantly deepened its understanding of human factors, medical error, and adverse events. This chapter provides an overview of these ongoing challenges and offers some suggestions regarding what to do about them.

NO DATA WITHOUT STORY, NO STORY WITHOUT DATA

The data disclosed in the Harvard Medical Practice Study were alarming. Behind each data point, however, there was a story. We know from experience that while data drives performance, stories drive engagement. In the spirit of "no data without a story, and no story without data," here we provide several stories that have helped to engage the industry in performance improvement.

Just months after "Error in medicine" was published in *JAMA*, Cal Sheridan was born a healthy baby boy in a large accredited hospital where over 5500 newborns were delivered each year. The date was March 23, 1995. As his mother Sue tells the story, "Cal was first noted to be jaundiced through visual assessment at 16.5 hours old, but a bilirubin test was not done. He was discharged from the hospital when he was 36 hours and was described as having head to toe jaundice, but a bilirubin test was not done. Neither was his blood typed nor a Coombs test performed."[3]

The Sheridan's received information about jaundice in a simple brochure that never mentioned jaundice can cause brain damage. They were assured that Cal's jaundice was normal and not to worry. On day four, Cal was still yellow, lethargic, and feeding poorly. A call to the newborn nursery resulted in Sue Sheridan being asked if she was a "first time mom" and then assured there was no concern. Not comfortable with that answer, Cal was promptly brought to the pediatrician who noted jaundice by visual assessment, but did not order a bilirubin test. The Sheridans were told to wait 24 hours to see if Cal would improve.

At 5 days of age, the pediatrician admitted Cal to the pediatric unit. Cal's bilirubin was tested for the first time and it was 34.6 mg/dL. Treatment was limited to phototherapy and that phototherapy failed Cal. On day six in the afternoon, Cal had a high-pitched cry, respiratory distress, and increased tone, and he started to arch his neck in a way that is characteristic of opisthotonos; these behaviors were all acute symptoms of kernicterus. Cal was suffering brain damage before the very eyes of his parents. Sue later noted, "I will be haunted by that memory and my failure to protect him forever."

Today, Cal has athetoid cerebral palsy throughout his body, neurosensory hearing loss, enamel dysplasia on his front teeth, crossed eyes, and other abnormalities. He cannot walk independently, his speech is impaired, he drools, and he has uncontrollable movements of his arms and legs.[3]

On the 1-year anniversary of "Error in medicine," 7-year-old Ben Kolb was hospitalized for elective ear surgery, a procedure that was to be quick and simple. The date was December 15, 1995. During surgery, Ben suffered a cardiac arrest and died the next day. When the incident was investigated, the hospital found that a terrible mistake had been made: Ben had inadvertently been given a highly concentrated form of epinephrine. The root of the problem was traced back to an unlabeled syringe of epinephrine that was mistaken as the local anesthetic (lidocaine). When poured into sterile containers used in the operating room, the two drugs looked exactly alike. While the staff had labeled the containers, they did not label the syringes. It was confirmed that the syringes thought to contain lidocaine actually contained epinephrine.[4]

In 2007, Alyssa Shinn, a preterm infant in Nevada received a lethal dose of zinc following an order for total parenteral nutrition (TPN). The automated compounder used for TPN required order entry of zinc in a mcg/kg dosing formulation, forcing the pharmacist to convert the physician's TPN order from mcg/100mL. While the pharmacist performed the calculation correctly, she inadvertently entered the zinc dose in mg, not mcg, resulting in a 1,000-fold overdose.[5]

These and many other stories bring to light the sometimes devastating consequences of medical errors. Adverse events that harm children may seem even more difficult to process and represent a tragedy not only to parents and family, but also to healthcare professionals who desire the same positive outcomes from medical care. Parents often deal with disbelief, extreme disappointment and often anger after placing their absolute trust in healthcare providers and encountering failure, while healthcare providers, themselves, often suffer as the "second victims" after harm occurs.

HOW BIG IS THE PROBLEM?

Over the past 2 decades we have gained an understanding of the scope of morbidity and mortality associated with medical care. The Harvard Medical Practice Study found that nearly 4% of hospitalized patients suffered an unintended injury caused by treatment that resulted in prolongation of hospital stay or disability at the time of discharge.[1] Subsequent studies provide further insight:

- Medication-related errors are estimated to account for about 7,000 deaths each year and increase a 700 bed hospital's annual operating cost by more than $3 million annually[6]
- Nearly 2 million patients annually acquire a healthcare-associated infection while being treated for another illness or injury, and nearly 88,000 die as a direct or indirect cause of this infection. United States

healthcare costs have increased by nearly $5 billion every year as a result of health are acquired infections.[7]

- According to CMS, approximately 1.24 million patient safety incidents occurred to hospitalized medicare patients over the years 2002 to 2004. These patient safety incidents were associated with more than 250,000 deaths and $9.3 billion in excess costs.[8]

To put this problem in context, the 1999 Institute of Medicine Report "To Err is Human" stated that more people die in a given year as a result of medical error than from motor vehicle accidents, breast cancer, or AIDs.[9]

In an era where healthcare costs continue to soar and millions are under-insured, the physical, socio-economic, and emotional toll of medical injury is staggering.

THE COMPLEXITY OF CARE

The provision of medical care is extremely complex. The prevention of disease, the diagnosis and treatment of new conditions, and the maintenance of patients with chronic conditions occur in a context with a baffling number of variables. Nothing is constant and few things are certain. Even with all the medical research that has been done over the past 100 years, there is not a high degree of agreement on what constitutes best practice; diagnosis and treatment are often performed under some degree of uncertainty; and medication monitoring, particularly in the outpatient setting, is quite challenging. For front-line practitioners, there are always new medications, new technologies, new procedures, and new research findings to assimilate. Patients are becoming increasingly complex and the diversity of the workforce grows at an increasing rate. Providing safe, reliable care has never been more challenging (Figure 3-1).

The pediatric patient's interaction with the healthcare system typically begins when the child is in utero and continues through transfer to adult medicine some 14 to 21 years or so later. In between, there are "well-baby" visits, trips to the emergency department for acute injuries and confounding conditions, sports and summer camp physical examinations, immunizations, care for chronic conditions like childhood asthma and diabetes, and rarely, one or more hospital admissions for acute illnesses. Some children will die of terminal disease (eg, Lesch–Nyhan syndrome) while others will be cured (eg, childhood leukemia), and still others will live long-productive lives with otherwise life-threatening conditions (eg, hemophilia) or minor health issues along their way.

While there are countless "touch-points" between the average pediatric patient, his/her family, and the healthcare delivery system, there are six major

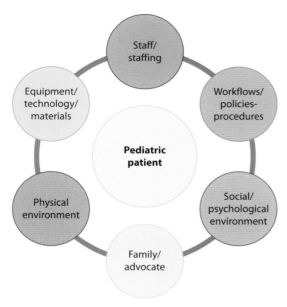

Figure 3-1 ■ Complexity of Care.

opportunities in the lifecycle of pediatric care for preventable harm due to human error and system design. These opportunities are during:

1. Newborn or neonatal care
2. Preventive care and screening (health maintenance or well child care)
3. Diagnosis of new conditions/illnesses
4. Medication management
5. Surgical/other invasive procedures
6. Treatment, not already specified

The life-cycle of pediatric care with a few examples of potential failure points are depicted in Figure 3-2. Those who provide care for the pediatric population know that children are not small adults. They have special needs based on their age, size, and developmental level. But it's much more complex than that. In the general pediatric outpatient office, the pace is often very fast. A pediatrician may see fourteen or more patients in a 3- to 4- hour session, many of whom have multiple needs, and all of whom require careful documentation of what was done (eg, immunizations, weight/height/head circumference checks, hearing and vision checks, ear washes, respiratory treatments, bladder catheterizations, oral and injected medications, anticipatory guidance). Mistakes happen and are often undetected for long periods of time. One such example occurred when a

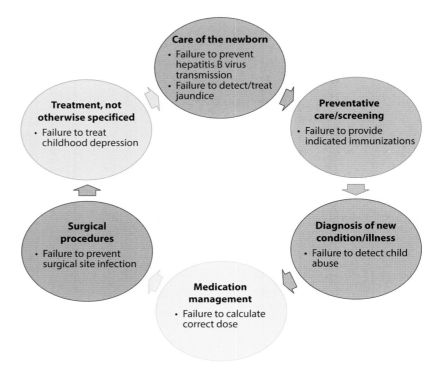

Figure 3-2 ▪ Lifecycle of pediatric care.

manufacturer changed its product preparation so that a vaccine had to be mixed with a diluent before administering. The packaging for the diluent looked similar to the prior vaccine packaging and a nurse administered straight diluent to a number of patients before the error was caught. While the diluent itself did not pose any risk of harm, the children who had received no vaccine were vulnerable to disease before the error was identified.

In the inpatient area, it is widely thought that the location of greatest risk to the pediatric patient is the neonatal intensive care unit (NICU). (see chapter 9) One study showed that adverse events (AEs) in the NICU occur at a rate of 74 events per 100 patients.[10] The most commonly reported AEs include intravenous catheter infiltrates, nosocomial infections, accidental extubations, intraventricular hemorrhage, and skin breakdown. Factors that increase the complexity of care in this setting include:

- The challenge to ensure that all staff have adequate experience and competency for tasks that may only be needed occasionally; eg, infant resuscitation, intubation, line placement, and ventilator management;
- Variation in practice in these settings based upon where staff trained and their personal preferences and experiences. This level of variation

leads to unnecessary complexity. Examples of unwarranted variation may include: prescribing custom total parenteral nutrition (TPN) when standard solutions will do; not using standardized order sets for vasoactive drips; and not using pharmacists for managing drug levels when research been shown that they are better at doing this than are physicians and nurses

In specialty areas, there are unique challenges specific to the pediatric population as well. For example, ordering and administering chemotherapy requires the use of treatment algorithms that often involve more calculations and have less margin for error than with an adult population. Adherence to the algorithms with adjustments as appropriate are critical to avoiding errors such as administering chemotherapy when it was contraindicated, or worse, administering it by the incorrect route; eg, intrathecal versus intravenous. In addition, services like pediatric cardiology and nephrology, for example, require specific knowledge and skills on the part of all healthcare team members, who must work as a high-performing team and provide care in acute settings to highly vulnerable infants and children.

Regardless of setting, the risk of harm in pediatric care can be compounded by inexperience, lack of education, drift in practice, and failure to follow-up.

One other risk to safety is availability of specialty care. A busy generalist must make decisions every day determining when it is necessary to seek a higher level of care for the patient in front of them. These decisions may lead to errors simply based on their scope of practice. The opportunity for a physician to consult with a specialist in real time can reduce these errors. Additionally, digital radiology makes it possible to consult with a radiologist remotely.

| THE CHALLENGE OF KEEPING PATIENTS SAFE

To underscore the challenge of keeping patients safe, even a very small error rate or near perfection, can have serious consequences in modern healthcare. The arithmetic is staggering. For example, in a teaching hospital, the average patient receives more than 30 different medications during hospitalization. Thus, an average sized (600 bed) teaching hospital may administer more than 4 million doses each year. If the medication ordering, dispensing, and administration process were 99.9% error free, there would still be over 4,000 errors a year in that hospital—if only 1% of these resulted in an adverse event, this seemingly low-error rate would cause 40 adverse events from medication alone.[11]

In healthcare, we know from experience that a large number of errors are caught by the people who make them; many others are caught by technology such as computerized physician order entry (CPOE), bar-coding, and radio-frequency tagged surgical sponges; and still other errors are caught by members of the care team including the patient and family reliably performing redundant checks (eg, a nurse doing an independent double check of a high alert medication; a physician requiring a write-down/read-back on a verbal order; a patient asking staff members if they've washed their hands).

Those errors that do reach the patient are often insignificant due to the amazing resilience of the human body or the characteristics of the ordered treatment itself (ie, relatively low toxicity, risk). A safe, reliable system design, however, doesn't rely on the resilience of the human body, or luck, or the ability of well-rested, fully alert, and cognitively focused practitioners to catch their own mistakes. Safe and reliable design (1) identifies, assesses, and eliminates conditions that produce human error and violations, (2) implements systems that detect and trap human errors before they cause harm, and (3) mitigates the impact of those errors that nevertheless make their way to the patient through early detection and timely response.

The remainder of this chapter will focus on understanding the causes of human error and violations to aid in the design of safer, more reliable systems.

ERRORS IN MEDICINE—SYSTEMS FLAWS, NOT CHARACTER FLAWS

To understand human error, one must understand what it is to be human. James Reason, cognitive psychologist and highly regarded error expert put it this way: "Correct performance and errors are two sides of the same coin. Human fallibility is not the result of some divine curse or design defect; rather it is the debit side of a cognitive balance sheet that stands heavily in credit. Each entry on the asset side carries a corresponding debit. Absent-minded slips and lapses are the penalties we pay for remarkable ability to automatize our current perceptions, thoughts, words, and deeds. If we were perpetually "present minded," having to make conscious decisions about each small act, we would never get out of bed in the mornings. The resource limitations of the conscious "workspace" that allow us to carry through selected plans of action in the face of competing situational demands also lead to information overload and leakage of memory items." He goes on to say, "Unsafe acts are like mosquitoes. You can try to swat them one at a time, but there will always be others to take their place. The only effective remedy is to drain the swamps in which they breed." In the case of errors and violations, the "swamps" are equipment designs that promote operator error, bad communications, high workloads, budgetary and commercial pressures, procedures that necessitate their violation in order to get the job done, inadequate organization, missing barriers and safeguards— all of these "latent factors" are, in theory, detectable and correctable before a mishap occurs."[12]

HUMAN ERROR AND VIOLATIONS: "MOSQUITOES IN THE SWAMP"

For the purpose of this text, consider errors and violations as behaviors that stray from the path of patient safety, which may include:

A. the unwitting deviation of action from intention (slips and lapses);
B. failure of intended actions to achieve desired goals (mistakes); or,
C. deliberate, but not unnecessary reprehensible deviation from those practices deemed necessary to maintain the safe operation of a potentially hazardous system (violation).

Some of the error-related behaviors noted above are rooted in the conduct of technical skills, others in the selection and execution of so-called "rules" (eg, algorithms, known pathways), and still others in the process of applying knowledge under infrequent, ambiguous, or unfamiliar circumstances.

Skills—based errors occur during the performance of routine tasks that people tend to do more or less on autopilot (very little conscious control). An example of a skills—based error in pediatrics might include missing a step in performing the "five rights" of medication administration before immunizing a child or failing to follow aseptic technique in maintaining a central line. For many tasks in pediatrics, however, it may be more challenging to have sufficient experience to ever be on autopilot.

Rule—based errors involve higher cognitive function wherein the individual encounters a problem and he tries to match it with a rule that successfully solved a similar problem in the past. An example of a rule-based error in pediatrics might include failure to ensure babies born to Hepatitis B surface antigen moms don't fall through the cracks or working a child up appropriately to rule out appendicitis. In the case of Cal Sheridan, it was failure to screen for hyper bilirubinemia.

Knowledge—based errors occur during infrequently encountered problems requiring careful consideration to think through a set of ambiguous indicators or factors. Examples of knowledge-based errors in pediatrics might include not considering all of the special needs of a child with a rare condition like Down syndrome. In the case of Alyssa Shinn, it was failure to recognize the formution of zinc required for TPN compounding, leading to a lethal calculation/conversion error.

In the context of providing safe, reliable healthcare, the errors described above may occur in the planning, storage, or execution phases of performing various medical tasks and procedures. From a pediatric patient safety perspective, however, understanding the taxonomy of error is not the goal; the goal is understanding how those errors are produced, preventing those that can be prevented, and identifying and mitigating the consequences of those that cannot.

Patient safety experts fundamentally believe that human errors are not the causes of medical harm, but the by-product of people trying to pursue success in resource-constrained, uncertain, and imperfect systems, what Jim Reason referred to as "the swamp." To reduce the risk of human error, one must "drain the swamp."

THE "SWAMP" OF HUMAN ERROR

The swamp that helps create and shape human error and violations of safe practice is more formerly called "latent factors." These are, as noted earlier, equipment designs that promote operator error, bad communications, high workloads, budgetary and commercial pressures, procedures that necessitate their violation in order to get the job done (eg, work-arounds), inadequate organization, and missing barriers and safeguards.

Latent factors are like resident pathogens that establish a set of conditions making it easier to commit both errors and violations. They arise from decisions made by designers, builders, procedure writers, and top-level management. James Reason explains that latent factors may lie dormant within the system for many years before they combine with active failures and local triggers to create an accident opportunity. Unlike active failures, whose specific forms are often hard to foresee, latent conditions can be identified and remedied before an adverse event occurs.[13]

The fact is that a high quality healthcare system is not solely safe; high quality care is timely, efficient, effective, equitable, patient-centered, and safe.[14] In other words, safety is not the only aim. Managers and leaders often face difficult decisions when balancing budgets and trying to run operations efficiently, and even highly competent leaders, sometimes make decisions with inherent trade-offs or unrecognized downsides. Errors and violations may be unknowingly produced by competing goals, demands, and priorities, as well as by the tools and materials staff use, the tasks they perform, and the operating environment in which they work. Simply put, healthcare providers are sometimes "set up" to make errors by the complex environment in which they work due to the limitations of being human.

As in other high-risk and highly complex industries, healthcare leaders have turned to the fields of cognitive psychology and human factors research to better understand risks and patient safety challenges associated with human fallabilities.

HUMAN FACTORS

Human factors leverage what we know about human behavior, abilities, limitations, and other characteristics to ensure safer, more reliable outcomes. Human factors focus on human beings and their interaction with each other, products, equipment, procedures, and the environment. Those with deep knowledge of human factors engineering examine activities in terms of their component tasks and then consider each task in terms of the following:

- Physical demands
- Skill demands
- Mental workload
- Team dynamics
- Environmental conditions

While relatively new to medicine, the science of human factors has been around since the 1920s, when most of the work in this area was focused on the selection and training of individuals. From about 1945 to 1960, human factors shifted away from focusing on individuals and were largely driven by military ergonomics (ergo = work, nomics = rules). The thoughtful and carefully constructed design of the aircraft cockpit is a great example of human factors from an ergonomics perspective.

From the mid-60s to present day, human factors are understood to include both the selection and training of individuals and ergonomic design, as well as a deeper appreciation and understanding of human to human interaction. An example of this is commercial aviation's crew resource management, with the goal of, (1) selecting and training highly competent individuals—create a team of experts; (2) designing great controls, instrumentation, and human-equipment interfaces for the individual experts to work within; and finally, (3) developing great communication, coordination, and collaboration among the individual experts—that is, move from a team of experts to expert teams.

Unfortunately, medicine does not have 50 years to develop the same track record as aviation safety. We must learn from aviation and other high reliability organizations who have applied human factors principles to practice to operate long periods of time between adverse events. One of the most significant lessons learned from these industries is that human error is not a cause of failure, it is the effect or symptom of deep trouble. Human error is also not random, it is systematically linked to an individual's tools, tasks, and operating environment.

Human factors engineers (HFEs) believe contributing factors in accident causation begin with management, including management's influence and control of: production pressure, policies, decision making, resourcing and staffing, employee selection and development, and structure.

They believe management in turn, impacts the following:

1. Physical environment
2. Equipment design
3. Work itself and
4. Social/psychological environment

These elements, in turn, interface with and affect the performance of the worker, who also comes to the workplace with their own set of unique qualities/characteristics (including age, experience level, intelligence, mental and physical health, and motivation).

Ultimately the worker performs a set of mental and/or physical tasks, which are subject to errors (eg, mistakes, slips, lapses) as well as procedural violations. Most of these errors (and violations) are inconsequential, and some of them are not. In addition, the patient/family plays a role in the process as well.

A visual display of this model might look something like this (Figure 3-3).

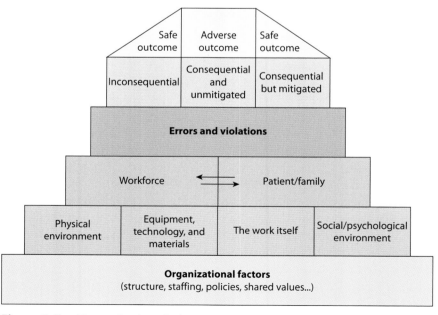

Figure 3-3 ■ The production of adverse outcomes.

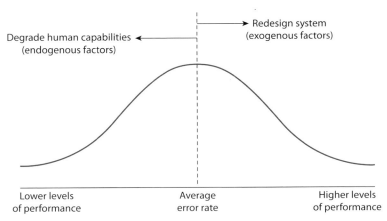

Figure 3-4 ▪ Human error performance.

HUMAN ERROR PERFORMANCE

Human factors engineering doesn't try to change the human condition—it tries to use its understanding of the human condition to change the conditions under which humans operate. Errors and violations are viewed as consequences rather than causes, having their origins not so much in the perversity of human nature as in "upstream" systemic factors.

One way to view human error performance in the context of human factors might be by using the model of a normal Gaussian distribution (Figure 3-4).

Across a large enough healthcare professional sample size, there is undoubtedly some nominal (or base) human error distribution rate associated with any cognitive or physical task we could imagine—performing simple calculations to program a medication pump, diagnosing and treating jaundice, marking the correct surgical site, remembering that a medication may produce ulcers which can lead to internal bleeding, or listening to the voice of a mother who says something is very wrong with her child. For the purposes of this analogy, assume the error performance has some normal, bell-shaped looking distribution associated with it.

If we want to improve that distribution, we need to re-design the system. If we want to degrade that distribution within any existing system and fixed group of healthcare professionals, we need to degrade human performance. Purposeful degradation of human performance is never done intentionally, of course, but human factors engineers and safety scientists would observe it done frequently.

When thinking about human factors infractions, think about design that either neglects to take into consideration the human condition, or worse yet, makes the human condition even more fragile than it already is.

The factors that can shift the performance of this curve to the left or to the right are largely known. The first set of factors to consider are exogenous factors, those that originate outside the body. Exogenous factors impact our propensity to err or intentionally violate a standard practice. These include the following:

- The design of the task or the workflow itself
- The type and amount of training provided
- The resources available to get the job done
- The time to get the job done
- The quality and usability of the equipment and materials used
- Whether policies and procedures are available, intelligible, workable, and correct
- The characteristics, attitudes, beliefs, and behaviors of the people doing the work
- The communications and information environment
- Environmental factors such as noise, lighting, temperature, interruptions and distractions, clutter, and available space
- The relationship with, and respect for, the patient and family—their voice, their preferences, their concerns
- External constraints (eg, regulatory) that impact the ability to perform as expected
- Whether or not, there is a mechanism in place to identify and trap errors before they have a chance to cause serious problems.

Endogenous factors, or those that are generated within our own human system, may also contribute to human error. They may be psychological, physiological, or both. Examples of endogenous factors which may increase our propensity to err include the following:

- Sleep deprivation—It has been shown that cognitive performance after 24 hours without sleep is equivalent to performing with a blood alcohol level of 0.10.[14]
- Stress—While stress may improve human performance in some areas, it can degrade it in others. Current research seems to indicate that stress may have its biggest negative effect on knowledge-based workers; that's healthcare workers! Stress is also a likely contributor toward tunnel vision, where one loses sight of the bigger picture and is unable to see the forest through the trees.
- Fatigue—By definition, fatigue is a decrease in physical and/or mental capability as the result of physical, mental, or emotional exertion which may impair nearly all physical or decision-making abilities, or balance. Some studies have shown that nurses who work shifts of 12.5 hrs or

greater are three times more likely to make an error than their colleagues working shorter shifts.[15]

Other endogenous factors that may adversely impact performance are fear, intimidation, and anger. The Joint Commission became so sensitized to this issue that they issued an alert specific to the impact of intimidation and other non-professional behaviors, or so-called "disruptive" behavior.

With an understanding of human factors and human error performance, it is obvious that human error is not a cause of failure, it is the effect or symptom of deep trouble; it is not random. It is systematically connected to the feature of people's tools, tasks, and operating environment. For those interested in improving patient safety performance, it is essential to look through a similar lens when assessing violations of safe practice. If "to err is human," to violate probably means you're still alive.

VIOLATIONS OF SAFE PRACTICE

Human error expert Jens Rasmussen emphasized that front line workers do not follow procedures in a strict and logical manner, but try to follow the path that seems most useful and productive at the time. Workers operate within an envelope of possible actions that are influenced all the time by wider organizational and social forces. He described pressure on individuals and systems to move toward the boundaries of safe operation. Furthermore, these violations can become more frequent and severe over time, so the whole system "migrates" to the boundaries of safety until an accident or recalibration occurs. These external pressures, coupled with individual rewards and benefits, may over time modify the work being carried out, lead to rules and recommendations being progressively ignored, and eventually greatly increase the possibility of disaster as the organization becomes accustomed to operating at the margins of safety.[16]

Violations of safe practice, in other words, like human error, are not explanations of adverse outcomes—they deserve explanations. While violations are often deliberate deviations from rules and standards, they can also come from a long, slow *drift* in practice. They may set in slowly over time, with operators becoming gradually more lax in their performance as tasks are completed, outcomes are met, and recognition is provided for a job well-done. The term "normalization of deviance"[16] has been used to describe such situations where individuals or teams repeatedly get away with a departure from established standards until their thought process is that repeated success in accepting deviance from established standards implies future success. Over time, the individuals/teams fail to see their actions as deviant. Any one who drives a car a bit over the speed limit, comes to rolling stops at stop signs, frequently finds themselves accelerating through yellow lights that are turning red, or even glances at their cell phone to see who is calling is guilty of this.

While many managers would like to draw a bright line between right and wrong choices individuals made in the aftermath of an adverse outcome with respect to compliance or adherence to safe practice, defining non-compliance is not so straightforward. The expected level of compliance, and therefore interpretations of non-compliance and violation, varies according to the type of instruction management has given, the nature of the work management has created, and the social and organizational context management has shaped. A good place to start with is the assumption that nobody comes to work in healthcare wanting anything less than the best for their patients.

The factors that shape an individual or team's propensity to violate are well-documented[17] but we don't need the literature to understand what is already known from observing our own behavior. Returning to the topic of driving habits: does anyone on the road these days always slow down at yellow lights; come to complete stops when turning right on red and at stop signs; drive the posted speed limit; use turn signals as required by law, minimize all unnecessary interruptions and distractions, including cell phones? The conditions which shape these driving behaviors include the following:

- Low probability of getting caught
- Inconvenience
- Lack of recognition of risk
- Authority or status to violate (self-perceived)
- Copying the behavior of others on the road
- No disapproving figure present in the car
- Group pressure

The same violation producing conditions that are present on the road, don't necessarily get checked at the doors of a hospital or clinic. They are pervasive throughout our society, in both our personal and professional lives. As our understanding of human factors is being leveraged to minimize the production of human error, so too must it be used to reduce the human propensity to violate.

ACCIDENT CAUSATION IN COMPLEX SYSTEMS

Even when medicine is error- and violation-free, it is inherently hazardous. Radiation and chemotherapy treatment of a child with cancer may save a life, but it is not risk free. The placement of a central line and an order for ventilator assistance for a neonate in the NICU may save a life, but it is not risk free. Even when a parent provides consent to all indicated immunizations for their child, they understand it is not completely risk free.

An adverse event is defined as an injury caused by medical management rather than the underlying medical condition itself. An adverse event may or may not be preventable. For example, in the aforementioned Harvard Medical Practice Study, Dr Leape concluded that 24% of the adverse events detected were judged unpreventable—in other words, they resulted from complications that could not be prevented with the current state of medical knowledge. He also found that 6% were only potentially preventable. This conclusion was made when no error or violation was detected but that a high incidence of this type of complication reflected low standards of care or technical expertise.

The focus of this chapter is largely on the 70% of adverse events that occur in hospitals (and other settings) that are preventable. While not immediately recognizing it at the time, Leape's review of human factors, cognitive psychology, and other "high reliability organizations" later helped him understand that most of the adverse outcomes that were preventable did not just result from a single human error or procedural violation. It takes many factors, all necessary and only jointly sufficient, to push a system over the edge of failure.

An accident model that has been found to be helpful in describing the concept of contributing factors being "necessary and only jointly sufficient" in pushing a system over the edge of failure, in causing a preventable adverse event if you will, is the Swiss Cheese Model of Accident Causation described by Jim Reason in his book *Human Error*.[12]

Reason asserts that the set-up for an accident to occur in a system begins with a fallible decision made by its top-level leaders. These decisions are then transmitted via line management and then ultimately to the point of production, or the point of care in our industry, where so-called pre-conditions or qualities of human behavior and production co-exist, including attributes like the level of skill and knowledge of the workforce, work schedules, technology, equipment, and maintenance programs, along with the individual and collective attitudes and motivation of the workforce which create its culture.

Ultimately, the commission of unsafe acts, which includes human error, violations, and often both, can be prevented or mitigated with a variety of defenses, but often these defenses have defects in them too.

The trajectory of accident opportunity begins with latent failures at managerial levels, proceeds with complex interactions as the impact of management's decisions gets closer to the point of care, and is neither stopped nor mitigated by one or more levels of defense that were designed to reduce the risk of harm associated with unsafe acts in the first place. The Swiss Cheese analogy here, as depicted in Figure 3-5, is that all of the holes or defects in the various levels of the system align to turn a variety of active and latent deficiencies into an adverse outcome.

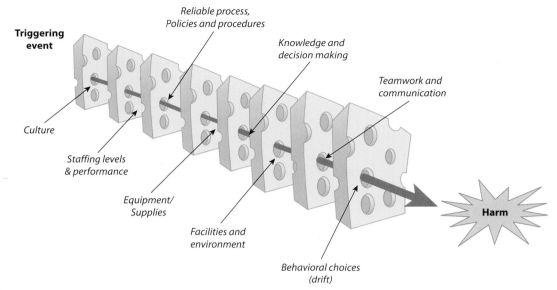

Figure 3-5 ▪ The Swiss-cheese model of accident causation. (Adapted, with permission, from Reason JT. *Human Error*. Cambridge, UK: Cambridge University Press, 1990.)

This graphic shows the complex layer of events that line up for an accident to occur in complex systems. Events are not a chance coincidence, nor the result of one incompetent provider in the system, but rather the result of an organization and its individuals operating in a vulnerable mode. Unless changes are made, other adverse events will occur, it is not a matter of if, but only when.

ERROR REDUCTION PRINCIPLES

Armed with an understanding of human factors, medical error, and the creation of preventable adverse outcomes, the good news is that significant performance improvement in pediatric patient safety is possible. While other chapters in this book will dive deeply into medication safety, teamwork and communication, leadership, and the importance of engaging patients and families, reductions of preventable errors and drift from safe practice begins with the following set of beliefs:

1. Most adverse events are preventable.
2. The primary cause of preventable injury is not bad people, but imperfect systems.
3. To prevent injury to pediatric patients, we need to redesign our systems.

This chapter concludes with twelve error-reduction principles that patient safety and quality improvement leaders should become familiar with. This list is not meant to be all inclusive, but it is a good start, and the reader will see references to these principles throughout the text:

1. Simplification: Simplify the structure of tasks to help minimize the load on vulnerable cognitive processes like working memory, and to reduce waste. Simplifying physician order entry for immunizations is one example of this principle in pediatric practice. In addition, at an organizational level, simplify the types of services to be provided, commensurate with the volume of patients served. For example, perhaps it is safer to focus on initial resuscitation and transfer of sick infants and children and not on hospitalization in low volume-hospitals. Simplify operations through the development of a reliable process of transporting them to a higher volume and acuity hospital.

2. Standardization: Create standard work processes, equipment, and materials to better assess and improve outcomes, orient and train staff, and improve ease of use. Standardization also requires clarification of roles and responsibilities regarding both routine and infrequent tasks so that everyone is absolutely clear about who is accountable for what. Standardizing how medication dosing will be done for pediatric patients is a good example of what this principle looks like in practice. Other examples include: (a) use of a reliable vendor to compound pediatric TPN solutions instead of having hospital pharmacists with limited experience perform this task; (b) standardizing criteria for ordering blood products; (c) using IV pumps that have pediatric specific "libraries" that make it less likely that the wrong dose of drug will be administered to the patient; and even (d) standardizing where these pumps are kept in order to prevent mingling of adult with pediatric pumps.

3. Avoid reliance on memory: Memory is a very weak aspect of human cognition. In particular, working or short-term memory is extremely limited in its capacity and so problem solvers are prone to lose items in what's called their "stack." Cognitive psychologists have shown that the number of discrete items of information human beings can hold in short-term memory is 7 ± 2. Humans compensate for the limited size of their working set by selective ignorance and chunking! This can be a fatal flaw in pediatric patient safety. Using checklists prior to central line insertion or surgery is an excellent example of reducing reliance on memory in pediatric care. Another example is integrating "best practice alerts" into the electronic medical record to prompt physicians and nurses to order the correct care.

4. Improve access to information: Improving access to information and intelligent decision-support can improve efficiencies, reduce reliance on memory, and minimize mistakes. This principle can be applied through high-tech (eg, automated medical records, with the entire medical record being accessible by the pediatric patient's family with appropriate consent; libraries created to prevent errors in infusions) and high-touch (eg, multidisciplinary rounding involving the pediatric patient's family) mechanisms in pediatric settings.

5. Take advantage of habits and patterns: Taking advantage of habits and patterns makes it easier to do the right thing and to minimize the risk associated with shortcuts, workarounds, and drift from safe practice. One example of taking advantage of habits and patterns is check for head of the bed elevation, as indicated, on the pediatric patient on a ventilator, during hourly nurse rounding.

6. Use constraints and forcing functions: In your home, a child safety device like a gate in front of a set of steep stairs is a constraint. A forcing function example could include tamper-free medication bottles. Exploit the power of constraints and forcing functions to make it hard to do the wrong thing such as making sure that tube connectors for enteral solutions are different from those for IV solutions.

7. Use visual controls to shape desired behavior: A new mother who is bonding with her child in a hospital may benefit from a visual control (in this case, a sign) on her door that indicates there are no interruptions.

8. Promote effective team functioning: Through enhanced training strategies (eg, simulation) and development of communication skills, teams can better leverage existing resources, minimize errors, and recover from harm. High performing teams also hold each other mutually accountable and are more capable in confronting each other's violations and drift from safe practice in the interest of patient safety. The use of simulation with feedback to improve neonatal resuscitations is one example of how to promote effective team functioning, as is encouraging debriefing for all neonatal resuscitations, even when they go well.

9. Deploy redundancies: Redundancies are independent safety nets that aim to detect and mitigate an error's ability to cause harm in a work-flow. Bar-coding medication is a redundancy that supplements the five rights of medication administration. CPOE with specific alerts or prompts that require the practitioner to take action is another form of redundancy. Used selectively, redundancies save lives.

10. Eliminate environmental factors that degrade human performance. Clutter, inadequate lighting, excessive noise, and needless interruptions

and distractions are not present in any high reliability organization (eg, commercial aviation, aircraft carrier operations, nuclear power) and they should not be present in ours.

11. Create systems that are better able to better tolerate the occurrence of errors and contain their damaging effects when they do occur. This includes using mitigation strategies such as bed alarms to lessen the impact of errors.

12. Enhance situational awareness, which is the ability for members of a team to know what is going on, know what is most important, and be able to reasonably predict what is going to happen next. Organizations like Cincinnati Children's use disciplined rounding and huddling processes to enhance and maintain situational awareness of their pediatric population. This allows the organization to proactively anticipate where the next problem may occur on any unit, and get to it, before it gets to them.

CONCLUSION

Most adverse events are not caused by simple human error or willful violations to the point of being reckless, but by some combination of error and drift where a staff member was following a path that seemed reasonable at the time. Pediatric patient safety is improved and sustained when organizations: (1) determine the best place for pediatric care to be provided based on their patient population, flow, and volume; (2) recruit, develop, and retain the best and brightest providers and create a learning system that continuously sharpens their technical and cognitive skills—this includes having continual exposure to peers who can hold each other accountable for current evidence-based practice; (3) create a culture of safety that includes placing a premium on teamwork, communication, adherence to safe practice and engagement of the pediatric patient and their family in the provision of safe care; and (4) design and sustain standard work in a way that acknowledges the human condition and continuously aims to improve the conditions under which humans work.

IN PRACTICE

Taking a practice, a workflow, or a set of processes as is, and making them significantly safer and more reliable, requires a systemic approach. This

(Continued)

(*Continued*)

shouldn't preclude any one individual, however, from taking responsibility for what is in their direct and immediate ability to influence or control tomorrow. Here are five vital behaviors of safe and reliable practice that can be implemented immediately:

1. Follow evidence- and consensus-based safety practices: Safety practices that are available, workable, intelligible, and correct, need to be followed. There are a number of protocols that have been developed in the aftermath of a single adverse outcome or through the analysis of trended data, but they only work when followed (eg, universal protocol; two patient identifiers; write-down, read-back; hand hygiene).

2. Ask for help when you need it: Asking for help to get something done safely is not a sign of weakness—it's a sign of strength. Everyone is busy, but no one should be too busy to put a patient at risk of harm.

3. Offer help when someone else needs it: Offering help is at the heart of team-based care. When someone else is struggling to do something safely, offer help immediately.

4. Speak up: In the absence of effective peer control and teamwork, "Drift Happens." When you choose to become a passenger in patient safety and don't put your safety concerns and perspectives on the table, your pediatric patients will get hurt. Every provider is 200% accountable: 100% accountable for the quality of the behavioral choices they make, and to protect the pediatric patient, 100% accountable for confronting drift when they see it in others.

5. Listen up: Patients and family members who have suffered preventable medical harm have time and again told us that either they did not feel listened to or were not "given voice." When they think about what could have made the biggest difference in averting the adverse event, it most often comes down to being listened to. In an effort to, above all else, do no harm—listen up!

FAQs

1. How can I apply the principles in this chapter to practice at my hospital or clinic? To make things right, for every patient, every day, will require a new way of thinking about errors in medicine, and a new approach to preventing harm. This journey begins with a deeper appreciation for error causation and prevention. We hope that this chapter provided a good foundation toward that end. By next engaging co-workers in the identification

and prioritization of patient safety challenges, the team can then use models such as that endorsed by the Institute for Healthcare Improvement that focus on the rapid application of "small tests of change." In other words, learn together by doing. Inviting patient and family members into the redesign of workflows and practices is another good way to develop "new ways of thinking."

2. It seems like the predominant response in medicine following an adverse outcome is to target individuals at the "sharp end" of care—the doctors, nurses, pharmacists, and other people providing care everyday. How can we shift from this "culture of blame"?

Rather than blaming people for human errors, safety experts recommend that we acknowledge human fallibility, and focus more on the conditions under which individuals and teams work. Then, workflow and defenses can be designed to avert errors, conditions that lend themselves to violations can be minimized, and mechanisms can be put in place to mitigate unsafe acts that may nevertheless occur. When the pediatric patient and family members are made part of the care team, the actualization of "first do no harm" becomes more and more possible each day.

REFERENCES

1. Leape L, Brennan T, Laird N, et al. The nature of adverse events in hospitalized patients. *NEJM*. 1991; 324(6):377-385.
2. Leape, L. Error in medicine. *JAMA*. 1994; 272(23):851-857.
3. CDC. Cal's story. Centers for Disease Control and Prevention. Available at: http://www.cdc.gov/ncbddd/jaundice/Cals-story.html.
4. http://www.paediatricchairs.ca/safety_curriculum/domain5_docs/StoryofBenKolb.pdf
5. ISMP Medication Safety Alert, Sept 6, 2007. Volume 12, Issue 18
6. Bates DW, Spell N, Cullen DJ, et al. The costs of adverse drug events in hospitalized patients. *JAMA*. 1997;277(4):307-311
7. www.cdc.gov/mmwr/preview/mmwrhtml/mm4907a4.htm accessed 5/29/2014
8. http://seniorjournal.com/NEWS/Health/6-04-03-MedicalErrors.htm
9. Kohn LT, Corrigan JM, Donaldson MS, eds. *To Err is Human: Building a Safer Health System*. Washington, DC: National Academies Press; 1999.
10. Sharek P, Horbar J, Mason W, et al. Adverse events in the neonatal intensive care unit: development, testing, and findings of a NICU-focused trigger tool to identify harm in North American NICUs. *Pediatrics*. 2006;118:1332-1340.
11. Leape L "The Preventability of Medical Injury," in Bogner M "Human Error in Medicine", CRC Press, 1994.
12. Reason J. *Human Error*. Cambridge, England: Cambridge University Press; 1990.
13. Committee on Quality of Health Care in America, Institute of Medicine. Crossing the quality chasm. *A New Health System of the 21st Century*. Washington, DC: National Academy Press; 2001.

14. Baker A, et al. Sleep disruption and mood changes associated with menopause. *J Psychosom Res*. 1997;43(4):359-369.

15. Rogers AE, et al. Health Affairs. 2004;23:202-213.

16. Vaughn D. *The Challenger Launch Decision: Risky Technology, Culture, and Deviance at NASA*. Chicago, Illinois: University of Chicago Press; 1996.

17. Reason J. *Managing the Risk of Organizational Accidents*. Burlington, VT: Ashgate Publishing Company; 1997.

PEDIATRIC MEDICATION SAFETY | 4

Medical errors represent a leading cause of morbidity and mortality, both in the United States and throughout the world.[1] Medication errors are by far the most prevalent type of medical error in all care settings, and for all patient populations,[2] and as noted in a seminal article on patient safety, the most common cause of iatrogenic adverse events.[3] As most medication errors are arguably preventable, strategies to promote medication safety are an essential component of patient safety and quality improvement initiatives. This chapter will address medication safety, with a focus on issues unique to the pediatric population.

DEFINITIONS AND EPIDEMIOLOGY

A medication error can be defined as "a failure in the medication process that leads to, or has the potential to lead to harm to the patient."[4] These failures may occur in the manufacturing and/or compounding of medications, or may occur during the medication use process, which encompasses drug prescribing, dispensing, administration, and subsequent drug monitoring. An adverse drug event (ADE) is a medication error that results in any injury (eg, physical, mental, physiological) to the patient. Fortunately, the vast majority of medication errors do not result in harm to patients. It has been estimated that one in seven medication errors have the potential to cause patient harm, with just one in 100 medication errors causing an injury.[5]

ADEs represent the largest single category of adverse events due to medical error experienced by hospitalized patients, accounting for nearly 20% of all injuries sustained.[6] As might be expected, ADEs are associated with increased morbidity and mortality, prolonged hospital length of stay, and higher healthcare costs.[7]

The Institute of Medicine (IOM) reported in January of 2000 that from 44,000 to 98,000 deaths occur annually in the United States from medical errors.[1] Of this total, an estimated 7,000 deaths occur due to ADEs.[1] In their 2007 report on medication error, the IOM estimated that between 380,000 and 450,000 preventable ADEs occurred annually in the hospitals of the United States.[2] Assuming an estimated 400,000 preventable ADEs annually, the projected cost of ADEs at that time was 3.5 billion dollars.[8]

Other studies on the incidence of ADEs in hospitalized patients have formulated significantly higher estimates. A meta-analysis of prospective studies estimated that 6.7% of the hospitalized patients in the United States will have a serious ADE, with an associated fatality rate of 0.32%.[9] If accurate, this would translate to greater than 2.2 million serious events, causing well over 100,000 deaths. This would position ADEs as the fourth leading cause of death in the United States. ADEs result in an estimated 700,000 emergency department visits annually, prompting an estimated 120,000 hospital admissions, and countless ambulatory care encounters.[10] All of these data are for adult patients.

Studies within the pediatric population indicate that the rate of medication errors may be higher in hospitalized children compared to adults.[11] Ferranti et al found medication errors to be three times higher in pediatric versus adult inpatients.[12] Examining medication errors in children hospitalized in two institutions, Kaushal and colleagues found a medication error rate of 5.7%, with a rate of potential ADEs of 1.1%—a figure three times higher than published rates for adults.[13] Twenty-five percent of the actual ADEs in this study were judged to be preventable. Data from other studies of pediatric inpatients suggest that medication error and ADE rates may actually be quite a bit higher. At a single tertiary pediatric center, Holdsworth et al reported ADE frequencies of 6 per 100 hospital admissions and 7.5 per 1,000 patient days, and potential ADEs of 8 per 100 admits and 9.3 per 1,000 patient days.[14] Nearly a quarter of the reported ADEs were judged as serious or life threatening. In a single pediatric center in Buenos Aires, Otero and colleagues found a medication error rate of 11.4%.[15] At a single pediatric tertiary center in the United States, Marino et al found a medication error rate of 24% in a tertiary children's hospital.[16] In all these studies, most of the errors occurred during prescribing.

Medication errors also occur in ambulatory, pre-hospital, and emergency care settings. In an effort to characterize the frequency and type of errors that occur in the ambulatory care setting, Abrahamson et al evaluated the prescribing practices of 78 office-based clinicians in two states over a 15-month study period.[17] The overall error rate, excluding illegibility of handwriting, was quite high, with one or more errors occurring in 28% of all prescriptions. Illegibility was enormously prevalent, with an error rate of 175 per 100 prescriptions written. Reviewers deemed that the vast majority of these errors could have been eliminated with the use of computerized provider order entry (CPOE) with clinical decision support (CDS). Data on pediatric ambulatory medication error rates are quite limited. A 2007 study by Kaushal et al investigating outpatient visits in Massachusetts pediatric primary care practices found 16% of all outpatient prescriptions were associated with an ADE, with 12% of the ADEs categorized as serious and 20% categorized as preventable.[18] In a follow-up study of medication error in pediatric outpatients, these investigators found that 50% of paper-based prescriptions contained an error, with 21% of prescriptions containing a potentially harmful error.[19] The most common types of error identified were inappropriate abbreviations and dosing errors. The most frequent root cause for error was illegibility. Data from specialty care clinics have reported even greater error rates.[20]

A study of medication administration by emergency medical services (EMS) providers in eight Michigan EMS agencies found frequent medications errors (defined as doses >20% from a weight appropriate dose) for commonly used medications, with approximately 1/3 of medications administered being incorrect.[21] Single institution studies of medication errors in the pediatric emergency care setting have reported rates ranging from 9% to 31%.[22-25] These studies report the experience at larger volume pediatric centers, where only a small percentage of U.S. children (9%–11%) receive emergency care. Using de-identified incident reports as the source for medication error reporting, Shaw and colleagues from the Pediatric Emergency Care Applied Research Network reported the medication event experience within their 18-pediatric tertiary center network.[26] They found that medication events constituted nearly 20% of all incident reports, with medication errors representing 94% of the reported events, and 13% of the errors causing patient harm. Reflecting upon the practice of pediatric emergency care in a non-tertiary center setting, Marcin et al studied medication errors experienced by high-acuity ill or injured children at four rural emergency departments (EDs) in Northern California, discovering an error rate of 39%, with 16% of these errors having the potential to cause harm.[27]

In addition to understanding the incidence of medication errors, and most importantly ADEs, it is useful to understand the burden of disease and the need for subsequent treatment in the pediatric population. Using data from the National Center for Health Statistics, Bourgeois et al determined there was an average of nearly 600,000 annual ADE-related visits for the time period spanning 1995–2005.[28] Seventy-eight percent of these visits occurred in ambulatory clinics, and 12% in EDs. Children 0 to 4 years of age had the highest incidence of ADE visits. The most common presenting complaints for all age groups were dermatologic (45%) and gastrointestinal (16.5%). The medication classes most frequently implicated were antimicrobials (27.5%), central nervous system drugs (6.5%), and hormones (6.1%). The highest rate of visits for ADEs resulted from antineoplastic and immunosuppressive agents, with

19.7 ADE-related visits per 1,000 outpatient visits associated with that medication class. Other studies using other national surveillance data sources have estimated close to 160,000 ED visits made by U.S. children annually due to an ADE.[29,30] Estimates indicate that 4.7% of all hospitalizations of children are the result of an ADE.[28]

The wide variations in reported rates of medication error and ADEs are likely due to several factors including differences in setting or institution type, medication use processes (eg, paper versus electronic prescribing), study design, and type of classification and methods employed for error identification. Whatever the true rate may be, medication errors, and particularly ADEs, represent a significant public health problem that is for the most part preventable.

WHY ARE CHILDREN AT GREATER RISK?: HOW ARE THEY DIFFERENT?

As described above, studies of medication error indicate that children bear an even greater risk for errors and ADEs. Pediatric patients are at increased risk for several reasons, including[31-33]:

- Drug pharmacokinetic parameters are different at various developmental stages
- Multiple calculations are needed to individualize doses based on age, weight, height, body surface area, or clinical indication
  - Early life (eg, neonates, premature infants) age-based dosing may be influenced by chronologic or gestational age
  - A wide dosing range exists for some drugs depending upon clinical indication and underlying patient disease
  - The 10-fold over- or under-dose is particularly prevalent in children
- Lack of available dosage forms and concentrations for pediatric and neonatal patients results in extemporaneous compounding
- Lack of published data and Food and Drug Administration (FDA) approved-product labeling addressing dosing, safety/efficacy, and clinical use of many key medications prescribed for pediatric patients
- Special domains within clinical practice pose an even greater risk for ADEs, such as transplantation, oncology, neonatology
- Limited patient ability to communicate to prevent an error or signal that an error has occurred

Of all the above, the factor that contributes most toward an increased risk of medication error and ADEs in children is the need for dosing calculations at multiple steps in the medication use process. It has been estimated that weight-based dosing error rates are nearly double that for non-weight-based dosing

(10.3% vs 5.9%).[34] The 10-fold dosing error is a particular concern in pediatric care and a direct descendant of flawed calculations. Doherty and McDonnell studied 10-fold errors over a 5-year period at a tertiary children's hospital.[35] Using a voluntary safety reporting database as their source, they found that 10-fold errors occurred at a rate of 0.062 per 100 total patient days. A relatively high percentage of these errors, 9%, resulted in harm to the patient. Opioids were the class of medications most frequently associated with these errors.

Fortescue et al rated the effectiveness of 10 strategies for reducing the rate of pediatric medication errors.[36] The three strategies with highest potential impact were:

1. Unit-based clinical pharmacists making rounds with the healthcare team (might have prevented 81.3% of medication errors).
2. Improved communication among physician, nurses, and pharmacists (might have prevented 75.5% of medication errors).
3. Use of computerized prescriber order entry (CPOE) with clinical decision support (might have prevented 72.7% of medication errors).

A survey in 2000 by the Institute for Safe Medication Practices (ISMP) and the Pediatric Pharmacy Advocacy Group (PPAG) found that such safety practices were not widely implemented during the prescribing, processing, dispensing, and administration of medications to pediatric patients.[37]

THE MEDICATION USE PROCESS

Prescribing

Historically, most errors (74%) and potential ADEs (79%) originate in the ordering phase.[13] Common prescribing errors that have been identified through pharmacist/nursing interventions include: wrong dose (over-dose/under-dose), wrong patient, wrong frequency, wrong duration, omission, wrong start time, wrong start date, and lastly, known allergy to prescribed medication. Prior to the implementation of computerized provider order entry (CPOE) and electronic prescribing, common sources of prescribing error included illegible or incomplete orders/prescriptions, and for hospital-based care, errors made by clerical staff transcribing handwritten orders into electronic order and dispensing systems. Verbal orders were (and still remain) another meaningful source of medication error and adverse events. Prescribing is an activity that is highly susceptible to the influences of various human factors, including fatigue, distraction, and of course, calculation errors. In fact, pre-CPOE studies of prescribing error noted that many prescribers, particularly trainees, lacked the ability to reliably calculate drug doses.[38,39]

Computerized Provider Order Entry and Clinical Decision Support

The development and implementation of electronic health records (EHR), and specifically CPOE, have been demonstrated to significantly reduce the incidence of both medical errors, potential ADEs, and adverse events in pediatric care.[20,36,40-43] Based on data from the Children's Hospital Association, in a nested matched case-control study, patients cared for in hospitals without CPOE were 42% more likely to experience a reportable ADE.[41] To date, data demonstrating improved pediatric patient outcomes as a result of CPOE have been limited.[20] Indeed, single center studies have, at times, demonstrated conflicting patient safety outcomes as the result of CPOE implementation.[44,45]

In addition to eliminating errors due to transcription and illegibility, most basic CPOE systems obviate the need for simple dose calculation. That said, CPOE systems have not eliminated medication error, and many commercial "off-the shelf" CPOE systems may fail to address critical unique pediatric dosing requirements for certain clinical indications, critical illness, or for specific states of physiologic impairment.[42,43,46] The addition of computerized clinical decision support (CDS), standardized order sets and checklists to CPOE systems has further decreased prescribing errors and ADEs.[42,42,46-50] Ferranti and colleagues describe the challenges of prescribing at the Duke Children's Hospital using a single university medical center CPOE architecture, and their development of a pediatric advanced dosing model.[43] Leu and colleagues similarly describe how the systematic updating of order sets during the implementation of a commercial CPOE improved care quality at the Seattle Children's Hospital.[49] Modest improvements achieved with CPOE alone have been further enhanced with the addition of CDS.[50]

At the Ann & Robert H. Lurie Children's Hospital of Chicago, medication events with potential for harm (≥D events on Safety Event Category Impact Scale, adopted from National Coordination Council for Medication Errors Reporting and Prevention, NCC MERP[51]), decreased from 0.08% to 0.002% (75% decrease) the month after CPOE implementation. This commercial CPOE system offered customized pediatric (and neonatal) CDS, including order sets, allergy and drug interaction alerts, and dosing guidelines for altered physiologic states and children of all ages. The event rate for potentially harmful events has been maintained at 0.003% for three years post CPOE implementation, an overall decrease of 70% for such events.

Due to data interfaces between electronic systems, and most importantly, due to the human-EHR interface, electronic prescribing systems are unable to prevent all medication errors, and may themselves be a source for error.[52,53] As an example, prescribers could enter an order for the right drug—but for the wrong patient. Prescribers may learn to "over-rely" upon CPOE, assuming that content provided is correct, and choose not to question a dosing recommendation offered. Most importantly, many prescribers are apt to not utilize available CDS,[20,42,52] as they may view the process as onerous or time-consuming, or if they view the advice or alerts offered to be meaningless. Likewise, prescribers frequently choose to ignore or over-ride CDS prescribing alerts, with reported over-ride rates as high as 92%.[54] In developing CDS systems, there may be a delicate balance between the level of dosing support and alerts provided, in an effort to avoid "alert-fatigue."[20,43]

Medication Reconciliation

According to the Institute for Healthcare Improvement, experience from hundreds of healthcare organizations has shown that poor communication of medical information at transition points is responsible for as many as 50% of all medication errors and up to 20% of adverse event (ADEs) in hospitals.[55] Studies of hospitalized adult patients have demonstrated that 60% experienced one or more unintended medication discrepancies during either admission or discharge, with nearly 20% of these errors being clinically important.[56] A review of the pediatric literature identified a broad range of reported frequencies, ranging from 22% to 72%.[57] This has led The Joint Commission and others, to focus on medication reconciliation to reduce the risk of errors during transition points. A Joint Commission National Patient Safety Goal (NPSG) requires hospitals to reconcile medications across the continuum of care.[58]

Medication reconciliation has been defined as the process whereby an up-to-date and complete list of a patient's medications is created, and then compared to medication orders generated during admission, discharge, and care transitions.[57] Steps in the medication reconciliation process are outlined below:

- **Obtain a medication history:** Obtain the most accurate list possible of the patient's current medications upon admission to the organization and before administering the first dose of medications (except in emergent or urgent situations). The list should include prescription and non-prescription medications, including the use of herbals and other supplements; the dose, route, frequency, and the time and date of the last dose. The medication history can be made by a physician, licensed independent practitioner (LIP), medical student, resident, nurse, pharmacist, or pharmacy student and should be completed in a timely fashion (ideally within 2 hours of hospital admission).
- **Reconcile and resolve discrepancies and prescribe the medications:** The review and documentation of prior-to-admission (PTA) medications and medication reconciliation upon admission is conducted in the patient's medical record, utilizing CPOE and CDS if available.

- **Reconcile again upon transfer and discharge:** Each time a patient moves from one setting to another, a review of previous medication orders alongside new orders and plans for care should occur, resolving any discrepancies. The sending LIP will enter a transfer order in the patient's medical record and the receiving LIP will reconcile medications. When the patient is discharged, the reconciled list of admission medications must be compared against the discharge orders, along with the most recent medication administration record. Any differences must be fully reconciled within the patient's medical record before discharge using CPOE and CDS if available.
- **Share the list:** Communicate a complete list of the patient's medications to the next provider of service when transferring a patient to another setting, service, practitioner, or level of care within or outside the organization. The discharge nurse should provide a copy of discharge medications and instructions for the patient, patient's family, and/or legal guardian.

As inpatient care poses the greatest risk for medication error and ADEs (greater patient and medication management complexity, risk for baseline and new medication interaction, acute illness impact on physiology and tolerance of errors, etc), it is sensible to initiate reconciliation efforts in this setting. The benefit of reliable communication of medication use should also occur in the ambulatory care setting[59] and at the interface (emergency department) between outpatient and inpatient care.

Processing/Verifying

With CPOE in place, pharmacists can focus on those components of the medication-use process where their clinical expertise can bring the greatest value to patients and clinicians, and not on issues such as deciphering illegible orders or monitoring the accuracy of order transcription from paper into electronic format. This allows pharmacists to thoroughly review orders for clinical appropriateness, review patients' medication history and assure that there are no potential drug interactions, that dosing and routes of administration are appropriate, and that there are no contraindications. As noted by Fortescue et al, the presence of pharmacists on inpatient rounds at a United States tertiary pediatric center significantly helped to prevent medication errors.[36]

Maat et al studied inpatient medication errors at a children's hospital in the Netherlands, with an existing CPOE system with "basic" CDS.[46] Over a 4-year study period, pharmacist interventions occurred for 1.1 % of the nearly 140,000 medication orders, a rate of 165 per 10,000 electronic prescriptions, with 80% of these interventions made for a dosing error that might have caused patient harm. The remaining interventions were for incomplete orders (eg, missing patient weight, medication dosage form or strength/concentration). Over-doses were more than twice as common as under-doses, and 11% of the incorrect doses reflected a 10-fold error. Dosing errors most frequently occurred in their immunology/hematology unit (31%), followed by the neurology and general medicine units. Not surprising was the finding that "free-text" prescriptions were five times more likely to require intervention by a pharmacist. Of interest, children aged 1 to 2 years had the greatest risk for an error requiring an intervention. The benefits of pharmacist review of electronic orders has been demonstrated in other centers, and in other hospital settings, such as the emergency department.[34,60]

ROLE OF A PHARMACIST

Although dispensing has traditionally been pharmacists' primary role in the medication-use process, pharmacists today are recognized as integral members of an interdisciplinary team with shared responsibility for safe and optimal patient care. Particularly in inpatient settings, pharmacists working alongside prescribers and nurses have helped prevent medication errors. The direct involvement of pharmacists throughout the medication-use process can minimize the risk of preventable ADEs, reduce morbidity and mortality, decrease costs associated with patient care, and improve patient outcomes associated with drug use.[61-64] The presence of a pharmacist on rounds as a full member of the patient care team in a medical intensive care unit was associated with a 66% decrease in preventable ADEs; nearly all (99%) of pharmacist interventions were accepted by prescribers.[61] Pharmacist participation in rounds on general medical units, where patients often have many comorbid conditions, has been shown to reduce preventable ADEs by 78%.[63]

Healthcare organizations should identify the patient care units in which pharmacists' presence will have the greatest impact on patient safety. Determining factors might include staffing patterns and expertise, the availability of medications on units, the types of patients served, the types of medications frequently prescribed and administered, the volume of new admissions and patient turnover, the typical volume of medication orders, and the type of drug distribution system used. Pharmacists should be present during peak hours when rounds are conducted and orders written.

At Lurie Children's Hospital of Chicago, pharmacists round daily with the pediatric intensive care unit, neonatal intensive care unit, hematology/oncology, bone marrow and solid organ transplant, and gastroenterology teams. Pharmacists contribute to the overall medication care plan including formal pharmacokinetic consultation for aminoglycoside antibiotics and vancomycin, parenteral nutrition components, tapering of narcotics, and providing overall clinical support in all medication-related decision making. Clinical pharmacists are available 24 hours a day, 7 days a week to verify all medication orders and entertain any medication related question. In addition to pharmacist interventions made on rounds, pharmacists enter retrospective interventions while reviewing and verifying medication orders. This intervention data are reviewed in aggregate and any trends are highlighted with medical staff.

DISPENSING

Formulations and Dosage Forms

Commercially available formulations are often not appropriate for pediatric patients and thus require dosage manipulation, which increases the chance of error.[31,34] For example, certain medications come only in tablet or capsule formulations that cannot easily be swallowed by infants or young children and in strengths that are not appropriate for pediatric dosing. Extemporaneous compounding of tablets/capsules into a solution or suspension is needed. This introduces the risk for calculation and/or measurement error, altered drug stability, and/or bioavailability, and errors related to repackaging, just to name a few. This holds true for injectable medications as well, whereas adult-based concentrations for many parenteral medications require further dilution for adequate pediatric dose administration. Again, this increases opportunity for error.[31,34]

In order to mitigate some of the potential for error with medication dispensing, several measures should be taken, including:

- Whenever possible, all medications should be prepared and dispensed by the pharmacy. Exceptions would be medications approved for storage in automated dispensing device (ADDs) for urgent and emergent administration.
- Stocking only one concentration of medication.
- Look-alike-sound-alike (LASA) medications should be stored separately and labeled with tall-man lettering.
- Dispensing area should be well lit, free of clutter, and most importantly, free of distractions.

In order to decrease waste, increase efficiency and focus efforts on safety, the Lurie Children's Hospital of Chicago pharmacy batches medications (both injectable and oral) into seven batches a day. This decreases the volume of medications prepared, checked, and delivered in any given time frame. This workflow allows pharmacists and technicians more time to focus on double checks and decreases wrong patient, wrong dose/volume, and wrong medication mix-ups.

Administration

Medication administration can be defined as the preparation, provision, and evaluation of effectiveness for all medications given to patients.[65] The integration of pharmacotherapy into patient care is a fundamental aspect of nursing care. Nurses are required to have an essential understanding of the medications they are administering in order to provide safe care and educate the patient and family while monitoring for adverse reactions and side effects. Utilization of resources, such as pharmacy staff, on-line formularies and institutional protocols, aids in the provision of safe medication administration. Safe medication practices are typically emphasized during the nursing orientation period when the new graduate nurse or a newly hired experienced nurse has a preceptor to guide them through the standards set by the institution for safe medication administration.

The National Coordinating Council for Medication Error Reporting and Prevention (NCCMERP) issued recommendations to improve the accuracy of medication reconciliation for hospitalized patients.[66] Included in these recommendations were a series of checks to be performed prior to the administration of a medication. Known since as the "rights," these checks include: the right medication, in the right dose, to the right patient, via the right route and dosage form, at the right time, with the right documentation.[67]

Stratton et al surveyed nurses to determine the source of medication administration errors. Distractions and interruptions were mentioned by 50% of the respondents. Other frequently noted sources included: suboptimal nurse to patient ratios, large volumes of medications requiring administration, and failure to double-check doses.[68] In a literature review on the issue of medication administration errors, additional contributing factors included communication, drugs with similar names, trailing zeros and decimal points, and lack of knowledge.[69]

High Alert and Look-Alike-Sound-Alike Medications

Although most medications have a wide margin of safety, a few drugs have a high risk of causing patient injury or death if misused. Special precautions are needed to reduce the risk of error with these medications. While all medications need to be reviewed prior to administration, high alert and LASA medications require special attention.[70,71] Each institution is required by The Joint Commission to create a list of high-alert medications.[70] The Institute for Safe Medication Practices offers annual updates of a list of high alert, or adverse event prone, medications.[72]

In order to decrease the potential for error, many institutions have created an independent double-check process for high-alert medications. The process includes a second nurse or licensed independent practitioner (LIP) who will perform an independent double check, with cosignatures required. The double check includes verification of the patient's name, medication syringe/bottle, dose, route, drug concentration, patient weight, expiration date, pump settings, and line attachments at the following situations/times: 1- before initial administration of the medication, 2- when IV bottle, syringe, or bag is changed, and 3- when the infusion set is changed. The expectation is that this double-check process also occurs with each patient handoff. By having two licensed professionals *independently* check the medication, the likelihood of catching errors anywhere in the process is high. Shaping this expectation and holding staff accountable for the independent double check can dramatically decrease the incidence of errors, specifically with high-alert medications. At Lurie Children's, policy and processes are in place to define safe and efficient ways of prescribing, dispensing, and administering medications that are considered "high alert" as well as medications that have similar names, which look alike or sound alike. Safety event data are reviewed annually and institution-specific lists are approved by the Medication Safety and Pharmacy and Therapeutics Committees. Figures 4-1 and 4-2 offer examples of high alert and LASA medication lists and some safety measures in place to prevent errors with these agents.

UTILIZATION OF TECHNOLOGY TO ENHANCE MEDICATION DISPENSING AND ADMINISTRATION SAFETY

The use of a pharmaceutical automated dispensing device (ADD) can improve the timeliness of medication administration, provide accountability for administering high-alert medications, support maintainance of supply levels, and assist leadership with fiscal data to assist in the budgeting process. ADDs can be customized to meet the needs of the patient care environment (emergency department vs operating room vs acute care unit vs ambulatory center vs intensive care unit [ICU]) and track usage by practitioner, which allows for greater accountability. ADDs can be configured to address necessary precautions for high alert and LASA medications (Figure 4-3).

Smart pump technology can assist the bedside nurse with high and low alerts for specific medications built into a drug library. Standardizing medication concentrations and creating service line modules (Example: ICU vs acute care units) can guard against programming errors by alerting the operator that the parameters programmed are out of range. On-going assessment of reports

HIGH ALERT MEDICATIONS
Chemotherapeutic Agents
EPINEPHrine (Infusions and Boluses)
Heparin (excludes: Flushes, Infusions with ≤1unit/mL Heparin)
Insulin
Potassium Chloride, Potassium Phosphate, Potassium Acetate (Concentrated Vials and IV Riders)
Neuromuscular Blockers (Cisatracurium, Pancuronium, Rocuronium, Succinylcholine, Vecuronium)
HYDROmorphone, Fentanyl, morphine (Epidurals, Infusions, PCAs, and IV Boluses)
TPN and Intralipids

- The High Alert Medications and Look-Alike/Sound-Alike Medication Policy will be accessible, via a link in EPIC® Order Entry and MAR, to all the medications on the High Alert List.
- The High Alert Medications and Look-Alike/Sound-Alike Medication Policy will be accessible, in Lexicomp® Special Topics and each individual Drug Monograph will be linked to the Drug Table.
- The High Alert Medications and Look-Alike/Sound-Alike Medication Policy will be accessible under Administrative Policy and Procedures via the Point.
- All High Alert Medications will require an independent nurse double-check and cosignature prior to administration and will show up with !! on the EPIC MAR.
- High Alert Caution Stickers will be placed in storage pockets/bins of all medications on the High Alert Medication List.
- High Alert Caution Stickers will be placed on bags/syringes of all patient-specific High Alert Medications dispensed.

Figure 4-1 ■ High-alert medications warranting special precautions to reduce risk for patient harm.

generated from Smart pumps can provide helpful information regarding the consistency of use and aid in the identification of education needs in order to maximize the functionality of the pump.

Barcoding medications (and patient ID bands) will assist the healthcare professional administering medications in making sure that the medication that is about to be administered is indeed on the patient's medication administration record (MAR) and is scheduled to be given at the designated time. The reading of barcodes may result in "false alarms," which can promote provider alert fatigue, this could cause clinicians to ignore true alerts. Professionals charged with building this technology into the providers' workflow should carefully consider what alerts should fire. Medications must be properly barcoded for this technology to be effective, so diligence at the time of labeling the medication is crucial to the success of this patient

Look-Alike Sound-Alike List

Ann & Robert H. Lurie
Children's Hospital of Chicago

cloBAZam	clonazePAM
DAUNOrubicin	DOXOrubicin
Depakote® (divalproex sodium) (delayed-release tablet)	Depakote ER® (divalproex sodium) (24 hour extended-release tablet)
ePHEDrine	EPINEPHrine
hydrALAZINE	hydrOXYzine
HYDROcodone	oxyCODONE
HYDROmorphone	morphine
humaLOG®	humuLIN®
oxyCONTIN®	oxyCODONE®
PHENobarbital	PENTobarbital
rifAMPIN	rifAXIMIN
sulfaSALAzine	sulfADIAZINE
vinBLAStine	vinCRIStine
VISIpaque®	OMNIpaque®

- **Look-Alike/Sound-Alike Warning Sticker/Label**
  1. On the medication shelf and/or container in the pharmacy.
  2. On the PYXIS pocket of the medication.
- Medication pairs are **Stored Physically Separated**.
- **Look-Alike/Sound-Alike Alert Warning** (medication specific)
  1. Displayed when entering order into the pharmacy computer system.
  2. Displayed on the MAR every time the medication is administered.
- Medication name written in **TALLman Lettering**
  1. On the medication shelf and/or container in the pharmacy.
  2. On the medication label in EPIC system.
  3. On the MAR.

Figure 4-2 ▪ LASA medication list and precautions taken to reduce error.

safety initiative. Barcoding reports will assist leadership in holding staff accountable for utilizing the technology. Establishing a desired threshold for compliance and clearly communicating the expectations to the staff are important elements to highlight when implementing or upgrading medication barcoding.

MEDICATION ADMINISTRATION OVERSIGHT

At the Ann & Robert H. Lurie Children's Hospital of Chicago, the group empowered to review medication administration is the Medication Safety Committee, which meets monthly to review events that had an impact on the patient. A subcommittee, the Medication Administration Committee, also meets monthly to review data mined from the electronic event

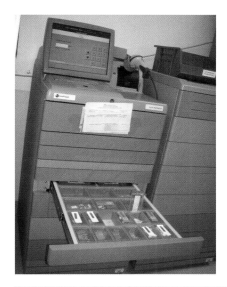

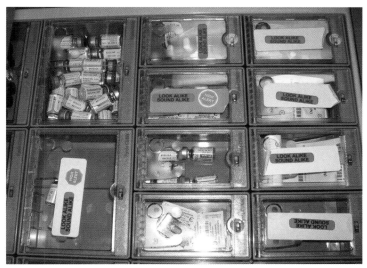

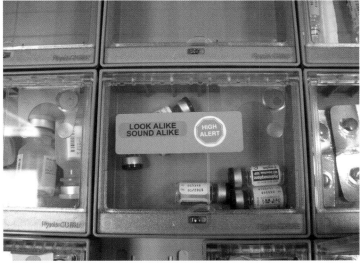

Figure 4-3 ▪ Organization and labeling of automated dispensing device drawers to reflect presence of high alert and LASA medications.

reporting system and barcoding data. This group also reviews medication administration and documentation processes in order to ensure compliance with regulatory standards. This is done by reviewing current practice, creating and initiating education for the end-users and monitoring compliance with established policies and procedures. Discussions revolve around safe medication administration practices across the institution and action plans are implemented to meet institutional and regulatory standards.

New medication administration policies and standards are brought to this group to review.

As an example, the process for administering boluses of medications or fluids from a Smart pump in the ICU setting was discussed as a potentially accurate, safe, and efficient way to deliver these agents in a timely fashion. Nursing leadership supported the adoption of this practice and identified a nursing administrator as the champion for this initiative, accompanied by the support of ICU physician leadership. Leadership support is vital to the successful implementation of new processes, clinical standards, or pathways. Therefore, identifying clinical leaders as change agents who can influence the practice of front-line staff is a critical component when implementing medication safety initiatives. The independent double-check process was identified as supporting reliably safe administration of boluses via the Smart pump. In planning for implementation of this new practice and staff education, simulation was identified as a strategy to educate and promote the required technical skills; this was done prior to the implementation of the new policy. Once in place, monitoring for staff compliance with the new policy ensued. Post-implementation evaluation for compliance with medication administration process/policy change is a critical component of process change, as issues often arise, including unintended consequences that need to be addressed. Re-education or reinforcement of these medication administration processes/policies may need to occur.

CHEMOTHERAPY SAFETY COMMITTEE

Many hospitals have found it helpful to create a multidisciplinary committee to specifically review chemotherapy-related safety events. Committee participants might include the quality manager or director of quality, physicians, advanced practice nurses, clinic and inpatient unit nurses, a nursing clinical educator, nursing director, clinical research associates, and pharmacists. Data should be shared with the organization's medication safety pharmacist and individual care providers. In addition, when both nursing and physician leaders support the work of this committee, outcomes can be shared more widely in forums such as division faculty meetings, hospital department meetings, and clinical staff meetings. Though the work of the Chemotherapy Safety Committee is primarily focused on the creation of chemotherapy safety guidelines for the treatment of children with malignancies, they also provide guidance for the use of cytotoxic agents in other patient populations. A Chemotherapy Safety Committee may also be responsible for the following:

- Orientation and education of care providers, including subspecialty trainee education and on
- Monitoring for compliance with hospital standards of care

- Reviewing and revising chemotherapy order sets within the EHR
- Reviewing related patient safety events
- Follow-up with individual care providers

ESTABLISHING AN EVENT REVIEW STRUCTURE

The use of an on-line event reporting system allows an institution to review all types of errors or near-misses that occur.[34,64,73] A reporting system can be invaluable when identifying trends in medication (or other patient safety) events that require a meticulous review in order to identify the root cause of the process failure that led to the event.[73] Often times, a multidisciplinary approach to examining the process will unveil aspects of medication prescribing, dispensing, and administration that can be built into a systems-based methodology designed to improve patient safety and prevent repeat errors or near-misses. Establishing a working group or committee to review and evaluate medication events that had a negative impact on the patient, including those near-misses that would have had a negative impact on the patient had they not been caught, will assist the institution in decreasing adverse medication events.

SAFETY EVENT REPORTING AND LEARNING FROM MISTAKES

Learning from errors and adverse events is key to improving processes, delivering high-quality care and improving medication safety. To encourage the reporting of medical errors, near misses and adverse events, many hospitals have implemented on-line anonymous safety event reporting systems (SERS). Implementation of a SERS promotes reporting of safety events in real-time, which then allows for immediate review of the reported event. Employees and healthcare providers are usually expected to submit an electronic report using the SERS within 24 hours of the event. When entering information about the event, the reporter is prompted to make a preliminary assessment regarding the potential level of impact using guides such as the Safety Event Category Impact Scale. The scale, as detailed below, has been adopted from the National Coordination Council for Medication Errors Reporting and Prevention (NCC MERP)[51] by many researchers and organizations, for use in classifying, measuring, and evaluating adverse events of all types.

- **A:** Circumstances that have the capacity to cause an event *(ie, near-miss)*.
- **B:** Event occurred but did not reach the patient/person.

- **C:** Event occurred and reached the patient/person but did not have an impact.
- **D:** Event occurred and reached the patient/person. Monitoring or intervention may have been required.
- **E:** Temporary impact on the patient/person may have occurred. Intervention required.
- **F:** Temporary impact on the patient/person may have occurred. Initial hospitalization or prolonged hospitalization required.
- **G:** Patient appears to have a permanent change in condition.
- **H:** Intervention may have been required to sustain life.
- **I:** Patient/person death.

Data and information gathered from the SERS is often managed by Patient Safety leaders in the organization and is used to identify system and process vulnerabilities or defects. Such information can be used by organization leaders to guide the selection of performance improvement projects, including failure modes effects analyses (FMEAs), and root cause analyses (RCAs) to improve clinical practices and processes of care.

IMPROVING MEDICATION SAFETY: A CASE EXAMPLE

Leadership is a critical function in promoting high quality, safe healthcare.[74] Research shows that leadership makes a major difference in the quality and safety of patient care. When a sentinel event occurs in a healthcare organization, inadequate or ineffective leadership is often one of the contributing factors. In fact, inadequate leadership was a contributing factor in 50% of the sentinel events reported to The Joint Commission in 2006.[75] At Lurie Children's Hospital, both leadership and front-line staff have placed emphasis on medication safety, making it a corporate goal in fiscal year (FY) 09. The goal was to initially decrease medication events with potential for harm (≥D events on NCC MERP Safety Event Category Impact Scale) by 20% in 1 year. At the end of FY09, the decrease was 55% with an overall event rate of 0.01% (Figure 4-4).

With the bar set at a 0.01% event rate for ≥D events, the goal going forward was to maintain this rate while implementing CPOE in FY10. While embarking on a whole new workflow for order entry, verification and nursing order acknowledgement and medication administration, it was determined that in order to preserve our event rate, we would need to do some proactive FMEAs. The areas targeted for CPOE FMEA included high-risk prescribing practices (insulin orders, medication reconciliation, drip titration, parenteral nutrition, and chemotherapy orders). With a successful CPOE implementation and proactive process improvements, the 0.01% goal was exceeded with a final FY10 event rate of 0.006% (Figure 4-5).

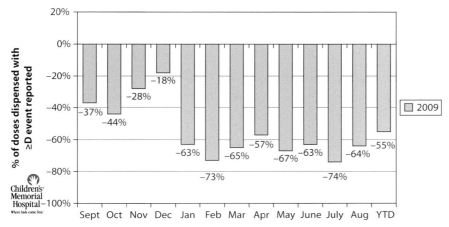

Figure 4-4 ▪ Percent of medication doses dispensed with >D event (NCC MERP Safety Event Category Impact Scale) reported, fiscal year 2009. The goal was to reduce events by 20%. By the end of the fiscal year, a 55% decrease was achieved, with an overall event rate of 0.01%.

In FY11, the goal was to continue to maintain this level of excellence in medication safety and allow for a full year post-CPOE implementation in order to assure that any unintended consequences were accounted for and corrective actions taken. The event rate for FY11 was 0.003% (Figure 4-6).

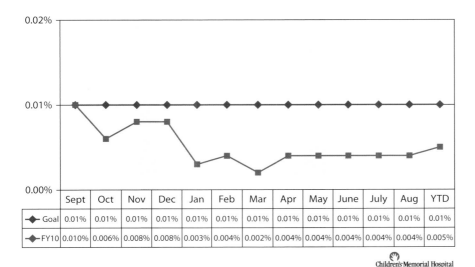

	Sept	Oct	Nov	Dec	Jan	Feb	Mar	Apr	May	June	July	Aug	YTD
Goal	0.01%	0.01%	0.01%	0.01%	0.01%	0.01%	0.01%	0.01%	0.01%	0.01%	0.01%	0.01%	0.01%
FY10	0.010%	0.006%	0.008%	0.008%	0.003%	0.004%	0.002%	0.004%	0.004%	0.004%	0.004%	0.004%	0.005%

Figure 4-5 ▪ Percent of doses dispensed with >D event (NCC MERP Safety Event Category Impact Scale) reported, fiscal year 2010. Red line reflects organization's error rate goal of 0.01%.

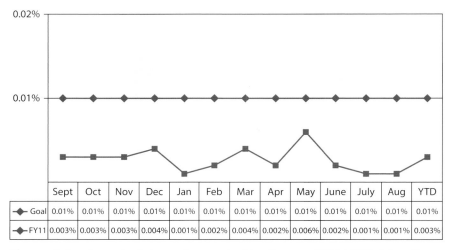

	Sept	Oct	Nov	Dec	Jan	Feb	Mar	Apr	May	June	July	Aug	YTD
Goal	0.01%	0.01%	0.01%	0.01%	0.01%	0.01%	0.01%	0.01%	0.01%	0.01%	0.01%	0.01%	0.01%
FY11	0.003%	0.003%	0.003%	0.004%	0.001%	0.002%	0.004%	0.002%	0.006%	0.002%	0.001%	0.001%	0.003%

Figure 4-6 ▪ Percent of doses dispensed with >D event (NCC MERP Safety Event Category Impact Scale) reported, fiscal year 2011. Red line reflects organization's error rate goal of 0.01%.

PLANNING FOR MEDICATION AND PATIENT SAFETY IN A NEW HOSPITAL

In 2012, the new challenge for the patient safety program would be continuing to maintain an already low rate (0.01%) of potentially harmful events while planning for and implementing a move to a new facility. Here again, the focus centered on simulation of some patient safety themes and a new environment. These included:

1. Neonatal intensive care unit (NICU) nursing double checks of drips/high-risk medications—with the NICU having private rooms at the new hospital, nursing double checks could become more challenging.
2. Pharmacy turnaround times—the verticality of new hospital layout (transition from nine to 25 floors) and reduced number of pharmacy satellites could pose turnaround time issues with regard to medication delivery.
3. Hematology/Oncology workflow of medication ordering-processing-dispensing-administering. The pharmacy satellite in the new facility is not located in a patient care area and is not in close proximity to either the ambulatory infusion center, formerly, the "day hospital," or clinic. The inpatient unit is located one floor below the satellite pharmacy, thus creating a need to develop a medication delivery

workflow. This is much different than the old hospital layout where the pharmacy was embedded between the day hospital and the clinic. Geographical placement of critical services must be considered when assessing the efficiency of the expected workflows for renovations or new structures.

4. ICU (CICU, PICU, NICU) medication ordering-processing-dispensing-administering—we would have an OR pharmacy satellite at the new hospital, but no PICU or NICU pharmacy satellites. All medications, including STATS will come from our main pharmacy (ninth floor), which is not in close proximity to the NICU (14th floor), CICU (15th floor), and PICU (16th floor). In addition, the tube stations will be located in more remote area and may require RN prompting when medication is tubed. Again, this is a much different workflow than what existed in the old hospital.

5. Code response simulation. The verticality of the building may have an unintended consequence of delayed response by code team members. This required consideration for optimal crash cart locations on each patient care unit, and enhanced basic life support readiness by front-line staff in all care areas.

These simulations, in addition to continued safety event review, process improvement and FMEAs assisted in sustaining the ≥D event rate of ≤0.01% throughout the year of the move with YTD rate of 0.003% for FY12 and 0.002% in FY13, where the goal was decreased to ≤0.008% (Figures 4-7 and 4-8).

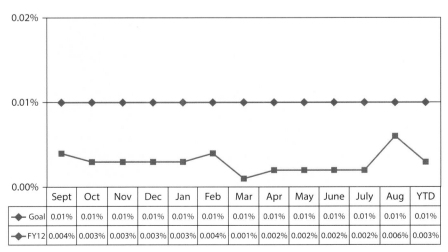

	Sept	Oct	Nov	Dec	Jan	Feb	Mar	Apr	May	June	July	Aug	YTD
Goal	0.01%	0.01%	0.01%	0.01%	0.01%	0.01%	0.01%	0.01%	0.01%	0.01%	0.01%	0.01%	0.01%
FY12	0.004%	0.003%	0.003%	0.003%	0.003%	0.004%	0.001%	0.002%	0.002%	0.002%	0.002%	0.006%	0.003%

Figure 4-7 ▪ Percent of doses dispensed with >D event (NCC MERP Safety Event Category Impact Scale) reported, fiscal year 2012. Red line reflects error rate goal of 0.01%.

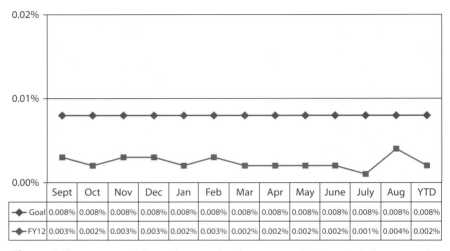

Figure 4-8 ▪ Percent of doses dispensed with >D event (NCC MERP Safety Event Category Impact Scale) reported, fiscal year 2013. Red line reflects error rate goal of 0.008%.

▌ WHERE DO I START?

For over a decade, the Institute for Safe Medication Practices (ISMP) and the Institute of Medicine (IOM) have been promoting the use of technology to enhance patient safety. The 1999 IOM report, "To err is human: building a safer healthcare system,"[76] estimated the annual costs of drug-related morbidity and mortality at $77 billion. IOM's 2002 report, "Crossing the quality chasm: a new health system for the 21st century."[77] urged health systems to place greater emphasis on the adoption of technology. This was followed in 2004 by another report, "Patient safety: achieving a new standard of care,"[78] which presented a detailed plan for development of data standards for collecting and classifying patient safety information. This report called for immediate access to complete patient information and decision support tools for clinicians and their patients. The 2006 IOM report. "Preventing medication errors,"[8] strongly supports greater use of information technologies.

So how does an institution begin to tackle implementation of technology in the medication use process? At Lurie Children's, the approach taken is depicted in Figure 4-9. New technology is not a remedy for medication errors, but it can provide safeguards that are not possible with a fully manual process. Whatever approach to technology integration an institution decides is best, it is important that baseline event data be gathered and system and process vulnerabilities be analyzed to guide the organization in selecting process improvement projects. Although technology cannot eliminate all errors, clinical decision support and automated redundancies can help prevent errors from reaching patients.

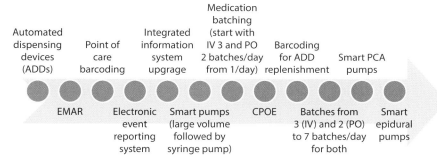

Figure 4-9 ■ Sequence for implementation of technology and related policies/procedures designed to improve medication safety at Lurie Children's Hospital of Chicago.

IN PRACTICE

- The medication use process represents the single largest source of medical error and adverse patient events in all healthcare settings. Children appear to be at a three-fold increased risk for medication errors compared with adult patients. Efforts to promote pediatric patient safety and improved care quality should therefore include a focus on medication error.
  - While these errors occur with a meaningful frequency in pediatric specialty care settings, a focus on pediatric medication safety is especially important for facilities and providers that primarily care for adults.
- Certain patient populations, healthcare settings/processes, and medications appear to bear an especially high risk for potentially serious medication errors and adverse events.
  - Neonates, children with special health care needs
  - Neonatal and pediatric ICUs, oncology unit, emergency department, resuscitation, care transitions
  - Opioids, look-alike sound-alike medications, chemotherapy, parenteral nutrition
- Three quarters of medication errors and adverse events impacting pediatric inpatients occur within the prescribing phase. Strategies that may prove useful towards the reduction of prescribing error include:
  - Computerized provider order entry (CPOE) with at least basic clinical decision support
- Dosing calculations represent the largest source of prescribing error in pediatric care; 10-fold dosing errors are especially common and dangerous in pediatric care.

(Continued)

(*Continued*)

■ Off-the shelf CPOE systems may require customization to address local practice and unique pediatric medication dosing and safety.
  • Unit-based pharmacist rounding with the healthcare team.
  • Improved communication among all disciplines involved with the medication use process.
  • Consideration of human factors (eg, fatigue, distraction) that impact safety in other aspects of patient care.
■ Medication reconciliation is an effective medication safety strategy and should occur at all transitions of care. This process should always engage participation by parents/caregivers of the pediatric patient.
■ Leveraging automation and the use of other technologies may further enhance patient safety during medication administration.
  • Automated dispensing devices
  • Barcoding systems for patient and medication identification
  • Smart pumps
  • Electronic medication administration record

FAQs

1. How can the data from event reporting systems and interventions be used in a timely and practical manner to educate staff re-medication safety?

   Having a dedicated clinician, who can review medication events in a timely manner and provide individual feedback to staff, as well as review data in aggregate to identify trends, is key to establishing a medication safety program. Individual follow-up should be done as quickly as possible so that details surrounding the event are captured. Event data should be shared regularly with pharmacy staff via huddles, staff meetings, and/or newsletters. In addition to these pharmacy-specific opportunities, medication event data and information about interventions should be shared with the multidisciplinary care team including nurses, physicians, and other care providers. Medication event data should also be shared regularly with hospital level committees such as the Medication Safety Committee, Pharmacy and Therapeutics Committee, and Medication Administration Committee.

2. How do you continue to challenge yourself in setting medication safety goals after achieving initial targets?

There are a few key elements that lead to success in achieving medication safety goals. First, focus on a goal that is measurable and sustainable. Second, be realistic. It is important to take into account other safety or operational initiatives that are taking place in the institution at the same time. Front-line staff are often overburdened and even overwhelmed by the number of mandates, initiatives, and improvement projects assigned to them. Lastly, start small and think big. For example, you might start with a goal of decreasing potentially harmful *inpatient* events related to narcotics, and then expand to other high-risk drugs. When improvements related to ADEs are maintained in the inpatient setting, you might expand the goal to include outpatient (emergency department, clinics, etc) and procedural (OR, Imaging, PACU, etc) areas.

3. What critical elements need to be in place to ensure successful implementation of an improvement project?

   Identifying the medication safety element that you want to improve upon requires a review of the literature and accreditation standards in order to structure a successful process. Having a leadership champion from the targeted group is essential. For example, if the initiative will target medication administration, a nursing leader should be a part of the task force charged with influencing change. If the initiative will target prescribing, a physician leader and an advanced practice nurse leader should participate on the process improvement task force. After establishing policy and educating the practitioners, monitoring for compliance and evaluating the process for any unforeseen fail-points are the keys to making the change long-lasting. Creating an accountability component can assist in accelerating the transformation of the process from a "change in practice" to the "standard of care."

4. Is it reasonable to assume that technology support is functional, or should this be reviewed?

   A thorough review of the technology employed by the institution in contrast to the technology needed to reach your medication safety goals is an important element of institutional assessment when strategically planning an organization-wide process improvement initiative involving safe medication delivery. Assess the medication administration record in the electronic medical record to determine if alerts are appropriate or additional alerts are needed. Identify opportunities to offer hyperlinks to policies and procedures that are linked to the administration of high-risk medications or complex protocols. Evaluate the medication barcoding system in place in order to request enhancements that assist in clinical decision making and alert the prescribers and pharmacists, as well as those administering medications, when appropriate. Explore expanding the use of medication barcoding to areas that do not have the ability to scan medications (ambulatory areas, surgical services, emergency departments, day infusion centers, etc). Investigate the functionality of the medication delivery systems to ensure that the practitioners are maximizing the utilization of the Smart pump technology. Updates to the pump libraries or upgrades may be required. Review the compliance data from the SMART pump vendor in order to assess areas that require re-education or greater accountability. Assess the functionality of the automated dispensing devices used throughout the institution with a focus on high alert and LASA medications. Establish a plan for evaluating the use of the override function to access medications.

5. Why is it important to periodically review hospital policies?

With technology updates, policies and procedures will most likely need to be reviewed and updated to reflect the changes in processes. Input from all disciplines involved in medication safety should be solicited. Education on the new standards should be followed up with an evaluation for effective change in order to determine if reinforcement is needed or if the new process is not a reasonable expectation for the providers, in which case a revamped process must be created.

REFERENCES

1. Kohn LT, Corrigan J, Donaldson MS. *To Err is Human: Building a Safer Health System*. Washington, DC: National Academy Press; 2000.
2. Aspden P, Wolcott JA, Bootman JL, Cronenwett LR. *Preventing Medication Errors: Quality Chasm Series*. Washington, DC: National Academy Press; 2007.
3. Brennan TA, Leape LL, Laird NM, et al. Incidence of adverse events and negligence in hospitalized patients: results of the Harvard Medical Practice Study. *N Eng J Med*. 1991;324(6):370-376.
4. Ferner RE, Aronson JK. Clarification of terminology in medication errors: definitions and classification. *Drug Saf*. 2006;29(11):1011-1022.
5. Bates DW, Boyle DL, Vander Vliet MB, et al. Relationship between medication errors and adverse drug events. *J Gen Intern Med*. 1995;10(4):199-205.
6. Leape LL, Brennan TA, Laird N, et al. The nature of adverse events in hospitalized patients. Results of the Harvard Medical Practice Study II. *N Engl J Med*. 1991;324(6):377-384.
7. Classen DC, Pestotnik SL, Evans RS, et al. Adverse drug events in hospitalized patients. Excess length of stay, extra costs, and attributable mortality. *JAMA*. 1997;277(4):301-306.

8. Institute of Medicine. Committee on Identifying and Preventing Medication Errors. *Preventing Medication Errors.* Washington, DC: National Academy Press; 2006.

9. Lazarou J, Pomeranz B, Corey PN. Incidence of adverse drug reactions in hospitalized patients: a meta-analysis of prospective studies. *JAMA*. 1998;279(15):1200-1205.

10. Budnitz DS, Pollock DA, Weidenbach KN, et al. National surveillance of emergency department visits for outpatient adverse drug events. *JAMA*. 2006;296(15):1858-1866.

11. The Joint Commission. Sentinel Alert, issue 39: Preventing pediatric medication errors. April 11, 2008. Available at: http://www.jointcommission.org/sentinel_event_alert_issue_39_preventing_pediatric_medication_errors/. Accessed 5.30.14.

12. Ferranti J, Horvath M, Cozart H, et al. Reevaluating the safety profile of pediatrics: a comparison of computerized adverse drug event surveillance and voluntary reporting in the pediatric environment. *Pediatrics*. 2008;121:1201-1207.

13. Kaushal R, Bates DW, Landrigan C, et al. Medication errors and adverse drug events in pediatric inpatients. *JAMA*. 2001;285:2114-2120.

14. Holdsworth M, Fichtl R, Behta M, et al. Incidence and impact of adverse drug events in pediatric inpatients. *Arch PediatrAdoles Med*. 2003;157:60-65.

15. Otero P, Leyton A, Mariani G, et al. Medication errors in pediatric inpatients: prevalence and results of a prevention program. *Pediatrics*. 2008;122(3):e737-e743.

16. Marino BL, Reinhardt K, Eichelberger WJ, Steingard R. Prevalence of errors in a pediatric hospital medication system: implications for error proofing. *Outcomes Manag Nurs Pract*. 2000;4(3):129-135.

17. Abrahamson EL, Bates DW, Jenter C, et al. Ambulatory prescribing errors among community-based providers in two states. *J Am Med Inform Assoc*. 2012;19(4):644-648.

18. Kaushal R, Goldmann DA, Keohane CA, et al. Adverse drug events in pediatric outpatients. *Ambul Pediatr*. 2007;7(5):383-389.

19. Kaushal R, Goldman DA, Keohane CA, et al. Medication errors in pediatric outpatients. *Qual Saf Health Care*. 2010;19(6):e30.

20. Abramson EL, Kaushal R. Computerized provider order entry and patient safety. *Pediatr Clin North Am*. 2012;59(6):1247-1255.

21. Hoyle JD, Davis AT, Putman KK, et al. Medication dosing errors in pediatric patients treated by emergency medical services. *Prehosp Emerg Care*. 2012;16(1):59-66.

22. Kozer E, Scolnick D, Macpherson A, et al. Variables associated with medication errors in pediatric emergency medicine. *Pediatrics*. 2002;110(4):737-742.

23. Fordyce J, Blank FS, Pekow P, et al. Errors in a busy emergency department. *Ann Emerg Med*. 2003;42(3):324-333.

24. Rinke ML, Moon M, Clark JS, et al. Prescribing errors in a pediatric emergency department. *Pediatr Emerg Care*. 2008;24(1):1-8.

25. Vila-de-Muga M, Colom-Ferrer MD, Gonzalez-Herrero M, Luaces-Cubells C. Factors associated with medication errors in the pediatric emergency department. *Pediatr Emerg Care*. 2011;27(4):290-294.

26. Shaw KN, Lillis KA, Ruddy R, et al. Reported medication events in a pediatric emergency network: sharing to improve patient safety. *Emerg Med J*. 2013;30(10):815-819.

27. Marcin JP, Dhamar M, Cho M, et al. Medication errors among acutely ill and injured children treated in rural emergency departments. *Ann Emerg Med*. 2007;50(4): 361-370.

28. Bourgeois FT, Mandl KD, Valim C, Shannon MW. Pediatric adverse drug events in the outpatient setting: an 11-year national analysis. *Pediatrics*. 2009;124(4):e744-e750.

29. Budnitz DS, Pollock DA, Weidenbach KN, et al. National surveillance of emergency department visits for outpatient adverse drug events. *JAMA*. 2006;296(15):1858-1866.

30. Cohen AL, Budnitz DS, Weidenbach KN, et al. National surveillance of emergency department visits for outpatient adverse drug events in children and adolescents. *J Pediatr*. 2008;152(3):416-421.

31. Levine S, Cohen NR, Blanchard NR, et al. Guidelines for preventing medication errors in pediatrics. *J Pediatr Pharmacolo Ther*. 2001;6:426-442.

32. Gupta A, Waldhauser LK. Adverse drug reactions from birth to early childhood. *Pediatr Clin North Am*. 1997;44:79-92.

33. Caldwell NA, Power B. The pros and cons of electronic prescribing in children. *Arch Dis Child*. 2012;97:124-128.

34. Mansur J. Medication safety for pediatric patients in the emergency department. In: Krug SE, ed. *Pediatric Patient Safety in the Emergency Department*. Oak Brook Terrace, IL: Joint Commission Resources; 2010.

35. Doherty C, McDonnell CM. Tenfold medication error: 5 years' experience at a university-affiliated pediatric hospital. *Pediatrics*. 2012;129(5):916-924.

36. Fortescue E, Kaushal R, Landrigan CP, et al. Prioritizing strategies for preventing medication errors and adverse drug events in pediatric patients. *Pediatrics*. 2003;111:722-729.

37. Institute for Safe Medication Practices. Medication safety alert. Hospital survey shows much more needs to be done to protect pediatric patients from medication errors. April 19, 2000. Available at: https://www.ismp.org/newsletters/acutecare/articles/20000419.asp. Accessed 5.30.14.

38. Potts MJ, Phelan KW. Deficiencies in calculation and applied mathematics skills in pediatrics among primary care interns. *Arch PediatrAdoles Med*. 1996;150:748-752.

39. Rowe C, Koren T, Koren. Errors by paediatric residents in calculating drug doses. *Arch Dis Child*. 1998;79:56-58.

40. Walsh KE, Landrigan CP, Adams WG, et al. Effect of computer order entry on prevention of serious medication errors in hospitalized children. *Pediatrics*. 2008;121(3):e421-e427.

41. Yu F, Salas M, Kim Y, Menachemi N. The relationships between computerized order entry and pediatric adverse drug events: a nested matched case-control study. *Pharmacoepidemiol Drug Saf*. 2009;18:751-755.

42. Caldwell NA, Power B. The pros and cons of electronic prescribing for children. *Arch Dis Child*. 2012;97:124-128.

43. Ferranti JM, Horvath MM, Jansen J, et al. Using a computerized order entry system to meet the unique prescribing needs of children: description of an advanced dosing model. *BMC Med Inform Decis Mak*. 2011;11:14.

44. Upperman JS, Staley P, Friend K, et al. The impact of hospital wide computerized physician order entry on medical errors in a pediatric hospital. *J Pediatr Surg*. 2005;40:57.

45. Han YY, Carcillo JA, Venkataraman ST, et al. Unexpected increased mortality after implementation of a commercially sold computerized physician order entry system. *Pediatrics*. 2005;116:1506-1512.

46. Maat B, Au YS, Bollen CW, et al. Clinical pharmacy interventions in pediatric electronic prescriptions. *Arch Dis Child*. 2013;98:222-227.

47. Stultz JS, Nahata MC. Computerized clinical decision support for medication prescribing and utilization in pediatrics. *J Am Med Inform Assoc*. 2012;19:942-953.

48. Broussard M, Bass PF, Arnold CL, et al. Preprinted order sets as a safety intervention in pediatric sedation. *J Pediatr*. 2009;154:865-868.

49. Leu MG, Morelli SA, Chung OY, Radford S. Systematic update of computerized physician order entry order sets to improve quality of care: a case study. *Pediatrics*. 2013;131:S60-S67.

50. Kadmon G, Bron-Harlev E, Schiller O, et al. Computerized order entry with limited decision support to prevent prescription errors in a PICU. *Pediatrics*. 2009;124:935-940.

51. NCC MERP. "Medication Errors Council Revises and Expands Index for Categorizing Errors: Definitions of Medication Errors Broadened," June 12, 2001. Available at: http://www.nccmerp.org/press/press2001-06-12.html. Accessed 5.30.14.

52. Sard BE, Walsh KE, Doros G, et al. Retrospective evaluation of a computerized physician order entry adaption to prevent prescribing errors in a pediatric emergency department. *Pediatrics*. 2008;122:782-787.

53. Koppel R, Metlay JP, Cohen A, et al. Role of computerized physician order entry systems in facilitating medication errors. *JAMA*. 2005;293:1197-1203.

54. Nightingale PG, Adu D, Richards NT, et al. Implementation of rules based computerized bedside prescribing and administration: intervention study. *BMJ*. 2000;320:750-753.

55. Institute for Healthcare Improvement. Reconcile medications at all transition points. Available at: http://www.ihi.org/resources/Pages/Changes/ReconcileMedications-atAllTransitionPoints.aspx. Accessed 5.30.14.

56. Vira T, Colquhoun M, Etchells E. Reconcilable differences: correcting medication errors at hospital admission and discharge. *Qual Saf Health Care*. 2006;15:122-126.

57. Huynh C, Wong ICK, Tomlin S, et al. Medication discrepancies at transitions in pediatrics: a review of the literature. *Pediatr Drugs*. 2013;15(3):203-215.

58. The Joint Commission. Improving America's Hospitals: The Joint Commission's Report on Quality and Safety 2007. Sentinel Event Root Cause and Trend Data. Available at: http://www.jointcommission.org/assets/1/6/2007_Annual_Report.pdf. Accessed 5.30.14..

59. Rappaport DI, Collins B, Koster A, et al. Implementing medication reconciliation in outpatient pediatrics. *Pediatrics*. 2011;128:e1600-e1607.

60. Frush K, Krug SE, American Academy of Pediatrics Committee on Pediatric Emergency Medicine. Patient safety in the pediatric emergency care setting. *Pediatrics*. 2007;120:1367-1375.

61. Leape LL, Cullen DJ, Clapp MD, et al. Pharmacist participation on physician rounds and adverse drug events in the intensive care unit. *JAMA*. 1999;19:130-138.

62. Bond CA, Raehl CL, Franke T. Clinical pharmacy services, pharmacy staffing, and the total cost of care in United States hospitals. *Pharmacotherapy*. 2000;20:609-621.

63. Kucukarslan SN, Peters M, Mlynarek M, et al. Pharmacists on rounding teams reduce preventable adverse drug events in hospital general medicine units. *Arch Intern Med*. 2003;163:2014-2018.

64. Kaboli PJ, Hoth AB, McClimon BJ, et al. Clinical pharmacists and inpatient medical care: a systematic review. *Arch Intern Med*. 2006;166:955-964.

65. Bulecheck G, Butcher H, Dochterman J, eds. Nursing interventions classification, 5ᵗʰ edition. St Louis, MO: Mosby/Elsevier; 2008.

66. National Coordinating Council for Medication Error Reporting and Prevention (NCC MERP). Recommendations to enhance accuracy of administration of medications. June 2005. Available at: http://www.nccmerp.org/council/council1999-06-29.html. Accessed 5.30.14.

67. Gonzales K. Medication administration errors and the pediatric population: a systematic search of the literature. *J Pediatr Nurs.* 2010;25:555-565.

68. Stratton K, Blegen M, Pepper G, Vaughn T. Reporting of medication errors by pediatric nurses. *J Pediatr Nurs.* 2004;19:385-392.

69. Lefrak L. Moving towards safer practice: reducing medication errors in neonatal care. *J Perinatal Neonat Nurs.* 2002;16:73-84.

70. The Joint Commission. Sentinel event alert, issue 11: High-alert medications and patient safety. Available at: http://www.jointcommission.org/sentinel_event_alert_issue_11_high-alert_medications_and_patient_safety/. Accessed 5.30.14.

71. Institute for Safe Medication Practices. Your high alert medication list: relatively useless without associated risk reduction strategies. April 4, 2013. Available at: http://www.ismp.org/newsletters/acutecare/showarticle.aspx?id=45. Accessed 5.30.14.

72. Institute for Safe Medication Practices. ISMP's list of high-alert medications. Available at: http://www.ismp.org/tools/institutionalhighAlert.asp. Accessed 10.01.13.

73. American Academy of Pediatrics Steering Committee on Quality Improvement and Management and Committee on Hospital Care. Principles of pediatric patient safety: reducing harm due to medical care. *Pediatrics.* 2011;127(6):1199-1210.

74. Molteni R, Krug SE. Hospital leadership and it's impact on the care of children in the emergency department. In: Krug SE, ed. *Pediatric Patient Safety in the Emergency Department.* Oak Brook Terrace, IL: Joint Commission Resources; 2010.

75. The Joint Commission. Sentinel event alert, issue 43: Leadership committed to safety. Available at: http://www.jointcommission.org/sentinel_event_alert_issue_43_leadership_committed_to_safety/. Accessed 5.30.14.

76. IOM Committee on Health Care in America. *To Err Is Human: Building A Safer Healthcare System.* Washington, DC: National Academy Press; 1999.

77. IOM Committee on Health Care in America. *Crossing the Quality Chasm: A New Health System for the 21ˢᵗ Century.* Washington, DC: National Academy Press; 2001.

78. IOM Committee on Data Standards for Patient Safety, Board on Health Care Services. *Patient Safety: Achieving a New Standard for Care.* Washington, DC: National Academy Press; 2004.

THE ROLE OF LEADERSHIP IN SAFE AND RELIABLE PEDIATRIC CARE | 5

The ability to deliver consistent high-quality care requires effective leadership, a culture of safety, good teamwork, consistent processes of care, and the ability to learn and improve. Leadership is the essential component that ties all these factors together, and is the differentiator between extraordinary care teams and those that are average. As culture and care delivery live at a clinical unit level, we will provide a practical framework that can be applied there or more broadly within a healthcare system.

A DEPARTMENT OR UNIT IS MADE UP OF CULTURE AND LEARNING

High-performing units or departments have two integral components: "culture" and "learning," and they have a particular relationship to each other in that, learning is built on and dependent on culture. Culture is the foundation out of which learning grows.

Learning, or more precisely a "learning system," is the combined effort of individuals working collaboratively toward a common set of goals, and in the process constantly and consistently reflecting on activities to learn and improve. Ultimately, learning is dependent on the relationships that individuals have with each other, and the best relationships are those in which defects or improvement opportunities can comfortably be made visible. Those relationships are shaped and determined by the milieu, or culture, in which the individuals work, determined in part by organizational factors such as leadership behaviors, how the individuals are chosen or hired, paid, encouraged

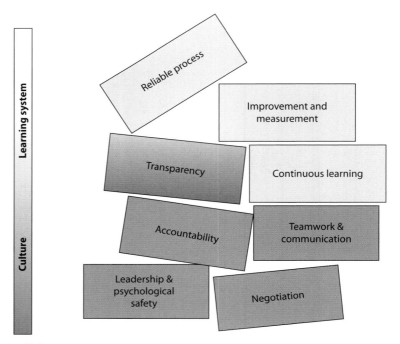

Figure 5-1 ■ A framework for excellence.

(or discouraged), by the agreed upon behaviors of the many individuals in that learning system, and by the attitude in the organization toward errors and human failure. Combined together, culture becomes "the way we do things around here."[1]

The components of culture are as follows:

1. Leaders and psychological safety
2. Teams and team behaviors including effective communication
3. An environment of organizational fairness, also described as a culture perceived as being just and with appropriate accountability.
4. Negotiation and the ability to constructively manage conflicts

The components of learning are as follows:

1. Reliable processes
2. Continuous learning
3. Measurement and improvement skills
4. Transparency

All eight components must be healthy to achieve stellar performance and the eight components are interdependent. Leadership, psychological safety, and negotiation are at the base of the structure. They are essential to building effective teamwork and to creating an environment of fairness. The learning system is built above these, and reliable process perches on top, slightly askew and at risk of teeter-tottering should any of the other components become unstable (Figure 5-1). A brief description of each is as follows.

Leaders refer to positions at multiple levels in healthcare environments, including the administrative leaders who head organizations, who tend to have the title "CXO" where the X may refer to executive, operating, medical, nursing, and financial officers. Other leaders include those titled with director and manager and include clinical and administrative roles. Clinical roles also include titles such as chair, chief, division head, and the like. All these positions and any others where position and title denote responsibility to manage a group of people comprise the **Leaders** referred to in the framework. These individuals, regardless of their place in their organization's hierarchy, and regardless of their focus on clinical, operational or business activities, have, as a primary responsibility, the generation and support of an environment of psychological safety. Psychological safety relates to the ability of any member of the care team to voice a concern when something is concerning or uncertain.[2] We all know about psychological safety on a personal level. The people we are always comfortable approaching when we have a question or a problem have established psychological safety; we know they will help us and treat us with respect. In other words, it is safe to have the conversation. Lack of psychological safety exists when we are hesitant to voice a concern or ask a question. Unfortunately, we have all had that experience. That hesitancy, or increased threshold to speak, creates risk for both patients and care givers as little problems can often become big problems.[3] Psychological safety exists in a work environment when questions, feedback, critique, and innovation are prized and supported.

Teams in this framework refer to any group of individuals who collectively work together, are thought of as a department or unit whether geographically co-located as in the members of an operating room team, or geographically dispersed as in the members of a home-care organization who travel out in the community. The group of individuals is a "team" if their ability to function well is enhanced by the relationships they have with each other, if knowing an overarching "game plan" is helpful to the completion of their work, if there is learning that they can do together that enhances their ability to work reliably and safely, and if the coordination of their activities has an impact on achieving an agreed upon overall goal.[4]

Organizational fairness, also described as "just culture" or appropriate accountability, refers to the policies and procedures that evaluate individuals when things go awry or people make mistakes. Organizational fairness exists when the policies and procedures place accountability appropriately, taking into account what is known about complex systems, human factors, and human fallibility, combined together so that decisions about censure are perceived by team members as fair. Organizational fairness extends to how effectively good policies and procedures are enacted and understood by leaders and team members; to how effectively organizational leaders navigate the pressures that come from outside groups such as the media, regulatory groups, and legal processes in the aftermath of an adverse event; and to how effectively leaders generate internal consistency, applying ethically sound practices in determining accountability.[5]

Negotiation in this framework refers to the skills, and training in those skills, that allows leaders and team members to effectively manage differences of opinion and conflict. The ability to focus on a common goal—the best interest of the patient—and depersonalize the conversation so it does not feel personal or judgmental is critically important for effective conflict resolution.[6]

Combined together, leaders and teams immersed in an environment of psychological safety and organizational fairness, who negotiate fairly and collaboratively, establish the ideal platform for a "learning system."

Learning systems in the context of this framework have a goal to achieve reliable and safe operational excellence. Reliability is the ability to achieve a specific result from a specific set of actions, so "reliable safe operational excellence" is the ability to apply a set of actions with confidence that the actions will yield the same result each and every time, that the result is perceived as excellent, and occurs safely. In healthcare "safely" means that things don't go awry causing harm to a patient or the providers involved in that patient's care.

Reliable process, then, is the goal of a good learning system, and reliable process develops through ***continuous learning***, the second component of the learning framework. Continuous learning means that the individuals and teams in the learning system reflect on their activities in such a way that defects of every kind are noted, discussed, and, in some manner, acted upon. Defects and improvement opportunities are imperfections that impair or degrade the processes of care and include everything from equipment malfunction to breakdowns in team function. Essentially, anything that doesn't go as planned, that doesn't unfold as smoothly as a team member would like, that leads to clinician confusion or error, or that in any way undermines perfect delivery of care is a defect. Continuous learning means that there is mindfulness in each individual to note defects, and mechanisms such as debriefings, that make the defects known and visible in the learning system.

Improvement and Measurement, the third piece of the learning system framework, refers to the skills necessary to evaluate defects and invent solutions that are applied to mitigate or eliminate them. Improvement presumes many skills from aim setting to performing tests of change; to measurement that showcases the impact of improvement on learning system processes.

Finally, *visibility and transparency* make up the last of the components, and refer to the willingness of leaders and team, and the wherewithal of manager and leaders, to show and discuss data in non-threatening ways, perceived by all members of the learning system as normal and expected, and used to focus attention on improvement that enhances performance.

SOCIO-TECHNICAL FRAMEWORK AND ORGANIZATIONAL EXCELLENCE

The components of learning and culture can be evaluated and placed on a spectrum from unmindful to generative that describes the Unit's ability to achieve reliable operational excellence. This spectrum, the Safe & Reliable Healthcare, allows these important elements to be evaluated and addressed within the care environment with regard to five progressive stages of cultural evolution (Figure 5-2). These stages, from least to most advanced, are as follows:

1. **Unmindful:** Traditional operation, cottage industry—"It's like we've always done." There is little or no awareness that change is needed.
2. **Reactive:** Awareness of issues but no active plans for training; respond in the aftermath of a crisis or adverse event. The organization/unit/team always seems to be reacting to events, playing catch-up and trying to recover, usually playing defense.
3. **Systematic:** The organization/unit/team does all the things they're supposed to do, complying with required or generally accepted initiatives. There are still avoidable adverse events and suboptimal outcomes despite the efforts. Some elements of systematic approaches to care are in place, but the application is not consistent.
4. **Proactive:** There is anticipation and thinking ahead—looking for trouble and often detecting problems quickly while they are small ones.

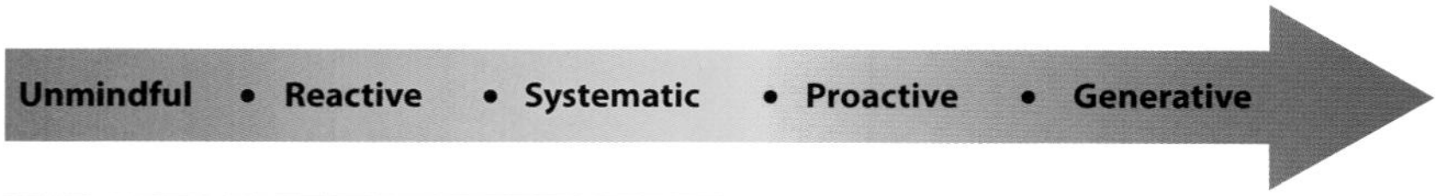

Unmindful • Reactive • Systematic • Proactive • Generative	
People	• Patient- and family-centered care • Senior leadership • Clinical leadership • Teamwork • Hiring
Process	• Improvement • Reportable data • High reliability
Technology	• Harm detection and mitigation
Organization	• Psychological safety • Organizational fairness
External environment	• Awareness & engagement

Figure 5-2 ▪ Safe & Reliable Healthcare.

Usually playing offense; strong culture norms driving very good outcomes. Always alert, thinking ahead.

5. **Generative:** Systematic processes exist to communicate effectively and support high levels of teamwork; high degrees of psychological safety combined with a pervasive awareness that failures can and do occur result in teams that think out loud, anticipate, and frequently avoid problems. Environment delivers optimal experience for patients and caregivers alike. Safety, continuous learning, and improvement are integral to everything the organization/unit/team does.

Each component of the framework for excellence can be evaluated along this evolution in thinking about reliability. For example, using this framework, clinical leaders might be described as follows in Figure 5-3.

THE ROLE OF LEADERS

Leaders play the most important role in shaping culture. They have three primary responsibilities in this regard:

1. They are the guardians of the learning system. As guardians, they must understand that a learning system is comprised of achieving reliable process through continual learning using improvement and measure-

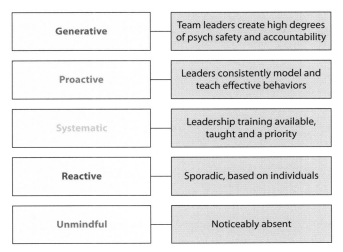

Generative	Team leaders create high degrees of psych safety and accountability
Proactive	Leaders consistently model and teach effective behaviors
Systematic	Leadership training available, taught and a priority
Reactive	Sporadic, based on individuals
Unmindful	Noticeably absent

Figure 5-3 ■ Increasing insights about safety and reliability. The evolution of clinical leadership.

ment made visible; they must have enough insight about each of the components that they can teach others, weigh in on the various aspects of learning, and shape the learning activity.

2. They determine the level of psychological safety that exists in the culture by defining the appropriate behaviors and the degree to which they model such behaviors.

3. They determine expectations about respect—the gift of giving respect, and the expectation by individuals that they will be treated with respect.

Leaders set direction and have vision. Managers are charged with shepherding others under their charge. Managers tend to have titles like administrator, director, manager, or charge, but this group includes any individual who is placed in a position of responsibility over others, with the expectation that they will manage the group. In the healthcare setting, all physicians, by definition, lead. The resident or fellow who is placed in charge of performing daily rounds becomes the de facto leader of a group of other physicians or a multidisciplinary group. In this position, they immediately become responsible for upholding the three primary responsibilities of leaders.

Some leaders, ie, the manager of a unit, are likely to be charged with other responsibilities such as maintaining a roster or schedule of personnel or managing a financial budget. These are necessary skills but come secondary to their primary responsibilities. Budget management and scheduling skills are of less use in a unit that is not a learning system.

Leaders and Psychological Safety

Psychological safety is the state of comfort by individuals to confidently:[7]

1. Ask questions especially when a team member is unclear about team goals or game plan, or when a team member believes that risk levels have increased.
2. Ask for feedback, especially when feeling unsure about their skill set or performance as part of a team.
3. Be appropriately critical or give voice to their sense of doubt or concern when something either looks or feels wrong.
4. Suggest innovative ideas (even whacky ideas when brainstorming).

Psychological safety presumes that questions, feedback, criticism, and innovation can be directed toward learning opportunities about both systems of work and the culture, and also when appropriate, respectfully directed toward other individuals or team members. The ability to speak up in those latter situations and maintain good working relationships is a key aspect of psychological safety and leadership.[8] If the fundamental understanding is that the group is working toward a common goal, then criticism or questioning of any action that undermines that process becomes less *ad hominum*, ie, a personal judgment, and more in service of the group as a whole.

James Reason, a cognitive psychologist whose career has been spent understanding the underlying factors behind catastrophic adverse events and the determinants of highly reliable human systems, coined the term "psychological safety." Amy Edmondson, a Professor at Harvard Business School, subsequently popularized the term in the American literature.

Psychological safety, or its absence, permeates every aspect of culture and learning because the learning system is dependent on uncovering and making defects visible and transparent, and psychological safety allows people to bring defects to the surface. A minority of defects comes to attention because they affect processes or outcomes significantly enough to command attention. The overwhelming majority of defects in a unit are overlooked by participants or are hidden, and come to attention only if individuals speak up about them. It is hard to fix problems that are not openly identified and addressed. The comfort about speaking up about defects is determined by the level of psychological safety felt by each individual. Leaders primarily shape psychological safety, although it is so fundamental that it ultimately is dependent on the values stated and manifested in the organization.

The leadership characteristic most likely to enhance psychological safety is intelligent and respectful feedback to individuals about their performance while in the unit. Feedback requires that leaders:

1. Be interested in learning about individual's actions and decisions prior to being judgmental.
2. Understand human factors—that lethal brew of human fallibility in complex environments that are the determinants of error and allow error chains to progress to the point they result in adverse events.
3. Be comfortable praising good work while also critiquing problems as is appropriate if work is inadequate or substandard.
4. Create an environment of high expectations while being perceived as accessible by members of the unit or team. This entails being explicit about desired team behaviors and expectations of habitual excellence.
5. Be fair and impartial when judgment is necessary.
6. Effectively manage conflict and the negotiation necessary to resolve differences of opinion in ways that feel fair, non-punitive, and support learning.

When leaders act accordingly, individuals learn that it is safe to speak up about concerns, ask questions when in doubt, ask for feedback when unsure, be appropriately critical when they perceive problems, and be willing to put themselves in the often uncomfortable position of innovating or experimenting.

The behaviors feed the learning system. Without them, the learning system is unable to reflect on itself, identify the defects that undermine its performance, and focus its improvement efforts appropriately.

COMMUNICATION IN LEARNING SYSTEMS

Effective communication between members of a team requires that the fidelity is high in the transmission from the provider to the receiver of information. Two team behaviors that help in ensuring high fidelity are structured communication and repeating back information received, often-called repeat-back or "closing the loop."

An example of structured communication is Situation, Background, Assessment, Recommendation (SBAR). SBAR is a communication mechanism that increases the likelihood of getting the necessary attention of the receiver, promoting executive thinking by the transmitter, and increasing the speed of problem solving.[9] SBAR is also an effective tool in managing conflict between individuals by exposing the logic in thought process and helping move from positional statements to an understanding of the interests of the individuals and the common goal of doing what is best for the patient. The communication is enhanced because the transmitter exposes their understanding of the facts in the Background, their logic about what the facts mean in the Assessment, and the relationship between the position and interests in the Recommendation.

SBAR sequentially exposes four components of a problem:

1. Situation—the "newspaper headline" that describes the problem requiring attention. Stated as such, it increases the likelihood of getting the attention of the receiver.
2. Background—the facts associated with the problem and providing context.
3. Assessment—promotes critical thinking, and requires the transmitter to analyze the facts and apply their knowledge and experience to the problem and to suggest alternative solutions. If the transmitter is too inexperienced or perplexed by the grouping of facts of the problem, the Assessment may be as simple as "I don't understand and I'm concerned."
4. Recommendation—the transmitter suggests a course, or possible courses of action to address the problem, ie, what needs to happen and when?

The repeating back of information received is another high-fidelity communication strategy. This can be especially useful in specific situations, such as:

1. The transmission of numbers.
2. Names—especially names of medications.
3. Summarization of patient histories.
4. After handing off care to another team member.
5. Assessing whether the communication has indeed been effective and there is a shared mental model.

Communication and Teamwork

Many teamwork-training programs are being applied to healthcare environments. Almost all of them are outgrowths from the crew resource management trainings started in the aviation industry[10] in the late 1980s. There are commonalities among these team training programs.

Effective teams are comprised of:

1. Individuals with different roles that synergize.
2. Individuals who know where and whom to go to for a specific skill set.

3. Leaders who manifest leadership skills known to, and expected by, the team, and team members who agree to abide by specific values and behaviors.
4. Known goals and a game plan to achieve them. Active discussion of risk (where can we go wrong?) and team limitations is quite valuable.

To be successful, teams must fundamentally be able to reliably and effectively engage in four activities:

1. Plan forward—when the team comes together.
2. Reflect back—when they are finished with their work and at appropriate times, during their work.
3. Communicate clearly—using specific and practiced communication behaviors.
4. Resolve conflict—using agreed-upon specific behaviors.

Essential behaviors for effective teams include the following (Figure 5-4):

1. To plan forward, teams brief, rebrief, pause, huddle, and round.
2. To reflect back, teams debrief quickly and collaboratively.
3. To communicate, teams agree to use structured communication models and read back, closing the loop.
4. To resolve conflict in the moment, teams use critical language—a specific term (Example: "I need clarity") that everyone agrees to. When stated, team members know to stop and talk every time to insure there is clear understanding about the goal, game plan, and levels of risk in the current processes.

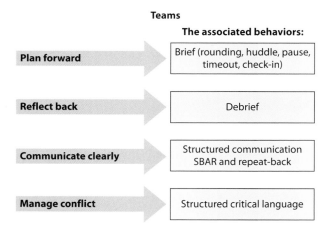

Figure 5-4 ■ The essential behaviors of teams.

NEGOTIATION, AN INTRINSIC PART OF TEAM FUNCTION

Conflict is an intrinsic component of all teams, the result of individuals having different perspectives about situations that arise, especially when having to manage the unexpected. Effective teams manage conflict at a variety of levels. In the moment when the team is actively engaged in team process, conflict management requires agreed-upon behaviors that increase the awareness of risk and lead to rapid actions that mitigate or eliminate that risk. As noted, one team behavior that requires simulation and practice is the use of "critical language," a statement that is understood by all to denote concern by the individual using the critical language, and usually means that the individual perceives an increase in risk requiring that others focus their attention and possibly their effort to decrease that risk. Risk increases when a team member can no longer identify their role and is unclear as to what exactly the plan of care actually is. Uncertainty also makes it harder to speak up and voice a concern. No one wants to look stupid, especially in a healthcare culture where people keep score by knowing the answers. The agreement that if anyone has concern or doubt the team will stop and respectfully recalibrate is a hallmark of high-performing teams, particularly in high-risk areas.

Alternately, the team member may believe that others are unaware of factors that they perceive have unacceptably increased risk to the team or its goal. Critical language can be used in this setting to stop activity so that team members can evaluate the concerns and current situation and respond appropriately.

A primary goal of negotiation is to reiterate the common goal, uncover and discuss the interests of the individuals involved in the disagreement, and help the individuals move away from taking fixed positions that hamper effective negotiation. Often individuals don't realize that they've taken positions, nor are they consciously aware of their underlying interests. Skillful negotiation helps clarify the underlying interests and link them to the desired outcome. Individuals approach conflict influenced by their personalities and also by the situational factors associated with the disagreement to be managed. Variably individuals will:[11,12]

1. Avoid—negotiating altogether
2. Accommodate to the other person's position
3. Compromise, seeking a middle ground between the perspectives of the individuals involved in the disagreement, in essence each giving something away.
4. Compete, actively trying to win over the other participant to their point of view or position

5. Collaborate, seeking to find new ground that expands the realm of possible solutions to benefit all participants, sometimes creating solutions greater than either individual imagined possible.

Effective leaders build the capacity for teams to negotiate well and resolve conflict by modeling the appropriate behaviors of respectfully focusing on a common goal and never letting the conversation become personal or judgmental.

APPROPRIATE ACCOUNTABILITY

Appropriate accountability, organizational fairness, and just culture are terms denoting that an organization is able, when something goes wrong, to differentiate between system accountability and individual accountability. Believing that you will be held accountable for actions beyond your control is demoralizing, especially if the rules delineating accountability are unclear or nonexistent. This situation arises in healthcare in a variety of ways. First, organizations frequently do a poor job of differentiating between system and individual accountability. For example, blaming a nurse for a medication error even though the hospital pharmacy buys medications from different pharmaceutical companies based on cost leading to confusing labeling and color-coding that predisposes to mistakes. Look-alike medications greatly increase the risk of inadvertently administering the wrong medication. Second, organizations may have reasonable mechanisms to assess system versus individual accountability, but adjust the response based on the severity of outcome from the adverse event. For example, a medication error without patient harm may be overlooked or even used as a learning experience, whereas the same error with patient harm leads to a punitive response. Third, organizations may treat disciplines differently, the classic situation in healthcare being that nurses are disciplined for mistakes while physicians' mistakes are variably ignored or discussed in rounds as learning opportunities or to embarrass.

A just culture with appropriate accountability exists when an organization adopts a sensible algorithm for assigning accountability and effectively applies the algorithm broadly (Figure 5-5). Managers use it daily to assess near misses and general activity, and risk management personnel apply the algorithm when serious adverse events occur and in the peer review process. Two commonly used algorithms come from James Reason's Incident Decision Tree, popularized in his book *Managing the Risk of Organizational Accidents*,[13] and David Marx's just culture work.[14] Simply put, everyone should be able to understand the rules and the rules must be fair. An organizational fairness algorithm developed by Allan Frankel and Michael Leonard builds on Reason's and Marx's works to produce a usable, simple model.[15]

How to use this chart: This chart should be used to categorize an individual caregiver's actions, not groups or systems. Evaluate each factor that influenced the caregiver's actions separately . When determining accountability, consider the context in which the action occurred.

1. First, exclude individuals with impaired judgement or whose actions might be malicious. (These cases must be managed using other appropriate avenues ie, employee assistance programs for substance abuse and psychosocial problems, legal authorities for cases with possible criminal intent.)	
Impaired judgment The caregiver's thinking was impaired - by illegal or legal substances - by cognitive impairment - by severe psychosocial stressors	**Malicious action** The caregiver wanted to cause harm.
• Discipline is warranted if illegal substances were used. • The caregiver's mindset and performance should be evaluated to determine whether a temporary work suspension would be helpful. • Help should be actively offered to the caregiver.	• Discipline and/or legal proceedings are warranted. • The caregiver's duties should be suspended immediately.

2. Second, use best judgment to categorize each action as either Reckless, Risky, or Unintentional based on the definitions in the chart. The categorization determines the general level of culpability and possible disciplinary actions; however, these general categories require further analysis as below prior to making a final decision.		
Reckless action The caregiver knowingly violated a rule and/or made a dangerous or unsafe choice. The decision appears to be self-serving and to have been made with little or no concern about risk.	**Risky action** The caregiver made a potentially unsafe choice. Their evaluation of relative risk appears to be erroneous.	**Unintentional error** The caregiver made or participated in an error while working appropriately and in the patients' best interests.
• The caregiver is accountable and needs re-training. Discipline may be warranted. • The caregiver should participate in teaching others the lessons learned.	• The caregiver is accountable and should receive coaching. • The caregiver should participate in teaching others the lessons learned.	• The caregiver is not accountable. • The caregiver should participate in investigating why the error occurred and teach others about the results of the investigation.

3. Third, perform a Substitution Test by asking at least three others with similar skills if they, in a similar situation, would act similarly, if the answer is "No" the individual is accountable. If "We do it all the time" system influence is substantial. If the answer are divided, evaluators should assign accountability with a goal to ensure perceptions of fairness by others.		
The system supports reckless action and requires fixing. The caregiver is probably less accountable for the action, and system leaders share in the accountability.	The system supports risky action and requires fixing. The caregiver is probably less accountable for the action, and system leaders share in the accountability.	The system supports error and requires fixing. The system's leaders are accountable and should apply error-proofing improvements.

| 4. Fourth, evaluate whether the individual has a history of unsafe or problematic acts. If they do, this may influence decisions about the appropriate responsibilities for the individual, ie, they may be in the wrong job. Organizations should have a reasonable and agreed-upon statute of limitations for taking these actions into account. |||

Figure 5-5 ▪ The fair evaluation and response chart.

The logic of the organizational fairness algorithm is as follows: When a serious adverse event occurs, the actions of the individuals involved should be evaluated separately. Each distinct activity should be evaluated separately. First, identify individuals for whom a just culture algorithm should not apply. The categories of individuals in this group include those whose sensorium is altered secondary to neurologic conditions like dementia or the use of mind-altering drugs, whether legal or illegal. The use of illegal drugs or alcohol at work is obvious, but so too is the use of legal medications that lead to a change in sensorium. For example, taking beta blockade for high blood pressure leading to sedation that results in an error causing harm. This group of individuals should appropriately be removed from their work and will need help, and illegal substance use may be subjected to criminal proceedings as appropriate. The second type of individual to be exempted from the algorithm is when their actions are malicious, or purposefully mean to cause harm. This is criminal behavior and should be treated as such.

Once these two groups are removed, the next step is to ascertain whether the actions by the individual would be considered reckless, risky, or simply error. Reckless behaviors are those performed where the individual appears disinterested in the risk incurred. Risky behaviors are those performed when individuals weigh risk incorrectly or are swayed inappropriately in their decision making. Errors are those events that occur in the course of diligently trying to do one's best but making a mistake in the process. A group of reasonable people evaluating most situations can generally assign actions to one of these three categories. Evaluating groups have the responsibility to gather as much information as needed to make a sensible assignment, and to err on the side of leniency when unsure.

Once assigned, the next step in the process is to apply Reason's Substitution Test—asking whether three individuals with similar skills in a similar situation would act in a similar fashion. If the answer is Yes, then likely the accountability is system based, meaning the environment sets up individuals to err. Occasionally, however, the substitution test identifies that an entire group has veered together into risky or reckless behavior. If the answer is No, then the individual is likely more accountable. In all of these situations, organizations should whenever possible tap, the individuals involved to help improve the system and educate others about the event and the learning generated from it. Lastly, an evaluation of the individual for a history of unsafe acts is reasonable to ascertain whether the person is in the wrong position in the organization.

Making a model like this live and breathe within an organization requires events and real cases, de-identified or made generic if necessary, be shared with front-line staff by leaders and managers to demonstrate there is a fair and consistent mechanism for looking at errors, and applying rules fairly. Most organizations have an existing algorithm today that is reasonably well understood by human resources and risk management. However, few organizations have effectively educated their middle managers and shown front-line providers that it is safe to discuss and learn from errors. The absence of such seriously impairs learning and improvement.

The power of leaders taking real events back to front-line caregivers and discussing them within this organizational fairness framework is the most effective mechanism to embed this model within the organization. It is important for front-line staff to be cognizant of the policies and practices that make it safe to learn from error. Having organizational leaders reinforce this message and demonstrate support for the ability to learn from these events in a way that is safe is critical. Otherwise, as occurs in most hospitals today, front-line caregivers don't know what the rules are, are hesitant to speak up, and the same undesired events continue to occur in the absence of fixing the underlying system failures.

LEARNING SYSTEMS

The *raison d'etre* of a robust safety culture, as described so far, is to create an effective learning system. Culture is the foundation for the learning system, and like the base of any architectural structure, determines the learning system's strength, permanence, and vitality.

As culture exists to create a learning system, learning systems exist to make processes reliable. The logic is that stable reliable processes reproducibly create reliable outcomes, and the goal is to apply clinical expertise so that we shape the processes to generate stellar reliable clinical outcomes. The concept is not theoretical. In healthcare, we have examples where application of these concepts has yielded excellent results through consistent and visible work on reliable process.[16–19] In the Toyota Production System (Lean) model, it is known as standard work.[20] Every clinician also knows that there is great value in being able to see patients on time in an outpatient clinic, give antibiotics consistently within 60 minutes prior to surgery, or discharge patients at the appointed time from the hospital. The lack of reliable process is wasteful, frustrating for patients and caregivers alike, and leads to unacceptably high levels of variation. Let's just consider the hospital discharge process. A patient may well have received outstanding care during their stay, and now they are ready to go home. The discharge is scheduled for 8 AM the following morning, and the family rearranges their day and takes off work. Unfortunately, the next morning everyone is kept waiting for hours until the physician shows up to sign the orders. No matter how wonderful the care has been, this is the last experience the family has, one of frustration and disappointment. This happens thousands of times every day in American healthcare. The lack of reliable processes causes numerous problems. High degrees of variation dictate that many patients will not receive the intended care and will suffer the consequences. This can make it challenging to know whether the patient is not responding to appropriate therapy or the lack of consistent application of clinical care. Suboptimal outcomes are the result, which is highly unacceptable.

In the absence of reliable process, the ability to consistently improve is precluded by the lack of a stable process that can be measured. High degrees of variation also lead to unpredictability, which increases clinical risk. For example, twenty-five obstetricians administering Pitocin to augment labor twenty-five different ways, means a nurse at the bedside may not be able to determine if a mistake has been made or one of a plethora of individualized formulas is being applied (eg, how do we know we're doing it right or doing it wrong?). This can easily translate into more newborn intensive care unit (NICU) admissions from uterine hyperstimulation or tachysystole and the subsequent effects. In high-risk domains like medicine, predictable and reliable processes make it much easier and much safer to deliver care. The hallmark of excellence is being able to do the basics consistently every time.

As described in the beginning of this chapter, learning systems are comprised of:

1. Continuous learning
2. Improvement and measurement
3. Transparency of the learning
4. Reliable performance.

An examination of these is as follows:

Continuous learning means collecting and documenting defects. In healthcare today, this tends to occur through audits and quality measurements, and haphazardly through management identifying problems and acting on them. Less frequently, but almost always in better-run units, managers systematically collect, document, and act on defects; and rarely, in the best of units, managers do so and make the process visible. Continuous learning entails the collecting of defects from all front-line providers in almost real time and the acting on those defects by the team, orchestrated by managers and directors.

The team behavior known as debriefing, where team members reflect on their activities and ask the three questions: (1) What worked well?, (2) What didn't work as we would have liked?, and (3) What would we do differently next time?, is the primary mechanism for continuous learning. Debriefing is not an event, it is a process to support an ongoing dialog of learning. In reality, all workers make note of problems and defects that arise during the performance of their duties, be they communication gaffs, clinical decision errors, equipment misadventures, personal slips or lapses, or poor teamwork. Most of the time the problems are subliminally acknowledged and lost, perceived as "the way things happen here". In the absence of a Learning System, caregivers resort to workarounds and first-order problem solving, ie, borrowing linen from an adjacent unit for the umpteenth time, as no one can seem to fix the problem. This is not only frustrating and risky, encouraging workarounds that potentially increase risk, but also demoralizing as front-line staff have repeatedly raised these issues and nothing ever happens, which translates to their belief that the organization doesn't care. That can quickly translate into "if they don't care, neither do I."

Continuous learning is the mindset, or mindfulness per Weick and Sutcliffe,[21] to take note of these episodes and defects. Debriefing is the act that collects and memorializes the collection of these episodes for future analysis.

In a robust learning system, managers and directors set clear expectations about debriefings, determining how frequently they should occur, who is to participate, and the questions to be asked. Managers showcase the importance of debriefing by making the findings visible on bulletin boards and the like, and frequently and actively update the information. Obviously, the collection of defects is useful only if actions are taken to address them, so tracking and showcasing improvement activity is a key aspect of supporting a continuous learning effort.[22]

▌IMPROVEMENT AND MEASUREMENT

Taking action on defects is a simple way of saying that managers and leaders must apply process-improvement techniques. These techniques have developed in other industries into impressively robust sciences with names such as Lean, Six Sigma, and the Model for Improvement, and all have been imported into healthcare with varying success. Fortunately, they all work when applied appropriately and have many aspects in common that can be extracted and applied without the often-confusing jargon that has developed with them. Following are some of the basic concepts.

The most basic concept of all is that processes can be divided into a series of very small actions, and each action is subject to testing (Figure 5-6). For example, an ambulatory clinic must ensure that there is an effective process for patients to know where to go when they arrive. As part of this effort, the front-desk secretary may test how effectively patients see a sign by placing the sign in different areas of the waiting room and asking patients if they notice it. This most basic of tests, a test of change, is comprised of four components: Planning, Doing, Studying, and Acting (PDSA). The PDSA cycle has an impressive pedigree, first conceptualized by Shewhart and then applied by Deming to the

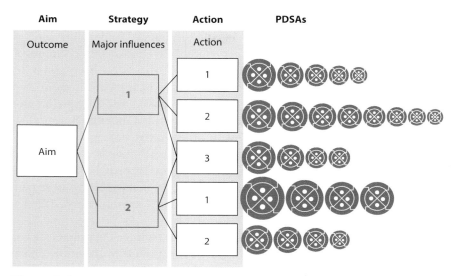

Figure 5-6 ▪ Aims, tests of change, and the strategy and actions that link them.

auto industry, and is now utilized by all industries. The rules are simple. A full PDSA must be a real change in the process; it is not a measurement nor is it a task that prepares for the change. In our example above, simply obtaining the new sign is a task, and, once placed, asking patients if they see the sign is a measurement. Those activities are necessary but the only real change and real test is when the sign is set up in a different place for patients so see. *Planning* comprises: (1) the tasks necessary to perform the test ("I'll tell my coworkers about this test and get a piece of colored paper"), (2) coming up with a theory about the change ("I think the sign will be visible in this spot"), and (3) a prediction about the likelihood of the change's success ("I think about 90% of the patients will see the sign"). *Doing* is actually performing, or when appropriate, simulating the change. *Studying* is evaluating and reflecting on the effect of the change ("Only half the patients saw the sign, and I watched them go by and they missed it because they had to look down at the stairs they were climbing"). *Acting i*s making changes to the process and is linked to *Planning* if another test is necessary.[23]

PDSAs are the fundamental building block of all process improvement and managers and leaders must know, and be able to identify and coach, each of the steps. Many small defects, such as a sign that patients don't see, are amenable to quick PDSAs leading to permanent changes that eliminate them. A series of tests will identify for the secretary what signage is most effective for the greatest number of patients. However, some defects are large and require many actions to ameliorate.

Decreasing readmissions to hospitals after discharge is such an example. In these many situations larger aims must be articulated, and can be done so in a prescribed and repeatable fashion applicable to almost all large improvement efforts. In every case, a baseline measure of the defect is necessary, ie, how many readmissions currently occur. From that baseline measure, an aim can be articulated identifying the improvement desired. For example, an aim might be that readmissions be decreased by 50% over 6 months. Note that all aims have a "what by when" phrasing. In other words, how much improvement is desired, (whether relative, ie percentage, or absolute ie, 5/month) and by what time period will the improvement occur. There is little science to selecting the two aspects of the aim, other than the perception by those participating that the goal is worthy and the time frame appropriately challenging but doable.

Baseline measurement, aims, and PDSAs are the three building blocks of improvement, and the aim, and PDSAs are the two ends of the entire effort. The filling between the overall aim and the small tests of change comes from intelligent people with clinical expertise defining the aspects of the process to target, and once the PDSAs have been performed and a worthy permanent change has been identified, obtaining the resources to support it. For example, a goal to reduce readmissions is likely to generate from knowledgeable physicians and nurses that patients who receive one-on-one coaching from advisors by telephone or equivalent tend to be readmitted less frequently. Therefore, a major factor in reducing readmissions is "appropriate patient coaching," and tests of change (PDSAs) can be designed to evaluate the impact of telephone calls versus computer interactions etc., performed variably by registered nurses (RN) versus lay coaches etc., daily versus every 3 days etc. Initial PDSAs would entail just one or two patients, and testing slowly refined and then enlarged to gain a greater understanding of the details leading to successful patient knowledge. Implementation occurs only after enough PDSAs have ascertained with a fair degree of certainty that daily conversations for 14 days after discharge with lay coaches using computer video interactions is workable in the particular setting being tested, at which point resources to hire lay coaches and obtain appropriate computers for patients are instituted.

Visible aims and PDSAs are the hallmark of effective managers, directors, and leaders. Leaders are the guardians of the improvement process just defined. Their actions must support this type of learning, and anything they do that undermines this learning is an abrogation of their leadership position. This explains why psychological safety is so important in the description of culture, and why leaders are charged with creating psychologically safe environments. Doing so is the only way to effectively create the milieu to not only embolden team members to speak up but also participate in the improvement efforts to identify aims and perform PDSAs.

TRANSPARENCY AND VISIBILITY

How do successful systems engage the teams, providers, and workers in the learning system? The mechanisms have been described: specific attributes of leaders combined with specific team behaviors in a psychologically safe and just environment. These are attributes of leaders and team members are essential, but for learning to occur, one additional component is required, making the entire process visible. Visual learning systems are a hallmark of many of the improvement sciences for a reason. Engaging the workforce requires setting expectations, ensuring that individuals feel that their voice is heard and acted upon, and showcasing the effectiveness of management and improvement. To achieve this, units must have specific locations where the process of improvement is formally discussed by leaders and team members, where the improvement effort is visually represented in such a way that those who view it can understand it, and see that it is dynamic and alive (Figure 5-7). This presumes that units identify times when these learning events occur and make them a priority to ensure that all can, and do, participate.

By analogy, the boards that showcase this effort are equivalent to how an electrocardiogram machine and oxygen saturation monitor placed on a patient depict in real time the physiology of the patient. Learning boards should be dynamic and depict the physiology of the unit's learning system, almost in real time. That means that a bulletin board, as we will describe below, is the place where managers and directors meet with team members to discuss not only the daily huddle about the schedule, but also the daily improvement activities, and

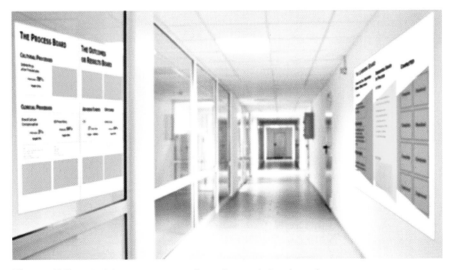

Figure 5-7 ▪ Visible management. Learning and aims boards.

the measures collected that relate to the chosen few aims of importance. The boards must be kept up-to-date with measures ideally collected by front-line providers; providers who do so are aware that the added effort pays dividends in the collective improvement that results, made visible on the learning board.

There are two types of bulletin boards. The first showcase the aims chosen by the unit and should highlight the improvement made over time using run charts or control charts. The second should showcase the results of debriefings by identifying the collected defects and those that have been acted on and resolved or mitigated.

The aims board should identify each aim including the what, by when, and the associated measures. For example, an effort focused on re-admissions might state the aims as "reduce re-admissions in X population by 50% within 6 months" and the measures might include # of readmissions and % of patients with one-on-one coaching. The # of re-admissions is a measure of outcome. The percentage of patients with one-on-one coaching is a measure of a process. The aims board should showcase changes in the processes and outcome over time using run charts (charts that show change over time), as well as highlighting the actions (PDSAs) taken to achieve the changes. The actions will sometimes yield good changes, but may also be detrimental to the effort. Showcasing all of these sequentially shows which improvements are useful. Adding in the names of providers who participated in each PDSA links improvement directly to the teams and individuals in the unit. In doing all the above, an elegant aims board makes learning visible and engages providers in the unit's improvement efforts.

The second board, the learning board, should have on it the collected defects identified from debriefings, but can also include defects identified by any other source available to the Unit, including, of course, patients. A rule of thumb for managers charged with the responsibility of producing these boards is that all comments from Unit participants must go up with the exception of *ad hominum* comments (ie, "Bob is a jerk"). Those issues should be taken up, as any good manager should do, by engaging the appropriate individuals in discussion to resolve differences and facilitate the resolution of conflicts.

The purpose of the learning boards is to take the insights of team members and act on them, thereby giving credibility to the all-important feeling by workers, "I feel like I'm being heard." Concurrently, acting on these defects is the mechanism to improve reliability, so the win-win combination in this effort cannot be overstated. Leonard Berry, in his evaluation of outstanding management, has pointed out that only through volunteerism is excellence achieved. Suffice to say that only when workers feel that their voice is heard will they be willing to volunteer their efforts. The process of debriefing and making the information visible is the mechanism to achieve this, and take note, once again psychological safety rears up as essential.

The learning board is comprised of three sections. Onto the first go the identified defects, each on its own card (or equivalent if an electronic board was developed). These defects move into the middle section when action is being taken to address them, and they move into the third section when they are resolved. All three sections are important, but the third appears to have the biggest impact on units. Seeing the small issues get resolved and the list mount up over time is tangible evidence of engagement and effective management. The list is a powerful motivator at all levels. Movement of each defect into the middle column occurs when the leader takes responsibility and performs actions to address the problem, the leader assigns responsibility to an appropriate team member, or a team member volunteers to solve a problem. Over time, if learning boards are implemented effectively, the tendency is for the actions to occur as a result of individuals volunteering to solve problems, and this evolution helps characterize the unit along the reactive to generative scale described earlier.

CONCLUSION

Learning systems are built on a healthy culture and entail continuous learning about defects, using process improvement made visible through learning and aims boards, all in pursuit of reliable process. Healthy cultures come from leaders who guard learning and create psychological safety and mutual respect; teams whose behaviors support effective forward planning, reflective debriefing, and in between clear communication and rapid resolution of conflict; and finally leaders and teams who work in an environment perceived by all as psychologically safe and fair.

IN PRACTICE

Taking a practice, workflow, or set of processes as is and making them significantly safer and more reliable requires a systemic approach. This shouldn't preclude any one individual, however, from taking responsibility for what is in their direct and immediate ability to influence or control tomorrow.

1. **Be an effective leader**. Effective leaders always set a positive, active tone, think out loud sharing the plan, and continually invite other team members into the conversation for their ideas and concerns. By setting a positive active tone and thinking out loud, they are sharing the plan and helping the team create a common mental model, or understanding of the plan of care. Inviting other team members into the conversation flattens the hierarchy or power dis-

(Continued)

(*Continued*)

tance, and makes the leader approachable. Both knowing the plan and an approachable leader make it much easier to speak up when one of the team members has a concern. Good leaders never assume that people will speak up; they always actively invite them to do so.

2. **Appreciate the critical importance of psychological safety.** Psychological safety concerns the willingness of individuals to voice a concern or speak up when they are unclear as to the plan of care. It is never OK for someone to be hesitant to speak up, yet it happens frequently in healthcare, a culture where people pride themselves on knowing the answer. Many avoidable adverse events happen because people are hesitant to speak up because they are concerned about looking dumb or due to the fact they were treated with disrespect the last time. Creating psychological safety is the primary role of leaders.

3. **Leaders have a profound impact on the ability of teams to learn from errors and near misses.** A model of organizational fairness that balances the need for individual accountability with not holding individuals responsible for system errors is fundamental for learning and improvement. Medicine is a culture that historically believed that skilled practitioners who try hard and pay attention do not make mistakes, which is quite unrealistic. Humans make mistakes at very predictable rates and complex systems often generate the potential for system errors. Having a simple model, that is fair and routinely used, to look at events with leaders modeling these behaviors is essential for learning. In the absence of these front-line discussions where leaders make it safe to learn from errors, the prospect of repeated similar events is quite high, and it feels quite unsafe for the front-line caregivers.

4. **Build a learning system.** Everyday there are opportunities to improve the quality of care and remove barriers to doing so. There is tremendous wisdom among front-line caregivers who do the work every day. Most often their insights and concerns are not well captured, as they do not receive feedback or see that the issues have been resolved. Reliable feedback and a transparent process of learning are essential for organizational learning and habitual excellence.

5. **Support effective teams.** Frequently, groups come together to work without clarifying the game plan for day discussing the groups' strengths and weaknesses. Brief to clarifying the goal ("We've got 35 patients to care for between us and are likely to get six admissions in the next 10 hours"), and identify the concerns to achieving the goal ("We've got three required meetings today that will slow us down. We need to coordinate our efforts around losing participation during the meetings.").

FAQs

1. What is the biggest challenge one will face when trying to implement leadership changes such as those described in this chapter?

   The biggest challenge in implementing the concepts described in this chapter is that few participants in the clinical healthcare environment understand the key components that lead to reliable operational excellence. Physicians are trained through an apprenticeship process and watch senior physicians using a huge variety of behaviors to achieve their personal goals. Specialty training has archetypes of behavior, but very few of the examples that trainees see exemplify the behaviors that successfully create effective teams, effectively manage conflict, or model the leadership that combines an expectation of excellence with the psychological safety that ensures learning. Nurses leaders, nursing regulatory groups, and nursing education stress the following of rules, and the expectation that not following rules will lead to punishment. Nursing is just beginning to incorporate an understanding of human fallibility into its accountability policies, the result being that many nurses work in situations where they are accountable for actions over which they have little or no control, a situation that leads to frustration and hopelessness. Physicians must learn the components that support reliable operational excellence. Nurses must learn about and apply human factors, human fallibility, and complexity science into their policies and practices.

REFERENCES

1. Schein E. Organizational Culture and Leadership, 3rd edition. San Francisco, CA: John Wiley and Sons; 2004. ISBN-13: 9780787968458.
2. Edmondson AC. Psychological safety and learning behavior in work teams. *Adm Sci Q.* 1999;44:350-383.
3. Bognár A, Barach P, Johnson JK, et al. Errors and the burden of errors: attitudes, perceptions, and the culture of safety in pediatric cardiac surgical teams. *Ann Thorac Surg.* 2008;85(4):1374-1381.
4. Leonard M, Frankel A, Federico F, et al. *The Essential Guide for Patient Safety Officers,* 2nd ed. Oak Brook, IL: IHI/Joint Commission Resources; 2013.
5. Wachter RW. *Understanding Patient Safety.* New York, NY: McGraw-Hill; 2012.
6. Stone D, Patton B, Heen S. *Difficult conversations: How to Discuss What Matters Most.* New York, NY: Penguin Books; 2000.
7. Edmondson AC. Learning from failure in health care: frequent opportunities, pervasive barriers. *Qual Saf Health Care.* 2004;13(Suppl 2):ii3-ii9.
8. Edmondson A. *Teaming: How Organizations Learn, Innovate, and Compete in the Knowledge Economy.* San Francisco, CA: Jossey-Bass; 2012.

9. Leonard M, Graham S, Bonacum D. The human factor: the critical importance of effective teamwork and communication in providing safe care. *Qual Saf Health Care*. 2004;13(Suppl 1):i85-i90.
10. Agency for Healthcare Research and Quality. TeamSTEPPS. Available at: http://team-stepps.ahrq.gov/. Accessed 18.08.2013.
11. Blake R, Mouton J. *The Managerial Grid: The Key to Leadership Excellence*. Houston TX: Gulf Publishing Co; 1964.
12. Thomas Kilmann Conflict Mode Instrument. Available at: http://en.wikipedia.org/wiki/Thomas–Kilmann_Conflict_Mode_Instrument. Accessed 18.08.2013.
13. Reason JT. *Managing the Risks of Organizational Accidents*. Aldershot, Hants, England; Brookfield, VT: Ashgate; 1997.
14. Marx D. *Whack-a-Mole: The Price we Pay for Expecting Perfection*. Dallas, TX: Your Side Studios Publisher; 2009.
15. Leonard MW, Frankel A. The path to safe and reliable healthcare. *Patient Educ Couns*. 2010;80(3):288-292.
16. Hanna L. *HBS Cases: Cincinnati Children's Hospital Medical Center*. Available at: http://hbswk.hbs.edu/item/6441.html?wknews=062810. Accessed 5/10/2014.
17. DiGioia A 3rd, Lorenz H, Greenhouse PK, et al. A patient-centered model to improve metrics without cost increase: viewing all care through the eyes of patients and families. *J Nurs Adm*. 2010;40(12):540-546.
18. Toussaint JA management, leadership, and board road map to transforming care for patients. *Front Health Serv Manage*. 2013;29(3):3-15.
19. Draycott TJ, Croft JF, Ash JP, et al. Improving neonatal outcome through practical shoulder dystocia training. *Obstet Gynecol*. 2008;112(1):1-7.
20. Kinney, C. Transforming Health Care: *Virginia Mason Medical Center's Pursuit of the Perfect Patient Experience*. New York, NY: CRC Press, 2011.
21. Weick KE, Sutcliffe KM. *Managing the Unexpected: Assuring High Performance in an Age of Complexity*. 1st ed. San Francisco, CA: Jossey-Bass; 2001.
22. Leonard M, Frankel A. *How Can Leaders Influence a Safety Culture?* The Health Foundation; 2012. Available at: http://www.health.org.uk/publications/how-can-leaders-influence-a-safety-culture/. Accessed 5/10/2014.
23. Langley GJ, Moen R, Nolan KM, Nolan TW, Norman CL, Provost PL. *Improvement Guide: A Practical Approach to Enhancing Organizational Performance*, 2nd Edition. San Francisco, CA: Jossey-Bass; 20xx. ISBN 978-0-470-19241-2.

TEAMWORK AND COMMUNICATION | 6

▋ INTRODUCTION

An effective healthcare team is of utmost importance to ensure safe, effective and efficient care for pediatric patients. Teamwork is particularly important when caring for children, as providers from various disciplines are performing different yet complimentary roles, all striving to provide high quality care, and at times in stressful situations. Failed communication and teamwork between providers, patients, and/or families are two of the most common attributable causes of medical errors.[1-3] Potential for error only increases when caring for children with complex medical conditions.

Providing healthcare to pediatric patients is often complicated by the inability of many children to express their symptoms and concerns, the elevated stress of caring for children, especially those who are critically ill or injured, caregiver involvement, and an increased margin for error. Rather than functioning as a skilled and integrated team, an entire group of healthcare providers may be focused on care of the patient, with each individual provider having different priorities or short-term goals which may conflict with one another. These conflicting priorities can be complicated by poor role clarity or a hierarchy that discourages open communication.

Communication errors or omissions are common and can have significant effects on patient care.[4] Lack of accountability and follow-up can further derail team efforts and may predispose a team to an unbalanced workload. Finally, in the busy medical environment, teams must develop strategies to deal with fatigue and distractions.

Overcoming barriers to teamwork in healthcare is a group effort, and necessitates acceptance from all disciplines. While some simple interventions may provide a positive impact, producing a culture change that focuses on teams rather than individuals, takes time, effort, and frequent coaching. By following the story of one child's illness, this chapter will discuss some strategies that have been successfully employed to address many of these challenges in hospitals and other complex work environments.

CASE SCENARIO #1

Setting: Pediatrician's Office

Ben is a 4-year-old boy who was climbing up onto a television cabinet to get a toy that was out of reach. Ben's mom heard a crash, and came running into the room to find him unconscious amidst the toppled cabinet and television. When she screamed his name and scooped him up, he groggily woke up crying, and after she was able to console him, he seemed to be back to himself. However, at lunch, he did not have much of an appetite and seemed to still be a bit sleepy, so his mom decided to take him in to see his pediatrician.

Upon checking in for a sick visit, the clerk notices that Ben "doesn't look quite right," so she ushers him back to an open examination room. As none of the examination rooms currently being used by Ben's pediatrician are available, the clerk puts Ben and his mother in an adjacent examination room, and tells a nurse that there is another patient to be seen.

The nurse makes a mental note of this, but is distracted by a request to prepare vaccines for a set of triplets. Meanwhile, the pediatrician continues to see the patients in the usual examination rooms. While Ben and his mother wait in their examination room, he becomes lethargic and begins to vomit, at which point his mother notifies a second passing nurse. At the insistence of Ben's mother, the pediatrician is called to the examination room, quickly recognizes Ben's concerning neurological status, and calls for emergency equipment. Both nurses leave the room to retrieve the office crash cart. The check-in clerk enters the room to see if there is anything she can do to help but doesn't ask the question out loud. One nurse brings the crash cart into the room and begins to look for vascular access. The pediatrician is looking through the cart for a pediatric oxygen mask while the second nurse is hooking up suction. Finally, the check-in clerk realizes that no one has called for an ambulance to take the child to the emergency department (ED). She leaves the room to place the call but does not let the team know she is doing this. At the same time, one of the nurses also takes out his cell phone and calls 911 for transport. Fifteen minutes later, an ambulance arrives with a basic life support crew. The office phone is ringing but no one is available to answer it as everyone is now in Ben's room participating in his care or waiting for instructions. The caller is the local 911 dispatch center trying to determine if there is still a need for a second ambulance for transport.

DISCUSSION

Several characteristics of the healthcare office environment predispose its teams to communication errors and teamwork failures. The increasing complexity of care and rapidity of workflow compresses huge amounts of information transfer into short periods of time. Also, healthcare providers of different disciplines often have their own tasks to complete, and any given provider may not be aware of the full clinical scenario. In this case presentation, a typically busy clinic day is interrupted by an unanticipated patient who needs urgent medical attention and the communication about his unexpected arrival and acuity are lost to distraction and assumptions. The lack of a predetermined plan for identifying patients needing timely attention is evident in this scenario. As is often the case, a parent must advocate for the child who cannot advocate for himself.

While EDs are accustomed to triaging acutely ill and injured patients, clinics and office-based practices are often focused on routine workflow and rely heavily on scheduling. Yet any medical setting must be prepared for an emergency, and have a plan to quickly address patient needs. In this case, Ben is placed in a room separate from the typical examination room rotation. While it is sometimes necessary, working outside the normal protocols and expected workflow of any medical environment increases the risk for an error. As such, it is important to ensure that the entire team is aware of alterations to normal workflow, and the reason for the change. As the presence of a patient requiring urgent resuscitation is not a frequent occurrence in this care setting, familiarity with team member roles and overall team performance would be improved by periodic practice or drills.

Achieving a shared understanding of patient care goals goes well beyond effective communication. In addition to a universal understanding of the goals of care, team members must also have situational awareness of circumstances in their work areas which may affect patient care and workflow.[5,6] Had the check-in clerk, both nurses, and the pediatrician all been aware of Ben's presence and shared their understanding of the urgency of his symptoms, it is likely that Ben would have been evaluated, treated, and transported earlier. This could have been accomplished by the use of a huddle, a quick touch-base group update that can be used to keep the team informed of changes in their environment and patients' status. Pre-determined triggers for a huddle such as an unexpected patient or a patient that "doesn't look right" are essential. If calling a huddle becomes routine practice, the team will share a better understanding of what is currently happening in their part of the clinic, providing role clarity for tasks and anticipating next steps and having a "shared mental model" for the care of the patient and the status of the rest of the clinic. In addition, the lack of situational awareness extends into Ben's care. Becoming fixated on a task (the nurse preparing vaccines), lack of role clarity (who calls for an ambulance, who retrieves the code cart) can prevent the designation of a team leader who is aware of the whole picture that is occurring and allows for overlap of tasks and poor resource management.

Learning Points

- Interdisciplinary communication may be hindered by interruptions, different priorities and tasks. Developing triggers for implementation of huddles can help maintain situational awareness among the team.
- Any deviation to expected workflow increases risk for errors and omissions.
- All healthcare settings can benefit from a clear plan to identify and address those patients who may need immediate attention.
- Periodic drills for unexpected critical events may serve to improve communication and teamwork.

CASE SCENARIO #2

Setting: Emergency Department

Upon arrival to the ED, Ben is only minimally responsive to pain. He is immediately sent to get a computed tomography (CT) scan of his head, but becomes apneic in the scanner and a code blue is called. The emergency team rushes in to intubate the patient.

The ED resident physician is the first physician in the room, and immediately takes over bag-mask ventilation. He also establishes himself as team leader. The ED attending enters the room but does not interrupt the resident. The resident calls out the medicines and equipment he wants to use for intubation. The respiratory therapist disagrees with the resident's requested endotracheal tube size, and speaks to the attending, who confirms the respiratory therapist's choice of endotracheal tube.

The team becomes slow to respond and confused as they are unclear which physician is the team leader in this situation. The resident calls out for the first dose of rapid sequence induction medications before the respiratory therapist is prepared with the intubation equipment, and the patient begins to desaturate during prolonged bag-mask ventilation. Then, as the resident realizes that a different endotracheal tube size had been prepared than what he initially asked for, he and the respiratory therapist argue, before the attending physician steps in and directs them to continue with the intubation with the prepared tube. The ED charge nurse is very uncomfortable with the interactions between the team members. She knows that all of the proper emergency medicines are not yet prepared for the procedure, but is afraid to speak up.

As the resident performs direct laryngoscopy, Ben becomes bradycardic. No atropine is readily available in the room, so a dose of epinephrine is ordered by the attending. However, the nurse delivering meds is unfamiliar with caring for children, and she delivers a full adult dose. Ben then becomes markedly tachycardic and hypertensive, which is initially perceived by the members of the team to be secondary to pain. The resident orders additional sedation medicines, which lead to subsequent hypotension necessitating volume resuscitation.

Ben's airway is finally secured, he becomes hemodynamically stable, and is able to complete the CT scan. The scan demonstrates a large epidural hematoma, and Ben is rushed to the operating room (OR) for evacuation of the blood collection.

DISCUSSION

Teams vary in composition, size, and skill levels. Regardless of these elements, teams function best when members have a clear understanding of roles. Unambiguous roles for team members maximize resource allocation and reduce negative redundant work efforts. Clear roles also allow for easy delegation of tasks by the team leader.

In this case, lack of role clarity causes several conflicts and delays during the intubation process. The ED resident tries to both manage the patient's airway and run the resuscitation, and therefore, neither task gets his full attention. His physical placement at the head of the bed and his attention to the airway likely prevent him from surveying the entire room and maintaining an adequate understanding of the entire clinical scenario. He also does not understand the role or appreciate the expertise of the respiratory therapist. Similarly, the nursing staff is unclear about who will be preparing and delivering the medicines during the code. The lack of clarity about team leadership causes a direct conflict regarding the endotracheal tube size. This conflict further contributes to an unwillingness of team members to speak up with any concern, as there is not an agreed-upon process for challenging an unsafe condition in the name of patient safety.

While it is important for individuals to have clear roles on a given team, these roles should also be flexible for a given task. This is particularly true of the team leader role. The concept of situational leadership describes the ability for different team members to step into the team leader role, depending on which is best suited for a specific task or scenario. While the physician is often the default team leader for directing patient care, there are times when the bedside nurse or others will be best suited to direct the team efforts. It is unrealistic to expect that the most senior person on the team must always be the team leader. There are times when the least tenured provider in the room actually has more experience or skill in a particular procedure or scenario. Senior team members can play an important role by encouraging the skill development of the more junior member of the team.

One of the most challenging barriers to clear team roles, particularly in academic medical centers, is constantly changing team membership. Staff may experience high turnover, trainees rotate on and off the team, personnel change shift to shift, and yet the pace of work and demands on the team do not waver. Something as simple as knowing the names of the other team members can significantly help the flow of communication.[7] Being able to ask something to an individual by using his/her name, gives that team member a clear role, along with personal ownership of that task.

Use of a "time-out," a specific type of briefing, has become the standard of care for confirmation of team readiness before procedures, to ensure situational awareness among the team.[8,9] Even in an emergent situation like the case scenario presented here, a brief time-out prior to medication delivery could have clarified the plan and ensured a safer, smoother intubation. In this case, the intubation process was started before the entire team was prepared, even though there were questions about the appropriate equipment, and not all necessary medications were available. Each of these things, along with further role clarity, could have been easily clarified with a team time-out, lasting only seconds.

Having clarity on team leader and team member roles should not establish an incontestable hierarchy. The leader will direct efforts and help solidify a vision of care, but a culture of safety dictates that any member of the medical team has both the right and responsibility to speak up with concerns or questions. Each team member brings their own unique knowledge, experience, and perspective to any given clinical scenario. In this case, the ED charge nurse was aware that not all of the necessary medicines were ready, yet she was uncomfortable challenging the authority of the attending physician. If a team member feels uncomfortable speaking up when he or she has a safety concern or suggestion, it handicaps the overall capability of the team. Yet it can be difficult for team members to challenge the team leader's decisions during a time of critical importance, perhaps due to their own uncertainty, presence of the patient or family, a chaotic environment, or even their general respect for that leader.

Like huddles, trigger words can also be very useful to focus communication during a period of critical importance. In this case scenario, the ED charge nurse sensed that the team was not prepared, but felt uncomfortable in contradicting the attending physician. The concept of "psychological safety" describes a culture in which any provider feels safe to speak out with safety concerns. Psychological safety is necessary to ensure optimal communication among a team, and can easily be hindered when an individual feels that their opinion is not respected by other team members, or is of secondary importance to the team leader. One strategy to help overcome the perceived hierarchy described in this case is the use of pre-determined trigger words. Healthcare teams agree on easily recognizable words or phrases which will have a targeted meaning for all team members. Trigger words are of particular use when body language fails to warn other team members of a concern, or when the listener is distracted or focused on a specific task. Any provider can say the pre-determined word or words, and everyone in the room will know that they need to pause and consider the situation. Examples may include "I am concerned," "is the attending aware of this," "stop," and "is this safe?" Team STEPPS® teaches a graduated response of trigger phrases, in the format of "C.U.S.": "I am **C**oncerned," "I am **U**ncomfortable," and "this is a **S**afety issue."[10] An additional phrase such as "I need clarity" should be developed and practiced to act as a "hard stop" for the entire team, allowing everyone to ensure that they are proceeding in a safe and coordinated manner.

Feedback to individuals is a team responsibility, and should be provided regularly. In the same way that frequent small steering corrections are needed to drive a car, frequent informal feedback between team members can keep a team on-track and help optimize behaviors. One form of feedback that could have been useful in this specific clinical scenario would be the use of closed-loop communication. Had the nurse delivering medicines repeated back what she heard regarding the epinephrine (including medicine name, dose, and route), it is likely that the dosing error would have been recognized and corrected before delivery of the medicine.

Individuals are often uncomfortable giving critical feedback to one of their peers and even more so to one with a status of authority. However, if continuous feedback becomes imbedded in the team culture, then constructive feedback can be delivered safely and shared frequently. In this case scenario, the respiratory therapist should have raised a concern regarding the endotracheal tube size directly with the resident who was the ordering provider. Immediate feedback to the resident not only allows for a learning opportunity, but helps establish a team mentality between the two providers. However, if conflict persists, it is appropriate to involve a third provider, such as the attending physician. Ideally, this discussion to resolve the conflict should involve both of the original parties along with the third, rather than a separate discussion with a supervisor. In the healthcare environment, medical errors can be initiated or amplified by such parallel conversations, as they fracture the shared mental model of the team. These separate conversations can often initiate competing orders or processes by team members who are unaware of the second discussion.

Feedback is most effective when it is *timely, brief,* and *specific to behaviors* that can be changed. One of the most effective methods to accomplish group feedback is to participate in debriefings as soon as possible after significant events.[11] In gathering the entire team together, providers can discuss what went well and what could be done better next time. It is important to include all team members in these discussions, and to maintain a focus on providing optimal care for the patient. Avoiding blame or intimidating comments regarding behaviors helps foster an open discussion among all team members. In this case scenario, a debriefing by the ED team following the intubation could have highlighted the issues of role clarity, team preparedness prior to starting the procedure, conflict resolution, and miscommunication regarding the medication dose. The debriefing process also gives a chance for the entire team to devise solutions that may prevent future team breakdowns.[12]

Learning Points

- Role clarity streamlines a team's efforts and minimizes conflict.
- Use of time-outs prior to procedures can help clarify the plan for all team members and ensure a coordinated effort in patient care.
- Pre-defined trigger words empower any team member to speak up at any time if he or she identifies an unsafe behavior or condition.
- Closed-loop communication enables immediate feedback about what the receiver received from an information exchange.
- Debrief as soon as possible after an event to provide important feedback to the team and to identify opportunities for improvement.

▌ CASE SCENARIO #3

Setting: Pediatric Intensive Care Unit, Patient Handoff From the Operating Room

The evacuation of the epidural hematoma goes well, but the surgeon notes a surprising amount of oozing after removal of the clot. Ben is slow to wake up from anesthesia, and given the late hour, it is decided to leave him intubated and deliver him to the pediatric intensive care unit (PICU) for subsequent extubation as soon as he awakens.

Exhausted after a long day of surgeries (and a newborn baby at home), the neurosurgery resident gives a quick report on the surgery and leaves the PICU. The anesthesiologist gives a similar brief report on the case and rushes back to the operating room (OR) for another emergency case. Not included during the hand-off is a report of the residual oozing after clot evacuation, a contact number for the surgeons, or the expected course for the night (including the plan to extubate). Also, at no point during the handoff does the receiving PICU team have a chance to ask questions to the OR team.

A few hours later, the PICU resident notes that Ben is beginning to wake up and become uncomfortable. She orders a sedation infusion, with the plan of extubating Ben in the morning, once the attending arrives. Later that night, however, Ben becomes hypertensive and bradycardic, and the bedside nurse notes a unilateral, dilated, non-reactive pupil. While mannitol is given for potential cerebral herniation, several calls are made to the neuro surgery resident who operated on the patient, with no response. The PICU resident continues bedside medical management, until the charge nurse insists that the PICU attending be called. The neuro surgery attending is also subsequently called as a repeat CT scan shows a recurrent epidural hematoma with adjacent subarachnoid hemorrhage, midline shift, and potential herniation with compression of the brainstem. Ben is once again rushed to the OR for evacuation of the hematoma.

DISCUSSION

Most people consider themselves to be effective communicators. When individuals wish to convey a thought, they provide what they feel is necessary to describe the concept that exists in their mind. The reality is that effective communication is best measured by what is received, rather than by what is given. Therefore, development of a shared understanding between providers is maximized by focusing on those at the receiving end of communication. In this case, the PICU team receiving the patient clearly did not obtain the information they needed to appropriately care for Ben.

A shared mental model is achieved when the communicator and the listener reach the same vision and understanding of not only the information being transferred, but the entire clinical scenario. While the PICU team did not receive any erroneous information from the OR team, there were several key pieces of omitted data that may have adversely affected Ben's care. Had the PICU team known about the unusual oozing, it may have led to further evaluation for a coagulopathy. Similarly, his time to return to the OR may have been dramatically shortened if the PICU team was able to easily contact the neurosurgical team.

Patient handoffs are particularly vulnerable to communication omissions and errors. It is not possible to convey every detail about a patient during a brief handoff, yet it is imperative to provide the necessary information to care for the patient. Handoffs are often complicated further by providers of different disciplines or specialties, who may have their own terminology and priorities for care. The handoff provider must also balance conveying known data, suspected diagnoses, and anticipated (but unknown) future course.[13] Despite the potential pitfalls, patients are typically passed off between providers more than 20 times during the course of a hospital stay,[14] a number that increases with case complexity and limitations on residency trainee duty hours.

Structured communication is one of the most important techniques which assists both the purveyor and receiver of information, particularly for communications that occur frequently. For the communicator, this method provides a framework to deliver information in a logical flow, and which reduces omissions by acting as a checklist of the important topics to cover. For the receiver of information, structured communication increases predictabiity and allows one to anticipate where in a narrative specific pieces of information will be delivered. This helps eliminate internal distractions and as information is processed, they listener will know what to expect and when, thus increasing the likelihood of accurate transfer of information.

Several examples of structured communication have demonstrated improved information transfer between providers during patient handoffs or discussions.[15-17] While these different methods have not been compared it is likely that the most important intervention to improve handoff communication is providing a consistent method, specifically tailored to and agreed-upon by the unit for conducting all handoffs.[15,18] Furthermore, education on handoff techniques have been associated with improved patient outcomes.[19,20]

Distractions and fatigue are common but significant barrier to communication among medical teams.[21] Fatigue will typically increase the number of omissions by the provider delivering information, and decrease both the attention and retention on the part of the information receiver. Distractions and interruptions can have the same effect by disrupting the flow of information or diverting the attention of the listener.[21] Foremost, team members must be responsible to ensure that they arrive on duty well rested and ready for work. Similarly, attention should be paid to providers' schedules to optimize the balance between shift length, time away from work, and minimizing the number of patient handoffs. Structured communication can assist both the provider delivering information, by decreasing omissions, and the receiver of information, through a standard approach of information delivery. Also, the concept of a "sterile cockpit," borrowed from the aviation industry[22] can help decrease interruptions and distractions.[23-25] Using this model, there is an understanding among the entire medical team that no interruptions will transpire during times of critical communication, including handoffs, except for emergencies. It is important to develop triggers for what defines an emergency requiring a break of the sterile cockpit.

In this case scenario, a script or checklist for the neurosurgeon and the anesthesiologist to follow during their handoff would have helped ensure that all important data were transferred, even though the handoff providers were fatigued (and likely not thinking clearly) or distracted (by the need to rush for the next emergency case). Fortunately, data support that scripts such as these improve data transfer without significantly increasing sign out time.[26,27]

Anticipatory guidance is another important, but commonly omitted, element of patient handoff. In addition to the transfer of known patient data, anticipatory guidance affords for the provider who knows the patient best to give their subjective view of the patient's anticipated trajectory status.[28] Including the handoff provider's sense of what the patient will do over the next shift not only allows the receiving provider to anticipate potential events, but also helps to provide a context for the patient's level of illness that may not have been conveyed by patient data alone. This guidance can be particularly helpful if there is a transition of care between providers of different specialties or disciplines. A surgeon handing a patient off to a medical team can provide key suggestions for continued post-operative care. Similarly, a physician may be able to provide a nurse a greater context of the patient's illness or expected course, just as a nurse may be able to provide details to a physician which may significantly affect the plan of care.

Any communication exchange should conclude with an opportunity for questions by the receiving provider. This allows for time to clarify any unclear data or inaccuracies, as well as revisiting any omissions that may have occurred. The chance to ask questions ensures that communication is not unidirectional (ie, one-sided). If the provider handing off the patient will be continuing in the patient's care, it is also important to have contact information for future questions or updates.

In this case scenario, no anticipatory guidance is given regarding the extubation plan. Had Ben not remained sedated, his neurologic examination may have given clues to the repeated bleed prior to the physiological signs of impending brainstem herniation. Similarly, had there been a clear plan to leave Ben sedated, the ICU team and neurosurgical team could have jointly developed a plan to better monitor his neurological status or intracranial pressure.

The hierarchy inherent in a teaching hospital may also contribute to a delay in care in this case scenario, when repeated attempts are made to reach the neurosurgery resident prior to contacting the supervising neurosurgeon. While there are data that support the safety of trainees making autonomous decisions,[29-31] there also needs to be a mechanism to quickly notify the attending physician when the trainee may be making poor decisions, does not respond in a reasonable time, or when decision time is critical. Similar to the prior case scenario, a pre-determined trigger phrase could be used by the charge nurse to clearly express her concern and stress the need to include the attending physician in clinical decision making. However, bypassing trainees should be used sparingly, as excluding any team member from clinical decision making can not only belittle that trainee's role to the team, but can lead to duplicate and/or conflicting efforts.

Learning Points

- The goal of any information exchange should be a shared mental model between the participating providers and/or team members.
- Structured communication during patient handoffs supports consistent and complete delivery of patient data. This structure also helps providers cope with fatigue and distractions.

- Anticipatory guidance during handoffs provides context beyond basic patient information.
- Patient handoffs should be a two-way conversation, and always conclude with a chance for the receiving provider to ask questions.

CASE SCENARIO #4

Setting: Pediatric Intensive Care Unit, Daily Rounds

The next morning on rounds, the same PICU resident summarizes the night's events for the PICU team. Fortunately, Ben has done well following the second surgery. The clot was removed, and there was markedly less oozing after a mild coagulopathy was corrected with fresh frozen plasma. Ben returned to the PICU intubated, but with an intracranial pressure monitor in place. At this point in rounds, Ben's mother volunteers that Ben had also had a lot of bleeding after a tonsillectomy about 1 year ago, and the team decides to initiate an evaluation for clotting disorders.

There is also discussion about the right time to extubate Ben, given his multiple surgeries and potential neurological insult from the subarachnoid bleed. The PICU attending uses this opportunity to teach about evaluation for extubation readiness and the importance of neurologic monitoring, during which time the nurse steps away to get some medicine from the medication room. The final decision is made to turn off the sedation infusions, with the plan to extubate as soon as he wakes.

Unfortunately, the nurse does not see the order to turn off sedation infusions, and therefore Ben remains sedated until the late afternoon, when the respiratory therapist remarks that Ben is not waking up as expected. At this point, the PICU team realizes the miscommunication, turns off the sedation infusions, and several hours later, is able to extubate Ben.

DISCUSSION

Daily inpatient rounds are a key time for optimizing communication. Rounds are unique in that they are often the only time of the day that providers of different disciplines and levels of training are gathered together to discuss patients. This collaboration allows the opportunity for physicians, nurses, pharmacists, and other ancillary staff to discuss all the many aspects of the current clinical scenario. Almost universally, providers are aware of different aspects of each patient's current status. Patients, parents, and family members will often share details with nurses that they will not mention to physicians, nurses typically can provide the most accurate update of the patient's minute-to-minute status, and physicians may be aware of different test results and consultant recommendations that will drive the global plan of care. Similarly, trainees may be up-to-date on the details of a patient's status, while supervising physicians may have the best understanding of the overall disease process and trajectory. As such, it is essential to include input from all providers to fully understand the patient's individual clinical picture. Finally, in the era of duty-hour reform, daily rounds are increasingly being used as a vehicle to handoff patients from the nighttime to the daytime staff, and many of the principles discussed previously with handoffs can be applied to the rounding process.

Healthcare providers from different disciplines often not only have varying priorities in their care delivery,[32] but may be trained to use different terminology and scripts. While physicians will often think of a patient in terms of a list of systems or medical problems, a nurse may describe the same patient through a narrative of their disease progression. Even within the same discipline, providers of different specialties (ie, general pediatricians, intensivists, surgeons, etc.) will encounter the same barriers. Functionally, this may result in team members speaking to each other in what seems like a foreign language, or at the very least, an alternate clinical dialect. Once trainees of different experience and skill levels are added, this communication barrier is only compounded. When conducted in a multidisciplinary fashion, daily rounds provide an opportunity for different providers to meet, discuss the patient, and develop a comprehensive plan of care.

Several studies have demonstrated improved communication using structured communication and multidisciplinary input on rounds, often focusing on daily goals and using communication facilitators such as checklists.[24,33-39] Direct improvements in patient care were noted in some of these studies, including reductions in severity adjusted mortality, length of stay, medication errors, and nosocomial infection rates. The authors of each of these studies have acknowledged the important role of teamwork in the successful implementation of their structured communication process.

The outcome of daily rounds, the formation of the day's medical plan, also speaks to the importance of this activity. Utilization of all the different providers present on rounds can be key to developing a comprehensive plan of care. Similarly, ensuring psychological safety, where each provider feels empowered to speak up regarding concerns, helps identify pitfalls in a given plan and can assist with early recognition of the patient who is at greatest risk for decompensation. Including families and patients on rounds may also provide important details, and often provides the family a much better understanding of the patient's current status and plan.[40-43] At the conclusion of rounds, the goal should be for all providers, the family, and the patient to have a shared understanding of the plan of care. If the entire medical team is "on the same page," the resulting coordinated effort will minimize redundancies and optimize the team performance, ultimately ensuring the best possible care.[42,44]

In this case scenario, prolonged discussion, time for bedside education, and team disassociation (the nurse leaving the bedside) all contribute to a breakdown in shared agreement of the patient care plan. Prolonged group discussion of a complex plan may be necessary for some patients, and bedside teaching is an important aspect of education in teaching hospitals. Similarly, in the ongoing busy medical setting, there are times when a provider must step away from rounds (or other group discussions). However, it is important to conclude all discussions with a brief, clear summary of the plan, and to make sure all providers are aware of this plan, with the chance to ask questions. The sterile cockpit concept can be utilized for rounds to minimize distractions and interruptions.[25]

Another method to optimize a shared mental model among providers is the use of huddles. At the conclusion of daily rounds on all patients, a brief huddle between all essential providers can be used to "run the list," quickly reviewing the main goals for each patient and identifying priority tasks. This is particularly helpful to review any updates on patient status that may have come up during the rounding process, and can assist with efficiency of workflow and patient bed flow.[6,45]

Learning Points

- Gatherings of the multidisciplinary team (such as on inpatient daily rounds) are key times to optimize communication.
- Communication facilitators, such as checklists, can assist with shared agreement among providers, and can improve patient outcomes.
- Family and patient centered rounds improve information transfer and increase both safety and satisfaction with care.
- The final plan should be restated or summarized after any prolonged discussion, with all team members present. Multidisciplinary huddles are one method to quickly ensure agreement among providers.

| CASE SCENARIO #5

Setting: Pediatric Intensive Care Unit, the Next Day

During her patient presentation on rounds the next day, the PICU resident summarizes Ben's current medications, including levetiracetam for seizure prophylaxis, given the subarachnoid hemorrhage. The relatively new bedside nurse knows that levetiracetam is not ordered for Ben, but thinks this is likely a minor omission, and does not feel it is her place to speak up and correct the physician.

That afternoon, Ben is noted by his bedside nurse to have some eye fluttering, which quickly advances to a generalized tonic-clonic seizure. The PICU team is called to the bedside, and orders medicines to control the seizure. When Ben continues to seize after two doses of lorazepam, the resident orders an intravenous fosphenytoin load.

As Ben's primary nurse is busy ensuring that Ben maintains his airway, a nurse from the next bedspace prepares the fosphenytoin and starts infusing it through Ben's one available intravenous line (IV). Unfortunately, this assisting nurse does not realize that dexamethasone (prescribed for some mild post-extubation stridor) has also been infusing through that line, and the incompatible medicines quickly crystallize, causing the IV to infiltrate the vein.

Fortunately, Ben's seizure resolves after a dose of intramuscular lorazepam that is given while the PICU team is trying to reestablish IV access. Ben is then started on levetiracetam as initially planned, and has an unremarkable remainder of his PICU course without further seizures or hemorrhage. He does, however, require wound management for the IV infiltrates from the crystallized fosphenytoin.

DISCUSSION

Once again, Ben suffers because of a miscommunication during rounds. Hierarchy may play a role in the bedside nurses' unwillingness to speak up regarding the reported levetiracetam order. While fear may not be the primary reason for this nurse not speaking up, she still does not see herself as a critical member of the team. Staff should be encouraged and empowered to provide correct, accurate information, as well as their professional opinion. As is demonstrated here, medical decisions made on incorrect data can have significant consequences for the patient.

High-functioning teams develop a culture that allows for mutual support among team members.[46] At any given time, a team member may be unable to complete one of their usual tasks; this could be due to a busy clinical scenario, or due to circumstances unrelated to the clinical environment, such as a team member's personal illness. Whatever the circumstances, the healthcare team will only be able to complete the task at hand if another team member can step forward to provide assistance where needed. Ideally, trust will exist among team members that will allow a provider to freely ask for help whenever needed. However, strong situational awareness by the team will allow for realization of the task that needs to be done before a provider has to ask for help.

In this case scenario, the bedside nurse was busy ensuring her patient could maintain a clear airway, yet the child also needed an intravenous antiepileptic. The quick recognition of this need, and the willingness to join in and deliver the medicine, shows good teamwork, and mutual assistance. However, a communication failure still leads to a poor outcome when the IV medications precipitate, delaying the medicine administration and causing an infiltrate. This "helper syndrome" can easily occur when a team member steps in to help with a task, but isn't aware of the whole clinical situation (in this case, that dexamethasone was running through the IV). Similar mistakes can occur with other assumptions, such as picking up a syringe prepared by someone else and giving the wrong vaccine, sending the wrong paperwork with blood product ordering, or incorrectly documenting history on the wrong patient's chart.

Having team members assist each other is necessary to ensure timely delivery of care, and if providers are aware of the inherent communication errors that may arise during such assistance, then they can take measures to minimize this risk. Closed-loop communication will allow the initial provider to give continuous feedback to the team member. In this scenario, if the assisting provider had clearly stated his planned action (ie, "I am going to give fosphenytoin through the IV in the right hand"), it would have provided a chance for the primary bedside nurse to recognize the potential issue of drug compatibility, and raise an alert to the helper.

Learning Points

- Multidisciplinary input should be encouraged to develop a complete and robust plan of care.
- Mutual assistance is an important strength of high-functioning teams, but adequate communication must occur to avoid errors by the assisting provider.

CASE SCENARIO #6

Setting: Pediatrician's Office

After several days, Ben has returned to his baseline neurological status, and is doing well enough to be discharged from the hospital. Clinic appointments are made for follow-up with Ben's pediatrician and the neurosurgeon. Ben is discharged on levetiracetam for seizure prophylaxis and oxycodone as needed for a residual headache.

On follow-up with his pediatrician the next day, Ben is again noted to be unusually sleepy, even though his mother reports that he was completely normal until she had given him some oxycodone for a headache before leaving the house. The ambulance is once again called. Unfortunately, the pediatrician has not received any information about Ben's hospital stay, but after some investigation while the ambulance is en route, she discovers that Ben's mother has given Ben 1 teaspoon of oxycodone, instead of the prescribed 1 milliliter (a five-fold dose error). After a few hours in the ED and a dose of naloxone to reverse the opiate, Ben recovers from his medication overdose, and is discharged home.

Two weeks later, Ben's pediatrician receives the discharge summary faxed from the hospital. She follows up on the outstanding laboratory values detailed in the discharge summary, and finds an abnormal von Willibrand's factor level, placing him at risk for bleeding. She passes this information on to the family, counsels them on its meaning and long-term implications, and notes it in his permanent record.

DISCUSSION

As discussed previously, handoffs between providers, particularly when they involve a change of environment, are a high-risk time for communication errors. The transition to home is no exception. While the patient is typically close to their baseline state of health upon discharge, it remains important for the patient, the family, and the patient's medical home provider to receive information about what transpired during the hospitalization, and how it may affect future health status and medical care.[28,47] This transition can be more challenging when patients have not reached their previous state of health upon discharge from the hospital, and families and patients must learn new care-taker responsibilities, often in the face of psychosocial stressors and potentially grieving for the loss of prior health.

In this case scenario, Ben's mother is assuming care from the medical team, with guidance from his pediatrician. As a bridge to care at home, parents must be given all of their child's necessary medical information and taught to care for any new medical needs. While Ben is not a medically complex child, there is a simple miscommunication regarding his medication dosing causing the potential for serious harm. One of the best methods to ensure understanding by parents or patients is the teach-back technique. After an education session, having the family or patient "teach back" what they have learned is an effective method to gauge the information that they have received and understood.[48,49] This not only ensures that the learner (family) has received the important information, but it also highlights the knowledge deficits to be targeted for reeducation or reinforcement. In the case of teaching a skill, having the family or patient demonstrate this skill is the best way to measure receptive learning. In Ben's case, had his mother demonstrated to a nurse or pharmacist how she would deliver his oxycodone, her error likely would have been caught before leaving the hospital. Some centers are also using pharmacists to help with medicine reconciliation at admission and discharge,[50] to assure clear communication regarding medication dosing.

While Ben's parents must assume his daily care upon discharge from the hospital, his pediatrician must also be given the proper handoff to resume her role as his primary care physician. The transition to the home environment and the primary care provider has become more challenging as an increasing number of children are cared for by hospitalists and specialists while in the hospital, and fewer pediatricians and family medicine physicians are routinely rounding on their patients in the hospital. Unfortunately, most primary care providers do not receive discharge summaries or direct communication regarding a hospitalization prior to the first follow-up visit after hospitalization.[47,51,52] Use of computer-generated discharge summaries and providing families with copies of the discharge summaries are methods which have increased information transfer to primary care physicians.[47] However, institutions must be aware of potential deficiencies in handoffs from inpatient to outpatient physicians, and should develop strategies to optimize handoff delivery as care is transitioned. Verbal handoffs (ie, direct phone calls to primary care physicians) followed by written documentation should be considered for particularly complex patients.

Learning Points

- Information is commonly lost in the transition from inpatient to outpatient settings. Institutions should develop strategies to address safe handoff to primary care physicians.
- Parents and caregivers are integral for the care of children, and must be included in transfer of care.
- The "teach back" method is an effective way to assess the knowledge gained by the patient and family.

ACHIEVING HIGH-FUNCTIONING TEAMS

When things are at their best, any team can be greater than the sum of its individual parts. This is of particular importance in the healthcare environment, where no provider works alone to care for patients. Pediatric patients present unique challenges, given distinctive disease processes, evolution of developmental and physiologic stages, their inability to effectively communicate disease symptoms and concerns, and the unique role of parents and family. As such, it is particularly important to advocate for the safe and effective care of this fragile population.

High-functioning healthcare teams also share a few key characteristics. These teams are adaptable and maintain their performance despite changing circumstances and team composition. This quality is achieved through a shared vision of care, mutual trust among team members, a collective situational awareness, and constant improvement. A focus on patient safety must also be in the forefront, often as a reflection of a culture of safety in the larger organization. Teams share a common vision of care, know their individual roles, communicate clearly, and trust each other. Safety, quality, and efficient care are provided when teamwork is optimized.[53]

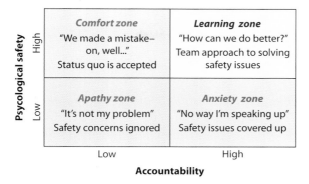

Figure 6-1 ▪ Learning from errors: matching high psychological safety with high accountability. (Data from Edmonson AC. The competitive imperative of learning. HBS Centennial Issue. *Harvard Business Review*. 86(nos. 7/8), 2008.)

Another key feature of high-functioning teams is the ability and commitment to learn from prior errors. This is accomplished not only by monitoring for errors, but also through the development of psychological safety and accountability. Figure 6-1 demonstrates how lack of psychological safety among team members and low accountability can each lead to teams repeatedly making the same mistakes. Only when team members take ownership of patient care and proactively discuss errors in a safe and productive forum, can teams develop strategies to prevent recurrent errors.

Individuals working together as teams wishing to improve their team performance must integrate teamwork principles and techniques into daily practice. Team STEPPS curriculum offers an evidence-based framework to optimize interdisciplinary teamwork and reduce patient harm. The framework for Team STEPPS offers specific leadership and staff actions and leverages identified knowledge, skills, and attitudes (KSAs) among all patient-care team members (Figure 6-2). Fostering the KSAs is critical and can be most challenging as it takes time to develop and incorporate them into the "DNA" of the team and the organization. Though challenging, once the KSAs are part of the culture, teams and organizations can expect decreased patient harm, increased adherence to best practices, increased information transfer accuracy, "glitch" capture and correction, increased patient and staff satisfaction, and improved equipment and staff utilization efficiencies. Strong leadership and accountability, the development of common goals, and fostering mutual support and trust among team members instills a shared vision and promotes team unity.[54]

In the case story presented in this chapter, our patient's disease and hospital course of treatment are marred by commonly occurring medical errors

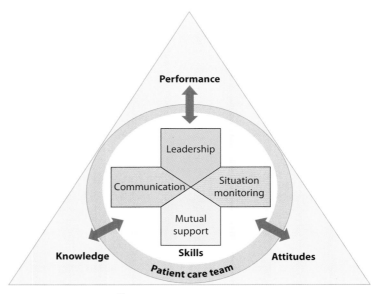

Figure 6-2 ▪ *TeamSTEPPS*™ framework of knowledge, skills, and attitudes to optimize team performance. (Adapted from TeamSTEPPS: Strategies and Tool to Enhance Performance and Patient Safety. Accessed July 7, 2013 at http://teamstepps.ahrq.gov/abouttoolsmaterials.htm)

that are attributable to breakdowns in communication and teamwork. While Ben will make a full recovery, each of the seemingly minor errors detailed during his course of treatment has the potential to contribute to significant harm, and most importantly, is preventable. Just as is done with other areas of patient safety, it is imperative on healthcare providers and health systems to monitor teamwork breakdowns and formulate processes to minimize future errors. Several safety inventories are available to monitor global team culture and target areas for improvement.[7,55-61]

Given the many barriers to teamwork and communication, it may be surprising that more medical errors are not caused by miscommunication. Undoubtedly, there are daily errors that are missed and many that cause no patient harm. However, it is a testament to the dedication and vigilance of bedside providers that miscommunication does not cause more patient harm. Multiple techniques exist to assist with accurate, timely, and complete information transfer, such as Team STEPPS and the I—PASS resident handoff bundle.[62,63]

Individuals recognized as effective communicators have often been taught some of these techniques, or in many cases, discovered them independently. Our challenge lies in ensuring these team techniques are taught, practiced, and sustained by all members of healthcare teams.

IN PRACTICE

To achieve a shared mental model among team members:

- Utilize structured communication methods to assist with critical information transfer.
- Empower all providers to actively participate in formation of the plan of care.
- Assess understanding by focusing on the receiver of information.

To optimize team efforts:

- Promote situational awareness through briefings and huddles.
- Emphasize role clarity and a clear team leader for any given task.
- Establish a culture of mutual assistance and trust among team members.
- Develop a culture of continuous feedback including closed-loop communication and debriefings.

To establish a culture of safety:

- Maintain primary focus on the patient.
- Eliminate hierarchy that limits communication among team members and provide a process for providers to raise concerns.
- Endorse that patient safety is everyone's responsibility.

FAQs

1. What are the best strategies to reach a shared mental model of care?

    Optimize opportunities to gather the team, however briefly, to achieve situational awareness and planning for the next set of tasks. Planned huddles and briefings can accomplish much of this task in less than 60 seconds. Any significant discussion should be concluded with a clear statement of the final plan. Repetition of key points or call-back by providers may be necessary, but the brief moments taken to ensure team agreement are easily accounted for by the gains in team efficiency and safety.

2. How can we increase team members' comfort in speaking up?

    Active communication during tasks is a good indicator of teamwork, open communication, and culture of safety. Team members should not only be encouraged to speak up, but it should be made clear that speaking up with safety concerns is an expectation of all team members. Furthermore, times of structured communication (eg, time-outs, huddles, debriefings, patient handoffs, daily rounds) should be designed to allow input from all providers.

3. What strategies can be used for team members who refuse to be "team players," or who demonstrate disruptive behaviors?

While the desire to provide optimal care is generally present among all healthcare providers, some individuals either lack communication skills or believe that they can behave outside of accepted norms. Many of the strategies discussed in this chapter (structured communication, trigger words, read-backs) may be used to assist with communication for those who have difficulty conveying their message. Furthermore, it is important to educate the entire team of the importance of psychological safety and to provide clear feedback to those team members acting outside of the accepted norms for that team. There should be no tolerance of continued disruptive behaviors. This is an expectation that should be made early (ideally during the hiring process). Furthermore, it is important that accountability is the same for providers of different roles; ie, behavior that would result in the firing of a nurse should not be tolerated from a physician. In the case that disruptive behaviors persist, it is important to realize that providers' technical skill sets can almost always be found elsewhere.

4. What are the most critical elements for communication breakdown?

We can identify a few key elements that place teams at risk for communication errors: patient handoffs, distractions, fatigue, working outside of established norms, multitasking during extremely stressful circumstances, and a lack of psychological safety.

SUMMARY OF LEARNING POINTS FROM CASE STUDIES

Case Study	Learning Points
1. Pediatrician's office	• Interdisciplinary communication may be hindered by interruptions, different priorities, and tasks. Developing triggers for implementation of huddles can help maintain situational awareness among the team. • Any deviation to expected workflow adds risk for errors and omissions. • All healthcare settings can benefit from a clear plan to identify and address those patients who may need immediate attention.

(Continued)

SUMMARY OF LEARNING POINTS FROM CASE STUDIES *(Continued)*	
Case Study	Learning Points
2. Emergency department	• Role clarity streamlines a team's efforts and minimizes conflict. • Use of time-outs prior to procedures can help clarify the plan for all team members and ensure a coordinated effort in patient care. • Pre-defined trigger words empower any team member to speak up at any time if he or she identifies an unsafe behavior or condition. • Closed-loop communication enables immediate feedback about what the receiver received from an information exchange. • Debriefings as soon as possible after an event provides important feedback to the team and identifies opportunities for improvement.
3. Pediatric intensive care unit; patient handoff from operating room	• Role clarity streamlines a team's efforts and minimizes conflict. • Use of time-outs prior to procedures can help clarify the plan for all team members and ensure a coordinated effort in patient care. • Pre-defined trigger words empower any team member to speak up at any time if he or she identifies an unsafe behavior or condition. • Closed-loop communication enables immediate feedback about what the receiver received from an information exchange. • Debriefings as soon as possible after an event provides important feedback to the team and identifies opportunities for improvement.
4. Pediatric intensive care: daily rounds	• Gatherings of the multidisciplinary team (such as on inpatient daily rounds) are key times to optimize communication. • Communication facilitators, such as checklists, can assist with shared agreement among providers, and can improve patient outcomes. • Family and patient centered rounds improve information transfer and increase both safety and satisfaction with care. • The final plan should be restated or summarized after any prolonged discussion, with all team members present. Multidisciplinary huddles are one method to quickly ensure agreement among providers.
5. Pediatric intensive care unit, the next day	• Multidisciplinary input should be encouraged to develop a complete and robust plan of care. • Mutual assistance is an important strength of high-functioning teams, but adequate communication must occur to avoid errors by the assisting provider.
6. Pediatrician's office	• Information is commonly lost in the transition from inpatient to outpatient settings. Institutions should develop strategies to address safe handoff to primary care physicians. • Parents and caregivers are integral for the care of children, and must be included in transfer of care. • The "teach back" method is an effective way to assess the knowledge gained by the patient and family.

(All opinions expressed in this paper are those of the authors and do not necessarily reflect the official opinion or position of the Department of Defense.)

▎REFERENCES

1. The Joint Commission National Patient Safety Goals. Available at: http://www.jointcommission.org/PatientSafety/NationalPatientSafetyGoals/.
2. Special report on sentinel events. Joint commission on accreditation of healthcare organizations. *Jt Comm Perspect.* 1998;18(6):19-33, 36-42.
3. Leape LL, Berwick DM. Five years after to err is Human: what have we learned? *JAMA.* 2005;293(19):2384-2390.
4. Bagnasco A, Tubino B, Piccotti E, et al. Identifying and correcting communication failures among health professionals working in the emergency department. *Int Emerg Nurs.* 2012;21(3):168-172. doi: 10.1016/j.ienj.2012.07.005.
5. Bleakley A, Allard J, Hobbs A. 'Achieving ensemble': communication in orthopaedic surgical teams and the development of situation awareness—an observational study using live videotaped examples. *Adv Health Sci Educ Theory Pract.* 2013;18(1):33-56.
6. Brady PW, Muething S, Kotagal U, et al. Improving situation awareness to reduce unrecognized clinical deterioration and serious safety events. *Pediatrics.* 2013;131(1):e298-e308.
7. Sexton JB, Helmreich RL, Neilands TB, et al. The safety attitudes questionnaire: psychometric properties, benchmarking data, and emerging research. *BMC Health Serv Res.* 2006;6:44.
8. Blike GT, Christoffersen K, Cravero JP, Andeweg SK, Jensen J. A method for measuring system safety and latent errors associated with pediatric procedural sedation. *Anesth Analg.* 2005;101(1):48-58.
9. Braaf S, Manias E, Riley R. The 'time-out' procedure: an institutional ethnography of how it is conducted in actual clinical practice. *BMJ Qual Saf.* 2013;doi:10.1136/bmjqs-2012-001702.
10. TeamSTEPPS™. Stratagies and tool to enhance performance and patient safety. Available at: http://teamstepps.ahrq.gov/abouttoolsmaterials.htm. Accessed July 7, 2013.
11. Makary MA, Holzmueller CG, Sexton JB, et al. Operating room debriefings. *Jt Comm J Qual Patient Saf.* 2006;32(7):407-410, 357.
12. Johnson HL, Kimsey D. Patient safety: break the silence. *AORN J.* 2012;95(5):591-601.
13. Siemsen IM, Madsen MD, Pedersen LF, et al. Factors that impact on the safety of patient handovers: an interview study. *Scand J Publ Health.* 2012;40(5):439-448.
14. DeFrances CJ, Hall MJ. 2005 National hospital discharge survey. *Adv Data.* 2007;(385):1-19.
15. DeRienzo CM, Frush K, Barfield ME, et al. Handoffs in the era of duty hours reform: a focused review and strategy to address changes in the Accreditation Council for Graduate Medical Education Common Program Requirements. *Acad Med.* 2012;87(4):403-410.
16. Koenig CJ, Maguen S, Daley A, et al. Passing the baton: a grounded practical theory of handoff communication between multidisciplinary providers in two Department of Veterans Affairs outpatient settings. *J Gen Intern Med.* 2013,28(1):41-50.

17. Petrovic MA, Martinez EA, Aboumatar H. Implementing a perioperative hand-off tool to improve postprocedural patient transfers. *Jt Comm J Qual Patient Saf.* 2012;38(3):135-142.

18. Solet DJ, Norvell JM, Rutan GH, Frankel RM. Lost in translation: challenges and opportunities in physician-to-physician communication during patient handoffs. *Acad Med.* 2005;80(12):1094-1099.

19. Mueller SK, Call SA, McDonald FS, et al. Impact of resident workload and handoff training on patient outcomes. *Am J Med.* 2012;125(1):104-110.

20. Pesanka DA, Greenhouse PK, Rack LL, et al. Ticket to ride: reducing handoff risk during hospital patient transport. *J Nurs Care Qual.* 2009;24(2):109-115.

21. Aggarwal R, Undre S, Moorthy K, et al. The simulated operating theatre: comprehensive training for surgical teams. *Qual Saf Health Care.* 2004,13(Suppl 1):i27-i32.

22. Federal Aviation Administration. The sterile cockpit rule; FAR 14CFR121.542. In: United States Government Printing Office; 1981.

23. Kreckler S, Catchpole K, Bottomley M, et al. Interruptions during drug rounds: an observational study. *Br J Nurs.* 2008;17(21):1326-1330.

24. Rehder KJ, Uhl TL, Meliones JN, et al. Targeted interventions improve shared agreement of daily goals in the pediatric intensive care unit. *Pediatr Crit Care Med.* 2012;13(1):6-10.

25. Baron R. The cockpit, the cabin, and social psychology. Available at: http://www.airlinesafety.com/editorials/CockpitCabinPsychology.htm.

26. Petrovic MA, Aboumatar H, Baumgartner WA, et al. Pilot implementation of a perioperative protocol to guide operating room-to-intensive care unit patient handoffs. *J Cardiothor Vasc Anesth.* 2012;26(1):11-16.

27. Catchpole KR, de Leval MR, McEwan A, et al. Patient handover from surgery to intensive care: using Formula 1 pit-stop and aviation models to improve safety and quality. *Paediatr Anaesth.* 2007;17(5):470-478.

28. Toccafondi G, Albolino S, Tartaglia R, et al. The collaborative communication model for patient handover at the interface between high-acuity and low-acuity care. *BMJ Qual Saf.* 2012;21(Suppl 1):i58-i66.

29. Claridge JA, Schulman AM, Sawyer RG, et al. The "July phenomenon" and the care of the severely injured patient: fact or fiction? *Surgery.* 2001;130(2):346-353.

30. Numa A, Williams G, Awad J, Duffy B. After-hours admissions are not associated with increased risk-adjusted mortality in pediatric intensive care. *Intens Care Med.* 2008;34(1):148-151.

31. Reriani M, Biehl M, Sloan JA, et al. Effect of 24-hour mandatory vs on-demand critical care specialist presence on long-term survival and quality of life of critically ill patients in the intensive care unit of a teaching hospital. *J Crit Care.* 2011;27(4):421.e1-e7. doi: 10.1016/j.jcrc.2011.10.001.

32. Quan SD, Morra D, Lau FY, et al. Perceptions of urgency: Defining the gap between what physicians and nurses perceive to be an urgent issue. *Int J Med Inform.* 2013;82(5): 378-386.

33. Jain M, Miller L, Belt D, et al. Decline in ICU adverse events, nosocomial infections and cost through a quality improvement initiative focusing on teamwork and culture change. *Qual Saf Health Care.* 2006;15(4):235-239.

34. Leape LL, Cullen DJ, Clapp MD, et al. Pharmacist participation on physician rounds and adverse drug events in the intensive care unit. *JAMA*. 1999;282(3):267-270.

35. Narasimhan M, Eisen LA, Mahoney CD, et al. Improving nurse-physician communication and satisfaction in the intensive care unit with a daily goals worksheet. *Am J Crit Care*. 2006;15(2):217-222.

36. Pronovost P, Berenholtz S, Dorman T, et al. Improving communication in the ICU using daily goals. *J Crit Care*. 2003;18(2):71-75.

37. Weiss CH, Moazed F, McEvoy CA, et al. Prompting physicians to address a daily checklist and process of care and clinical outcomes: a single-site study. *Am J Respir Crit Care Med*. 2011;184(6):680-686.

38. DuBose JJ, Inaba K, Shiflett A, et al. Measurable outcomes of quality improvement in the trauma intensive care unit: the impact of a daily quality rounding checklist. *J Trauma*. 2008;64(1):22-27; discussion 27-29.

39. Agarwal S, Frankel L, Tourner S, et al. Improving communication in a pediatric intensive care unit using daily patient goal sheets. *J Crit Care*. 2008;23(2):227-235.

40. Kuo DZ, Sisterhen LL, Sigrest TE, et al. Family experiences and pediatric health services use associated with family-centered rounds. *Pediatrics*. 2012;130(2):299-305.

41. Muething SE, Kotagal UR, Schoettker PJ, et al. Family-centered bedside rounds: a new approach to patient care and teaching. *Pediatrics*. 2007,119(4):829-832.

42. Rosen P, Stenger E, Bochkoris M, et al. Family-centered multidisciplinary rounds enhance the team approach in pediatrics. *Pediatrics*. 2009;123(4):e603-e608.

43. Wu AW, Sexton JB, Pronovost PJ. Partnership with patients: a prescription for ICU safety. *Chest*. 2006;130(5):1291-1293.

44. Avansino JR, Peters LM, Stockfish SL, Walco GA. A paradigm shift to balance safety and quality in pediatric pain management. *Pediatrics*. 2013;131(3):e921-e927.

45. Turner P. Implementation of TeamSTEPPS in the emergency department. *Crit Care N Quart*. 2012;35(3):208-212.

46. Brock D, Abu-Rish E, Chiu CR, et al. Interprofessional education in team communication: working together to improve patient safety. *BMJ Qual Saf*. 2013;22(5):414-423.

47. Kripalani S, LeFevre F, Phillips CO, et al. Deficits in communication and information transfer between hospital-based and primary care physicians: implications for patient safety and continuity of care. *JAMA*. 2007;297(8):831-841.

48. Howard T, Jacobson KL, Kripalani S. Doctor talk: physicians' use of clear verbal communication. *J Health Commun*. 2013;18(8):991-1001.

49. Kornburger C, Gibson C, Sadowski S, et al. Using "teach-back" to promote a safe transition from hospital to home: an evidence-based approach to improving the discharge process. *J Pediatr Nurs*. 2013;28(3):282-291.

50. Hume AL, Kirwin J, Bieber HL, et al. Improving care transitions: current practice and future opportunities for pharmacists. *Pharmacotherapy*. 2012;32(11):e326-e337.

51. van Walraven C, Seth R, Austin PC, Laupacis A. Effect of discharge summary availability during post-discharge visits on hospital readmission. *J Gen Intern Med*. 2002;17(3):186-192.

52. van Walraven C, Seth R, Laupacis A. Dissemination of discharge summaries. Not reaching follow-up physicians. *Can Fam Phys*. 2002;48:737-742.

53. Armour Forse R, Bramble JD, McQuillan R. Team training can improve operating room performance. *Surgery.* 2011;150(4):771-778.

54. King H, Battles J, Baker D, et al. Team STEPPS™: team strategies and tools to enhance performance and patient safety. *Advances in Patient Safety: New Directions and Alternative Approaches.* Volume 3: Performance and Tools. Rockville, MD: AHRQ, 2008;3.

55. Ballangrud R, Hedelin B, Hall-Lord ML. Nurses' perceptions of patient safety climate in intensive care units: a cross-sectional study. *Intens Crit Care Nurs.* 2012;28(6): 344-354.

56. Profit J, Etchegaray J, Petersen LA, et al. The Safety Attitudes Questionnaire as a tool for benchmarking safety culture in the NICU. *Arch Dis Child Fetal Neonat Ed.* 2012;97(2):F127-F132. doi: 10.1136/archdischild-2011-300612.

57. Pronovost P, Holzmueller CG, Needham DM, et al. How will we know patients are safer? An organization-wide approach to measuring and improving safety. *Crit Care Med.* 2006;34(7):1988-1995.

58. Pronovost PJ, Sexton JB, Pham JC, et al. Measurement of quality and assurance of safety in the critically ill. *Clin Chest Med.* 2009;30(1):169-179, x.

59. Sexton JB, Paine LA, Manfuso J, et al. A check-up for safety culture in "my patient care area". *Jt Comm J Qual Patient Saf.* 2007;33(11):699-703, 645.

60. Baker DP, Amodeo AM, Krokos KJ, et al. Assessing teamwork attitudes in healthcare: development of the TeamSTEPPS teamwork attitudes questionnaire. *Qual Saf Health Care.* 2010;19(6):e49.

61. TeamSTEPPS Teamwork Perceptions Questionaire (T-TPQ) Manual. Contract HHSA2902006000193 Task Order #3 2010, 1-17. Available at: http://teamstepps.ahrq. gov/Teamwork_Perception_Questionnaire.pdf as of 07.07.2013.

62. Starmer A, Spector N, Srivastava R, et al. I-pass: a mnemonic to standardize verbal handoffs. *Pediatrics.* 2012;129(2);201-204.

63. Spector N, Starner A, Allen A, et al. I-PASS Handoff Curriculum: Core Resident Workshop. MedEdPORTAL 2013. Available at: www.mededportal.org/publication/9311. Accessed July 7, 2013.

THE IMPORTANCE OF INFORMATION TECHNOLOGY IN PEDIATRIC PATIENT SAFETY

7

INTRODUCTION

Information technology is currently evolving at a rapid pace and its application in healthcare is no exception. Health information technology (HIT) has the potential for revolutionizing patient safety and improving healthcare quality. A series of Institute of Medicine (IOM) reports helped catalyze the view that HIT has the potential for improving patient safety and quality. The 1999 IOM Report "To err is human: building a safer health system" brought to the forefront the problem of medical errors and proposed HIT as a solution for reducing those errors.[1] This was further iterated by the IOM report "Crossing the quality chasm: a new health system for the 21st century" where one of the key recommendations was the application of health information technology to help redesign the healthcare system. It was recognized in this report that HIT had the potential for impacting all six aims of this report: safety, effectiveness, patient-centered, timely efficient, and equitable.[2]

HIT may have a particularly important impact in a specific area of high risk for pediatric patients: that of medication errors and adverse drug events (ADEs). Adverse drug events in pediatric patients are estimated to occur at a rate of 2.3 to 11.2 ADEs per 100 pediatric inpatients.[3-6] It is estimated that the rate of ADE in pediatric inpatients is approximately three times that in hospitalized adults.[3] Health information technologies such as computerized physician order entry and computerized clinical decision support have been proposed as an important strategy to reduce ADEs in pediatric patients.[3,7-10]

Electronic health records (EHRs) are defined as the computerized record system that contains the patient's data on their inpatient and outpatient visits. Key functionality of EHRs as defined by the Institute of Medicine are health information and data, results management, order entry/management, decision support, electronic communication and connectivity, patient support, administrative processes, and reporting and population health management.[11] Despite national calls for the adoption of EHRs, surveys of ambulatory physicians and hospitals show that 13% of ambulatory physicians have a basic EHR system and 4% have an extensive EHR system while 7.6% of hospitals have a basic EHR system and 1.5% of hospitals have a comprehensive electronic system.[12,13] In one survey of pediatric hospitals, 48.6% of respondents surveyed had an EHR system and 39% of respondents planned on implementing one within 2 years.[14] Another survey found that 10.5% of pediatricians who answered the survey had implemented an EHR.[15]

Improving patient safety and decreasing medical errors is a common driver for the implementation of HIT.[14] Multiple barriers exist for pediatric hospitals and general hospitals to implement these systems.[14,16] One large barrier is the cost to purchase EHRs. Hospital systems have spent millions to hundreds of millions of dollars on such systems, and the average cost of an EHR for an outpatient practice is estimated to be approximately $15,000 to $70,000 per provider.[17-21]

The passage of the Health Information Technology for Economic and Clinical Health (HITECH) Act as part of the 2009 American Recovery and Reinvesting Act (ARRA) provides incentives up to $25.9 billion for hospitals and outpatient practitioners to adopt HIT.[22] By providing these incentives, the government has decreased one of the significant barriers for adoption of EHRs, but there are others. Disruption in current patient flow and staff/office work flow, time requirements for training on a new IT system, and unanticipated glitches in the roll-out or use of the system are just a few examples. However, the advantages of a well-functioning HIT system are great, and the goal of HITECH is not to invest in information technology infrastructure, but to reward providers for improvement of the health of patients and their quality of care.[23] As one of the key hallmarks of HITECH, hospitals and outpatient providers must demonstrate "meaningful use" of EHRs to quality for incentives.[24]

The key components of "meaningful use" include implementation of key functionalities such as computerized physician order entry and electronic prescribing, electronic reporting of quality measures, and electronic exchange of health information.[24] These components will be discussed from the perspective of pediatric care providers, with an emphasis on the importance of HIT and its impact on pediatric patient safety.

COMPUTERIZED PHYSICIAN ORDER ENTRY

Computerized physician order entry (CPOE) or computerized provider order entry allows a provider to electronically enter orders including medication, radiology, or laboratory orders into the electronic health record, and the system transmits the orders to their respective departments. The advantages of CPOE include decreasing lost orders, eliminating ambiguities from illegible orders and transcription errors, and improving turnaround times for pharmacy, laboratory, and radiology orders.[25-27] When CPOE is integrated with clinical decision support systems, it can decrease duplicate testing or improve medication dispensing. Ambulatory CPOE, also called electronic prescribing (e-prescribing), allows for the prescribing of ambulatory prescriptions through EHR systems and electronic transmittal of the prescription to the outpatient pharmacy. The Centers for Medicare and Medicaid Services defines e-prescribing as "a prescriber's ability to electronically send an accurate, error-free, and understandable prescription directly to a pharmacy from the point-of-care."[28]

CPOE and e-prescribing are of great importance in pediatric care, as children are considered at a higher risk for medication errors than adults.[3,4,10] Ordering and prescribing medications in pediatrics are more prone to errors because there is not one standard dose as there is in adults. Medication ordering in pediatrics requires consideration of weight or body service area for each medication. A review estimated that errors are found in 5 to 27% of medication orders for children and a rate of 100 to 400 prescribing errors per 1,000 patients.[29] CPOE has been advocated as a strategy to reduce medication errors in pediatric patients.[3,7,9]

Early evidence from the Brigham and Women's Hospital showed a significant reduction in serious medication errors by 55% and preventable ADEs by 17% due to CPOE systems.[30,31] Early studies in pediatrics also suggested similar results with decreases in medication prescribing errors and ADEs after implementation of a CPOE system.[32-36] At the Children's Hospital of Pittsburgh, a study showed that CPOE decreased the number of harmful ADEs.[37] The publication of this paper, in which the authors found an associated increase in mortality after CPOE implementation in the pediatric intensive care unit at the same hospital, raised concerns that CPOE may increase mortality.[38] Further studies showed that other pediatric hospitals using the same vendor CPOE system had no increase in mortality in the pediatric intensive care unit,[39] and further, a decrease in overall mortality rate was seen after CPOE implementation in several pediatric hospitals.[40] The seemingly contradictory effects on quality and mortality of pediatric CPOE systems are discussed in more detail later in this chapter.

Multiple organizations including the American Academy of Pediatrics, the Agency for Healthcare Research and Quality, and Health Level Seven (HL7)

Table 7-1	PEDIATRIC SPECIFIC CPOE FUNCTIONALITY
Functionality	Description
Weight-based dosing	CPOE systems should calculate medication dosages by weight. Systems should allow for dosing by body service area or other calculated rates such as ideal body weight.
Weight checking	The system should determine if an entered weight is out of range for the child's age.
Weight unit conversion	The system should use only metric units or convert every weight entered as pounds into kilograms.
Dose-range checking	The system should check an ordered medication dose after it is entered to determine if it is in the recommended dose range.
Dose rounding	The system should round liquid volumes for pharmacists, nurses, or family members to easily draw up and administer these liquid medications.
Dose maximum	The system should round doses to the maximum adult dose if the weight-based calculated dose exceeds the adult dose.
Concentration to volume calculations	Pediatric medications can be available in different concentrations such as Amoxicillin 400 mg/5 mL or 250 mg/5 mL. The system should calculate the volume of a medication based on an ordered concentration and dosage.

have developed pediatric-specific functional requirements for CPOE and e-prescribing systems.[41-45] These requirements are listed in Table 7-1.

A key pediatric functionality to be considered in the design of CPOE systems is the ability to calculate medication dosages by weight or size for pediatric patients.[41] Systems should allow for calculation of medication doses by body surface area or other calculated rates such as ideal body weight. Additional weight-based functionality includes checking that the entered weight is current and that a weight entered into the system is considered within range for the age of the child. When implementing a CPOE system, consideration should be placed on minimizing errors due to entering incorrect units for weight into the system. Implementers should consider configuring the system to use only one unit, such as kilograms, or automatically converting weights entered in pound units to kilograms. Dose-range checking can then be done using pediatric references after an order or prescription is placed into the system. Many pediatric institutions have found that they have to customize commercial drug databases to accurately reflect pediatric drug dosing ranges. For example, many pediatric medications are provided in liquid formulations, and CPOE systems should allow rounding of doses to accommodate safe and easily administered volumes of medications.[46]

When implemented with pediatric functionality, CPOE has the potential to improve the safety and quality of care of pediatric patients. Because of the complexity of prescribing medications for pediatric patients, CPOE systems designed for the care of pediatric patients require considerations that systems designed solely for the care for adults may not need.

CLINICAL DECISION SUPPORT

Computerized clinical decision support (CDS) is defined as the use of a computer system to bring relevant knowledge to bear on the healthcare and well-being of a patient at the point of care.[47] The IOM report "Preventing medication errors: quality chasm series," recommends the use of HIT solutions such as CPOE linked with CDS to decrease medication errors.[48] Multiple meta-analyses and reviews of CDS have shown that CDS modestly improves medication errors and practitioner performance, but have not shown a difference in patient outcomes.[49-52] In one analysis comparing clinical and quality outcomes of EHRs with and without CDS systems, there was no association of EHRs with CDS and improved quality of care in the outpatient setting.[53]

Medication Clinical Decision Support with Computerized Physician Order Entry

CDS systems coupled with CPOE systems form the foundation of most medication safety systems in the EHR. These CDS systems can be implemented in two stages: basic and advanced. Basic decision support is defined as drug-allergy checking, basic dosing guidance, formulary decision support, duplicate therapy checking, and drug–drug interactions. Advanced decision support is defined as dosing support for renal insufficiency, guidance for medication-related laboratory testing, drug-pregnancy checking, and drug disease contra-indication checking.[54] Definitions and examples of medication-specific CDS functionality can be found in Table 7-2.

In a review of the pediatric literature on CDS for medication ordering, CDS improved some measures of ADEs and medication errors, but also resulted in a large number of overrides and showed no clear impact on patient care in other studies.[55] In pediatric inpatient,[33,37,56] neonatal and pediatric intensive care units,[57-59] and outpatient settings, multiple studies on medication CDS showed an improvement in ADEs and medication errors.

Table 7-2	MEDICATION-SPECIFIC CDS FUNCTIONALITY	
Functionality	Description	Examples
Drug-allergy checking	Verifies documented drug allergy and cross-reactive allergies with an ordered medication and medications within that class.	Alert for Penicillin allergy when Augmentin (Amoxicillin-Clavulanate) ordered; warning when Cephalosporin ordered for patient with Penicillin allergy.
Basic dosing guidance	Provides automated method to calculate doses based on recommended standard doses to guide clinicians in ordering doses.	Dosing calculator with recommended weight-based dosing; button with standard doses available.
Formulary decision support	Checks if an ordered medication is in compliance with hospital or insurance formularies and provides alternatives if nonformulary medication is ordered.	Order for Famotidine results in an alert that Famotidine is nonformulary and Ranitidine is the suggested therapeutic alternative.
Duplicate therapy checking	Ordering more than one drug in the same therapeutic class.	Warning that Morphine and Hydromorphone are ordered on the same patient.
Drug-drug interactions	Checks if an ordered drug will interact with any drugs that are ordered.	Alerts for when Coumadin and Aspirin are ordered together because it increases the bleeding risk.
Dosing support for renal insufficiency	Suggests an adjusted dose if there is evidence of renal insufficiency	Adjusts Gentamicin dosing based on renal function tests.
Guidance for medication-related laboratory testing	Suggests testing for a medication that requires laboratory testing to follow therapeutic levels of a medication and prevent them from reaching toxic or nontherapeutic levels of the medication in their system.	Vancomycin order results in suggestion of Vancomycin trough levels to be ordered as well.
Drug-pregnancy testing	Suggests a pregnancy test for any medications that could be teratogenic to a developing fetus.	Ordering a FDA category X medication such as Isotretinoin when the patient is pregnant.
Drug-disease contraindication checking	Alerts for a drug order that may be contraindicated in a disease.	Alert for when a patient with asthma is ordered a Beta Blocker.

Implementing these types of medication decision support systems can potentially improve patient safety during the ordering or prescribing of medications. However, there must be close monitoring of alerts to determine when there are so many signals that clinicians develop alert fatigue and begin to ignore the intended warning. Many systems allow thresholds to be set for these types of alerts as well as the intended targets. For example, drug–drug interactions may result in many alerts, but one can set the threshold to display only drug–drug interactions classified as high severity for ordering providers, to prevent alert fatigue but display all severity alerts to pharmacists. Alert fatigue will be discussed later in this section.

The Leapfrog Group for Patient Safety is a group representing large companies and purchasers of healthcare who advocate for best practices or "leaps" for improving patient care through incentives and advocacy. One of their key recommendations for improving patient safety is the implementation of CPOE with medication CDS. They have created as a component of their annual patient safety survey a CPOE evaluation tool. The CPOE evaluation tool tested many of the basic and advanced medication decision support functionalities including therapeutic duplication, single and cumulative dose limits, allergies and cross allergies, contraindicated route of administration, drug–drug and drug–food interactions, contraindications/dose limits based on patient diagnosis, patient age or weight, laboratory studies, or radiology orders.[60] In their initial findings, the mean score for detecting ADEs was 44%.[61] In tests specifically targeting pediatric hospitals, 42% of medication orders did not receive an appropriate warning and 33.9% of potentially fatal orders did not receive an appropriate warning.[62]

One potential reason the pediatric hospitals did not perform well on the Leapfrog CPOE evaluation tool is that much of the drug dosing content in commercial CPOE and CDS systems is derived from drug databases that are oftentimes not well designed for pediatric patients. Many pediatric hospitals have elected to customize their own databases to reflect pediatric-specific content, or they simply turn off the CDS alerts.

Pediatric Clinical Decision Support Systems

While studies on the impact of CDS on adult quality are more proliferative than studies on the impact of pediatric-specific clinical decision support, there is emerging evidence that pediatric CDS can improve the quality of care of pediatric patients. Most CDS interventions are targeted at providers; however, other CDS interventions have been targeted at patients.

A study in a network of urban primary care centers used CDS to reduce missed opportunities for vaccination and improve immunization rates. This CDS intervention improved immunization opportunities from 78.2% to 90.3%

at well-child visits and increased up-to-date immunization rates from 81.7% to 90.1% by 24 months of age.[63] A prospective, cluster-randomized study on CDS alerts targeting children with asthma demonstrated modest improvement in influenza vaccination rates (3.4%) in the intervention group as compared to the control group.[64] In another asthma cluster-randomized study, CDS was shown to improve provider compliance with National Asthma Education Prevention Program guidelines in urban and suburban pediatric practices. CDS was able to improve outcomes for pediatric asthma patients including an increase in rates of prescriptions for controller medications, updated asthma care plans, and spirometry improvements.[65]

In a study in a pediatric facility, CDS was created to improve the use of evidence-based guidelines to decrease the number of red blood cell (RBC) transfusions. The results demonstrated a significant decrease in red blood cell transfusions (and thus the risk and expense to the patient) in the pediatric ICU and pediatric wards.[66] In another cluster-randomized CDS study in outpatients, CDS was shown to improve the adherence to otitis media guidelines.[67]

While most CDS interventions target clinicians or providers, there is an emergence of CDS interventions targeted at patients and families. In one intervention, parents of children with asthma entered patient information including symptoms, medications, and unmet needs. Then the CDS system provided a plan of action for providers. In this trial, CDS led to a small increase in inhaled controller medications prescribed, but no change in other outcomes including parental satisfaction and information sharing.[68,69] In another CDS cluster-randomized study, decision support was designed to target clinicians and families to improve vaccination rates for the human papilloma virus (HPV) vaccine. In this study, decision support directed at different audiences resulted in different outcomes. CDS directed at clinicians were most effective in initiating the three shot series. Decision support consisting of automated phone call reminders directed at families was most effective in the completion of the full series. The combination of decision support directed at both clinicians and families helped improve the overall immunization rates of the HPV vaccine.[70]

Alert Fatigue

One key outcome for any CDS implementation that requires vigilance is tracking alert fatigue. If the alert frequency of CDS is too high without appropriate or helpful information provided to clinicians, they will become desensitized to the alerts and begin to ignore the warnings, leading to alert fatigue. The phenomenon of alert fatigue is well described in medication and other types of CDS. In one case report in a pediatric hospital, CDS alerts in one intensive care unit were described as leading to alert fatigue in a complicated transplant patient, resulting in several patient safety events.[71] One pediatric hospital took a systematic approach to document the alert rates and alter them to reduce their medication-related CDS warnings.[72] Strategies for the measurement of medication-related CDS alert fatigue are available in this guidebook.[73]

Clinical decision support has shown varying success in improving the quality of care and increasing adherence to best practices and evidence in pediatric patients. Some key considerations described in the literature for best practices for implementing CDS include workflow considerations, providing real-time data, and measuring outcomes.[74,75] Descriptions of the theory, practice, and implementation of CDS are well described in other textbooks.[47,76] Continued experience and research on the use of CDS in pediatrics will be required. As the practice of pediatrics becomes more complicated with the ever increasing amount of data that is generated for each patient in the EHR environment, CDS has the potential to improve patient safety and quality by embedding best practices and evidence into the workflow of the EHR to help guide pediatricians in their decision making.

BARCODE MEDICATION ADMINISTRATION

Barcode medication administration (BCMA) is an electronic system that is linked to an EHR CPOE system or an independent system that allows for the scanning of a patient's ID band and the medication to verify that the medication is linked to the correct order and is administered to the right patient. The BCMA process can help verify the "five rights" of the medication administration process: right patient, drug, time, dose, and route. Alerts or warning can be provided to notify nurses of an incorrect patient or time of administration of medications. While CPOE primarily targets providers and the ordering and prescribing phase of the medication management process, BCMA is further downstream in the medication management process and primarily targets nurses and the medication administration phase. When BCMA is linked to a CPOE system and an electronic medication administration record (eMAR), the system can fully integrate an electronic process from prescribing to administration of the medication. The CPOE order can be sent electronically to the pharmacy system and the eMAR, so that the correct dose and formulation can be dispensed. The nurse can then link the medication administration to the order in the eMAR by scanning the patient and the medication when it is administered. This is in contrast to paper processes where a medication order was placed on paper, a pharmacist transcribes it into a dispensing unit in the pharmacy, a nurse transcribes it into a paper medication administration record, and then the nurse documents the medication in the paper medication administration record when it is administered. This manual process is vulnerable to errors throughout the process including many opportunities for transcription errors.

The Veteran's Affairs Administration was one of the first institutions to implement BCMA in their hospitals.[77] One large academic facility was able to decrease dispensing errors and potential ADEs, completely eliminate their transcription errors, and significantly decrease their medication administration timing errors.[78,79] A hospital system that had a fully integrated CPOE, eMAR, and BCMA system demonstrated reduced prescribing errors and medication administration errors while improving patient verification. In this study, the time spent on medication administration was increased.[80] Like any electronic system, workarounds of BCMA have been described. [81]Overall, a review of the literature on BCMA showed a reduction in medications errors with no increase in time spent on medication administration.[82]

There are special pediatric considerations for BCMA systems in pediatrics: the size of the armband and barcode should accommodate all ranges of pediatric patients from premature neonates to adolescents; the barcode should be scannable through neonatal incubators; and barcodes should encode compounded medications and liquid medications in syringes, which are more common in pediatric care.[83] Another special neonatal consideration for BCMA systems is the ability to produce and scan barcodes for breast milk stored and prepared in the milk bank.[84] A survey of nursing perceptions of BCMA in a pediatric hospital showed improved safety in the medication administration process, but concerns related to the usefulness of BCMA, time efficiency, and ease of documentation as compared to the pre-BCMA period.[85] A study of the implementation of BCMA in a neonatal intensive care unit showed that BCMA reduced the relative risk of targeted, preventable adverse drug events by 47%.[86]

▌ AUTOMATED SURVEILLANCE OF ADVERSE EVENTS

The amount of data created by EHRs is growing at an exponential rate. There is great potential for the secondary reuse of data generated from EHRs to improve patient safety. One example is the use of EHR data to provide surveillance of adverse events. The use of information systems to identify adverse events was suggested soon after the introduction of computerized physician order and EHRs.[87] Early work focused on the use of information technology to detect nosocomial infections, ADEs, and adverse events.[88,89] These methods of automated detection used different HER-generated data as signals. For example, a combination of laboratory, pharmacy, and diagnosis code data can be used to detect ADEs. Studies have shown that these automated methods are more effective in detecting adverse events than traditional methods such as voluntary self-reporting.[90,91] In one study, the automated surveillance system detected ADEs at a rate 3.6 times that of voluntary reporting systems at a university hospital and 12.3 times that of voluntary reporting systems at a community hospital.[92]

The Institute for Healthcare Improvement (IHI) developed the trigger tool methodology to detect harm and adverse events without a complete chart review.[93,94] The initial use of the trigger tool in pediatrics has been in the detection of ADEs in pediatric inpatients and neonatal intensive care units.[5,95] An example of triggers adapted from the IHI list and the initial pediatric studies used to detect pediatric ADEs is shown in Table 7-3.[96] These triggers were initially developed for manual chart review. Recent work has begun to automate these triggers from EHR-generated data to increase detection of adverse

Table 7-3	**ELECTRONIC TRIGGER TOOL EXAMPLES**
Trigger Number	**Description**
T1	Diphenhydramine
T2	Flumazenil (Romazicon)
T3	Antiemetics
T4	Naloxone (Narcan)
T5	Sodium polysterene (Kayexalate)
T6	Anticoagulation lab values out of range
T7	Over-sedation, lethargy, falls, hypotension
T8	Rash
T9	Abrupt cessation of medication
T10	Unplanned transfer to higher level of care or resuscitation
T11	Serum glucose level of <50 or >200 mg/dL
T12	*Clostridium difficile*-positive or oral Vancomycin
T13	Rising serum creatinine (1.5 × baseline)
T14	Potassium level of <2.5 or >5.5 mEq/L
T15	Laxative or stool softener

Reproduced, with permission, from Tham E, Calmes HM, Poppy A, et al. Sustaining and spreading the reduction of adverse drug events in a multicenter collaborative. *Pediatrics.* 2011;128(2):e438-e445. Copyright by the AAP 2011.

events. Once the triggers are identified, a targeted review of the chart is performed to identify potential harm.

Some of the triggers listed in Table 7-3 will be easily adapted into the EHR. For example, medication triggers such as diphenhydramine, flumazenil, and naloxone can be detected from the eMAR and laboratory values such as high or low glucose and high potassium can be detected from the laboratory results. Other triggers such as rash or lethargy are more difficult to adapt to the electronic environment. Selection of the source of the electronic triggers in the electronic health record will potentially change the sensitivity of the triggers. In one study on the use of naloxone as the electronic trigger, different numerators, denominators, and rates were derived depending on which of the five different electronic sources of the triggers was used.[97] Four of the sources were directly from the EHR: medications charged, medications ordered, medications administered, and medication orders that were changed. The fifth source was from Pediatric Health Information Systems (PHIS), the national pediatric database that is derived from administrative and billing data.

Electronic trigger tools have expanded from detecting ADEs to detecting adverse events by adapting the IHI global trigger tool to pediatrics. A study using the paper IHI global trigger tool applied to pediatrics showed that it was effective in identifying adverse events.[98] Several studies are being conducted currently to validate pediatric specific global trigger tools adapted from the IHI global trigger tools and create electronic global trigger tools for pediatrics. Several large EHR vendors now provide packages and instructions on how to embed trigger tools in their EHRs.

Most current strategies for implementing electronic trigger tools include the creation of retrospective reports with the triggers as the criteria derived from EHR data. This allows for retrospective evaluation of the triggers for adverse events by a reviewer. This type of system allows the trending of triggers and adverse events over time to target quality improvement interventions to high-risk or high-impact areas identified through this trending. In a study of an automated hypoglycemia trigger over a 1-year period at a pediatric hospital, the automated surveillance system identified 1254 hypoglycemia triggers with 198 adverse events identified with a positive predictive value of 15.8%. By comparison, none of these hypoglycemic events were identified by the voluntary incident-reporting system.[99]

However, the retrospective review methodology does not allow for real-time interventions to prevent harm and adverse events. Another alternative strategy is to create real-time triggers that alert an end user to investigate if a trigger is an indication of an adverse event. With a real-time trigger, an end-user may be able to intervene to prevent or mitigate the harm to the patient. One example would be a real-time trigger of high vancomycin trough level that is sent to the pharmacist caring for patients on the medical floor. This real-time trigger would allow the pharmacist to intervene and adjust the dose of the medication to mitigate or prevent further renal injury to the patient from too high of a vancomycin dose. EHRs have different tools that potentially allow for the implementation of real-time triggers including the use of the CDS engine to build rules for real-time triggers or the use of clinical scoring systems.

A national collaborative of pediatric hospitals, the Automated Adverse Event Collaborative, has recently been established to facilitate sharing of lessons learned and exchange of data across member institutions. Monthly meetings of users of several different types of EHRs allow for the rapid dissemination of ideas and development of automated trigger tools for detection of adverse events in pediatrics.[100] The use of automated trigger tools in pediatrics continues to evolve and is currently in its infancy. Continued research in developing these methods will improve the safety and quality of care of pediatric patients in an EHR-environment.

UNINTENDED CONSEQUENCES OF HEALTH INFORMATION TECHNOLOGY

While health information technology holds many promises for improving patient safety, it also has the potential for causing patient harm. One of the earliest examples in medicine is the Therac-25 case. Therac-25 was a radiation therapy machine with a software design that led to miscalculations in radiation dosing, resulting in overdoses of radiation.[101] Several patients suffered radiation poisoning and several died from the radiation overdoses administered by the Therac-25 machines. Because of trust in the machines, human providers did not question the dosages calculated and given by the machines.

After initial studies touting the potential of CPOE and other HIT, there was a growing recognition that these technologies could lead to unintended consequences. Ash categorized unintended consequences of HIT leading to errors. She described two categories: errors in the process of entering and retrieving information and errors in the communication and coordination process.[102] Koppel described 22 different types of medication errors that were facilitated by CPOE.[27] Ash and her colleagues have published further research on the categories and described the extent of unintended consequences of CPOE.[103-105] Campbell describes eight categories of unintended consequences of CPOE including more or new work for clinicians, unfavorable workflow issues, never ending system demands, problems due to persistence of paper, negative changes in communication patterns and practice, negative emotions, generation of new kinds of errors, and unintended changes in institutional power structures.[104] This and other research led experts to begin questioning whether CPOE was helpful or harmful.[106]

One type of error due to the processing of entering and retrieving information described by Ash is a human computer interface that does not support the environment of healthcare where healthcare providers are constantly interrupted. This can lead to juxtaposition errors where a wrong medication may be selected because it is next to the intended medication. The interruptions can also lead to ordering the wrong medication or test on the wrong patient when multiple patient windows are open in one screen. Other types of errors include cognitive overload from emphasizing structured and complete data entry, structures of electronic templates requiring more work to complete than paper charts, fragmentation of information from moving between multiple screens or scrolling, and over-complete notes with extraneous data or information due to copy-paste functionality.[102]

Ash describes two types of errors in the communication and coordination process: misrepresenting clinical work as linear with predictable workflows and misrepresenting communication as information transfer. Examples of errors due to misrepresenting clinical work as a linear and predictable workflow include inflexibility of information technology solutions to adapt to exceptions, urgency in fulfilling emergent medications, workarounds to overcome the inflexibility of the system, and transfers of patients to different units or locations, leading to lost orders or information. Examples of errors due to the misrepresentation of communication as information transfer include loss of communication and feedback where a provider assumes that an order entered into the system will be automatically viewed by the nurse, and the nurse assumes that new orders will be available to them to view. Other examples include decision overload when a provider feels like an alert should not be directed at them, but then ignores an important alert because he has received so many inconsequential alerts.[102]

Unintended consequences and errors due to HIT have been described in pediatrics as well. Walsh described errors due to CPOE including duplicate medication errors, drop-down menu selection errors, keyboard entry errors, and order set errors due to choosing the wrong medication.[36]

The Pittsburgh CPOE Case

As described briefly earlier, one of the most cited cases of unintended consequences in pediatrics was the implementation of CPOE at the Children's Hospital of Pittsburgh. An initial report from Pittsburgh described how CPOE decreased harmful ADE rates.[37] The team from Pittsburgh further described their change management processes leading to what was viewed as a successful implementation of CPOE.[107] However, Han published a paper that demonstrated an increase in mortality in patients that were admitted via interhospital transport to their pediatric intensive care unit after the implementation of CPOE in Pittsburgh. The authors reported an increase in mortality rate from 2.80% pre-CPOE implementation to 6.57% post-CPOE implementation. Han also reported some of the inflexibility of CPOE systems for variable workflows that Ash described in the unintended consequences literature. For example, because they could not order medications and obtain medications until a patient had arrived in the unit and was registered into the system, it took two physicians to care for the patient. One physician placed orders in the CPOE system, while another resuscitated the critically ill child. Another example of a workflow inflexibility problem was that at times it took 10 clicks or 2 minutes to input one order because order sets were not prepared for the ICU.[38]

Subsequent editorials and letters to the editor on the Han paper have focused on the lack of preparation for the implementation such as the use of order sets and the use of off-the-shelf systems in the intensive care unit.[108-111] One editorial describes the implementation at CHP as a "stunning example of how pressure to deploy HIT stifled common sense and had deadly results" and described the 6-day implementation as an "audacious task."[111]

Del Beccaro replicated the Han study at Children's Hospital and Regional Medical Center in Seattle using the same commercial system as Pittsburgh and found that there was no increase in mortality in the ICU after they implemented CPOE at their institution. Their analysis showed that the mortality rate in the PICU prior to CPOE implementation was 4.22% and, after CPOE implementation, 3.46%, with no statistical difference between the 2 periods. They concluded that careful design, build, and implementation helped mitigate against the increased risk of mortality in the ICU.[39] An expert panel convened to discuss the different outcomes between Han and Del Beccarro to better understand how to prevent increased mortality from health information systems. Most of the expert informaticians on the panel concluded that the whole CPOE implementation process was flawed at CHP, which led to the increased mortality.[112] More recently, Longhurst described how the implementation of CPOE with the same commercial CPOE system as Pittsburgh and Seattle at the Lucille Packard Children's Hospital reduced the mortality of their inpatients. Their mean adjusted mortality rate decreased by 20% after the implementation of CPOE.[40]

EHR Harm Mitigation

Implementation of CPOE and other HIT solutions has the potential of unintended consequences and "e-Iatrogenesis," harm to the patient from information technology systems.[113] There is a growing recognition that safety and mitigation plans be instituted to monitor the safety of EHRs and other HIT. One suggestion is the creation of an EHR rapid response team consisting of leaders in clinical areas, information technology, informatics, patient safety, risk management, and public relations.[114] This team could quickly address and mitigate problems with the EHR leading to potential patient harm. There have been further calls for the development of local teams to analyze, mitigate, and report these EHR-related hazards to a national monitoring body.[115]

The IOM released a report in 2012 entitled "Health IT and patient safety: building safer systems for better care" to address the safety concerns of the unintended consequences of health information technology. In this report, the IOM committee described three threats to patient safety: poor user-interface design, poor workflow, and complex data interfaces. They also described the lack of system interoperability as a barrier that prevented improving patient safety and clinical decisions.[116] The IOM report provided multiple recommendations to improve the safety of HIT systems including the creation of a national reporting and surveillance system for EHR-related harms and deaths. The committee also recommended that if there was not a significant change driven by industry to improve the safety of HIT, then the Food and Drug Administration (FDA) should begin to regulate HIY products.

CONCLUSION

This chapter reviews several examples of health information technology that support the improvement of the quality of care and safety of pediatric patients including computerized physician order entry, CDS systems, barcode medication administration systems, and automated adverse event surveillance systems. The initial enthusiasm that HIT would dramatically improve patient safety has been tempered by the documented unintended consequences of HIT. Evaluation studies need to continue to be conducted to document the improvements and harms of HIT systems on pediatric patients. Furthermore, all those who care for children, and especially those in the pediatric patient safety and quality improvement fields, should continue to advocate for pediatric specific functionality to be built in health information technology. Otherwise, as Dr Andrew Spooner writes, in an editorial entitled "We are still waiting for fully supportive electronic health records in pediatrics:" "We could also take a more active role in creating a roadmap for how all EHRs ought to work in pediatric care ... But pediatricians should be able to make the case such that better child health functionality would improve the fortunes of all involved. If we cannot make this case, then we must continue to wait."[117]

IN PRACTICE

- When considering an IT system for a pediatric practice, be sure to assess the pediatric specific CPOE functionality such as weight-based dosing
- When implementing clinical decision support in your EHR, measure the response of clinicians to the alert to determine the outcomes of your intervention as well as to prevent alert fatigue
- While health information technology oftentimes improves the quality of care or patient safety, one must be on the lookout for any unintended consequences

FAQs

- What is the best source of information for a pediatric provider who is considering selection of an IT system for implementation in his/her office? The American Academy of Pediatrics Child Health Informatics Center and Council on Clinical Information Technology provides multiple resources for pediatric providers implementing an electronic health record including an EHR review site and an email listserv to ask questions to peers (http://www2.aap.org/informatics/chic.html). As part of the Health Information Technology for Economic and Clinical Health (HITECH) Act, the Office of the National Coordinate created Regional Extension Centers (RECs) to support providers in EHR implementations.
- What are some considerations that a pediatric provider should consider for implementing a clinical decision support alert in their EHR? Bates published an article "Ten commandments for effective clinical decision support" that provides guidelines on effective CDS implementation.[74] Many of the pediatric examples cited in the chapter describe their methods as well as lessons learned.
- What functionality for an EHR should pediatric providers as vendors for? The American Academy of Pediatrics has published several technical reports and policy statements that detail functionality needed in EHRs and health information technology to care for pediatric patients including special requirements for pediatrics,[41] inpatient systems,[42] electronic prescribing,[43,44] medical homes,[118] and personal health records.[119]

REFERENCES

1. Kohn LT, Corrigan J, Donaldson MS. *To Err is Human : Building a Safer Health System.* Washington, DC: National Academy Press; 2000.

2. Institute of Medicine (US). Committee on Quality of Health Care in America. *Crossing the Quality Chasm : A New Health System for the 21st Century.* Washington, DC: National Academy Press; 2001.

3. Kaushal R, Bates DW, Landrigan C, et al. Medication errors and adverse drug events in pediatric inpatients. *JAMA.* 2001;285(16):2114-2120.

4. Holdsworth MT, Fichtl RE, Behta M, et al. Incidence and impact of adverse drug events in pediatric inpatients. *Arch Pediatr Adolesc Med.* 2003;157(1):60-65.

5. Takata GS, Mason W, Taketomo C, et al. Development, testing, and findings of a pediatric-focused trigger tool to identify medication-related harm in US children's hospitals. *Pediatrics.* 2008;121(4):e927-e935.

6. Takata GS, Taketomo CK, Waite S. California pediatric patient safety initiative. Characteristics of medication errors and adverse drug events in hospitals participating in the California Pediatric Patient Safety Initiative. *Am J Health Syst Pharm.* 2008;65(21):2036-2044.

7. Kaushal R, Barker KN, Bates DW. How can information technology improve patient safety and reduce medication errors in children's health care? *Arch Pediatr Adolesc Med.* 2001;155(9):1002-1007.

8. Leape LL, Berwick DM, Bates DW. What practices will most improve safety? Evidence-based medicine meets patient safety. *JAMA.* 2002;288(4):501-507.

9. Fortescue EB, Kaushal R, Landrigan CP, et al. Prioritizing strategies for preventing medication errors and adverse drug events in pediatric inpatients. *Pediatrics.* 2003;111(4 Pt 1):722-729.

10. Kaushal R, Jaggi T, Walsh K, et al. Pediatric medication errors: what do we know? What gaps remain? *Ambul Pediatr.* 2004;4(1):73-81.

11. National Research Council. *Key Capabilities of an Electronic Health Record System: Letter Report.* Washington, DC: National Academies Press; 2003.

12. DesRoches CM, Campbell EG, Rao SR, et al. Electronic health records in ambulatory care—a national survey of physicians. *N Engl J Med.*2008;359(1):50-60.

13. Jha AK, DesRoches CM, Campbell EG, et al. Use of electronic health records in U.S. hospitals. *N Engl J Med.* 2009;360(16):1628-1638.

14. Menachemi N, Brooks RG, Schwalenstocker E, Simpson L. Use of health information technology by children's hospitals in the United States. *Pediatrics.* 2009;123(suppl 2): S80-S84.

15. Grinspan ZM, Banerjee S, Kaushal R, Kern LM. Physician specialty and variations in adoption of electronic health records. *Appl Clin Inform.* 2013;4(2):225-240.

16. Johnson KB. Barriers that impede the adoption of pediatric information technology. *Arch Pediatr Adolesc Med.* 2001;155(12):1374-1379.

17. Fleming NS, Culler SD, McCorkle R, et al. The financial and nonfinancial costs of implementing electronic health records in primary care Practices. *Health Affairs.* 2011;30(3):481-489.

18. Bodenheimer T, Grumbach K. Electronic technology: a spark to revitalize primary care? *JAMA.* 2003;290(2):259-264.

19. Blumenthal D, Glaser JP. Information technology comes to medicine. *N Engl J Med.* 2007;356(24):2527-2534.

20. Smith PD. Implementing an EMR system: one clinic's experience. *Fam Pract Manag.* 2003;10(5):37-42.

21. HealthIT.gov. How much is this going to cost me? Available at: http://www.healthit.gov/providers-professionals/faqs/how-much-going-cost-me. Accessed 06.01.2014.

22. The American Recovery and Reinvestment Act of 2009. Available at: http://www.recovery.gov/About/Pages/The_Act.aspx. Accessed 25.01.2010.

23. Blumenthal D. Launching HITECH. *N Engl J Med.* 2010;362(5):382-385.

24. Blumenthal D, Tavenner M. The "meaningful use," regulation for electronic health records. *N Engl J Med.* 2010;363(6):501-504.

25. Mekhjian HS, Kumar RR, Kuehn L, et al. Immediate benefits realized following implementation of physician order entry at an academic medical center. *J Am Med Inform Assoc.* 2002;9(5):529-539.

26. Sittig DF, Stead WW. Computer-based physician order entry: the state of the art. *J Am Med Inform Assoc.* 1994;1(2):108-123.

27. Koppel R, Metlay JP, Cohen A, et al. Role of computerized physician order entry systems in facilitating medication errors. *JAMA.* 2005;293(10):1197-1203.

28. Centers for Medicare and Medicaid Services. E-Prescribing. Available at: http://www.cms.gov/Medicare/E-Health/Eprescribing/index.html. Accessed 12.06.2013.

29. Miller MR, Robinson KA, Lubomski LH, et al. Medication errors in paediatric care: a systematic review of epidemiology and an evaluation of evidence supporting reduction strategy recommendations. *Qual Saf Health Care.* 2007;16(2):116-126.

30. Bates DW, Leape LL, Cullen DJ, et al. Effect of computerized physician order entry and a team intervention on prevention of serious medication errors. *JAMA.* 1998;280(15):1311-1316.

31. Bates DW, Teich JM, Lee J, et al. The impact of computerized physician order entry on medication error prevention. *J Am Med Inform Assoc.* 1999;6(4):313-321.

32. King WJ, Paice N, Rangrej J, et al. The effect of computerized physician order entry on medication errors and adverse drug events in pediatric inpatients. *Pediatrics.* 2003;112(3 Pt 1):506-509.

33. Holdsworth MT, Fichtl RE, Raisch DW, et al. Impact of computerized prescriber order entry on the incidence of adverse drug events in pediatric inpatients. *Pediatrics.* 2007;120(5):1058-1066.

34. Potts AL, Barr FE, Gregory DF, et al. Computerized physician order entry and medication errors in a pediatric critical care unit. *Pediatrics.* 2004;113(1 Pt 1):59-63.

35. van Rosse F, Maat B, Rademaker CMA, et al. The effect of computerized physician order entry on medication prescription errors and clinical outcome in pediatric and intensive care: a systematic review. *Pediatrics.* 2009;123(4):1184-1190.

36. Walsh KE, Adams WG, Bauchner H, et al. Medication errors related to computerized order entry for children. *Pediatrics.* 2006;118(5):1872-1879.

37. Upperman JS, Staley P, Friend K, et al. The impact of hospitalwide computerized physician order entry on medical errors in a pediatric hospital. *J Pediatr Surg.* 2005;40(1):57-59.

38. Han YY, Carcillo JA, Venkataraman ST, et al. Unexpected increased mortality after implementation of a commercially sold computerized physician order entry system. *Pediatrics.* 2005;116(6):1506-1512.

39. Del Beccaro MA, Jeffries HE, Eisenberg MA, Harry ED. Computerized provider order entry implementation: no association with increased mortality rates in an intensive care unit. *Pediatrics.* 2006;118(1):290-295.

40. Longhurst CA, Parast L, Sandborg CI, et al. Decrease in hospital-wide mortality rate after implementation of a commercially sold computerized physician order entry system. *Pediatrics.* 2010;126(1):14-21.

41. Spooner SA, and the Council on Clinical Information T. Special requirements of electronic health record systems in pediatrics. *Pediatrics.* 2007;119(3):631-637.

42. Kim GR, Lehmann CU, Council on Clinical Information T. Pediatric aspects of inpatient health information technology systems. *Pediatrics.* 2008;122(6):e1287-e1296.

43. Johnson KB, Lehmann CU, Council on Clinical Information Technology of the American Academy of Pediatrics. Electronic prescribing in pediatrics: toward safer and more effective medication management. *Pediatrics.* 2013;131(4):e1350-e1356.

44. AAP Council on Clinical Information Technology Executive Committee. Electronic prescribing in pediatrics: toward safer and more effective medication management. *Pediatrics.* 2013;131(4):824-826.

45. Agency for Healthcare Research and Quality. Children's electronic health record format. 2013. Available at: http://healthit.ahrq.gov/health-it-tools-and-resources/childrens-electronic-health-record-ehr-format. Accessed 14.06.2013.

46. Johnson KB, Lee CKK, Spooner SA, et al. Automated dose-rounding recommendations for pediatric medications. *Pediatrics.* 2011;128(2):e422-e428.

47. Greenes RA. *Clinical Decision Support : The Road Ahead.* Amsterdam, Boston: Elsevier Academic Press; 2007.

48. Institute of Medicine. *Preventing Medication Errors: Quality Chasm Series.* The Washington, DC: National Academies Press; 2007.

49. Kaushal R, Shojania KG, Bates DW. Effects of computerized physician order entry and clinical decision support systems on medication safety: a systematic review. *Arch Intern Med.* 2003;163(12):1409-1416.

50. Yourman L, Concato J, Agostini JV. Use of computer decision support interventions to improve medication prescribing in older adults: a systematic review. *Am J Geriatr Pharmacother.* 2008;6(2):119-129.

51. Pearson S-A, Moxey A, Robertson J, et al. Do computerised clinical decision support systems for prescribing change practice? A systematic review of the literature (1990-2007). *BMC Health Serv Res.* 2009;9(1):154.

52. Garg AX, Adhikari NKJ, McDonald H, et al. Effects of computerized clinical decision support systems on practitioner performance and patient outcomes. *JAMA.* 2005;293(10):1223-1238.

53. Romano MJ, Stafford RS. Electronic health records and clinical decision support systems: Impact on national ambulatory care quality. *Arch Intern Med.* 2011;171(10):897-903.

54. Kuperman GJ, Bobb A, Payne TH, et al. Medication-related clinical decision support in computerized provider order entry systems: a review. *J Am Med Inform Assoc.* 2007;14(1):29-40.

55. Stultz JS, Nahata MC. Computerized clinical decision support for medication prescribing and utilization in pediatrics. *J Am Med Inform Assoc.* 2012;19(6):942-953.

56. Walsh KE, Landrigan CP, Adams WG, et al. Effect of computer order entry on prevention of serious medication errors in hospitalized children. *Pediatrics.* 2008;121(3):e421-e427.

57. Cordero L, Kuehn L, Kumar RR, Mekhjian HS. Impact of computerized physician order entry on clinical practice in a newborn intensive care unit. *J Perinatol.* 2004;24(2):88-93.

58. Kadmon G, Bron-Harlev E, Nahum E, et al. Computerized order entry with limited decision support to prevent prescription errors in a PICU. *Pediatrics.* 2009;124(3):935-940.

59. Ferranti J, Horvath M, Jansen J, et al. Using a computerized provider order entry system to meet the unique prescribing needs of children: description of an advanced dosing model. *BMC Med Inform Decis Mak.* 2011;11(1):14.

60. Kilbridge PM, Welebob EM, Classen DC. Development of the leapfrog methodology for evaluating hospital implemented inpatient computerized physician order entry systems. *Qual Saf Health Care.* 2006;15(2):81-84.

61. Metzger J, Welebob E, Bates DW, et al. Mixed results in the safety performance of computerized physician order entry. *Health Affairs.* 2010;29(4):655-663.

62. The Leapfrog Group. Leapfrog Group Report on CPOE Evaluation Tool Results. June 2008 to January 2010. Available at: http://www.leapfroggroup.org/media/file/LFG_CPOE.pdf. Accessed 5/30/2014.

63. Fiks AG, Grundmeier RW, Biggs LM, et al. Impact of clinical alerts within an electronic health record on routine childhood immunization in an urban pediatric population. *Pediatrics.* 2007;120(4):707-714.

64. Fiks AG, Hunter KF, Localio AR, et al. Impact of electronic health record-based alerts on influenza vaccination for children with asthma. *Pediatrics.* 2009;124(1):159-169.

65. Bell LM, Grundmeier R, Localio R, et al. Electronic health record-based decision support to improve asthma care: a cluster-randomized trial. *Pediatrics.* 2010;125(4):e770-e777.

66. Adams ES, Longhurst CA, Pageler N, et al. Computerized physician order entry with decision support decreases blood transfusions in children. *Pediatrics.* 2011;127(5):e1112-e1119.

67. Forrest CB, Fiks AG, Bailey LC, et al. Improving adherence to otitis media guidelines with clinical decision support and physician feedback. *Pediatrics.* 2013;131(4):e1071-e1081.

68. Porter SC, Cai Z, Gribbons W, et al. The asthma kiosk: a patient-centered technology for collaborative decision support in the emergency department. *J Am Med Inform Assoc.* 2004;11(6):458-467.

69. Porter SC, Forbes P, Feldman HA, Goldmann DA. Impact of patient-centered decision support on quality of asthma care in the emergency department. *Pediatrics.* 2006;117(1):e33-e42.

70. Fiks AG, Grundmeier RW, Mayne S, et al. Effectiveness of decision support for families, clinicians, or both on HPV vaccine receipt. *Pediatrics.* 2013;131(6):1114-1124.

71. Carspecken CW, Sharek PJ, Longhurst C, Pageler NM. A clinical case of electronic health record drug alert fatigue: consequences for patient outcome. *Pediatrics.* 2013;131(6):e1970-e1973.

72. Beccaro MA, Villanueva R, Knudson KM, et al. Decision support alerts for medication ordering in a computerized provider order entry (CPOE) system: a systematic approach to decrease alerts. *Appl Clin Inform.* 2010;1(3):346-362.

73. Osheroff JA. *Improving Medication use and Outcomes With Clinical Decision Support : A Step-by-step Guide*. Chicago, IL: Healthcare Information and Management Systems Society Mission; 2009.

74. Bates DW, Kuperman GJ, Wang S, et al. Ten commandments for effective clinical decision support: making the practice of evidence-based medicine a reality. *J Am Med Inform Assoc.* 2003;10(6):523-530.

75. Sittig DF, Wright A, Osheroff JA, et al. Grand challenges in clinical decision support. *J Biomed Inform.* 2008;41(2):387-392.

76. Berner ES. *Clinical Decision Support Systems : Theory and Practice*. 2nd ed. New York, NY: Springer; 2007.

77. Johnson CL, Carlson RA, Tucker CL, Willette C. Using BCMA software to improve patient safety in Veterans Administration Medical Centers. *J Healthc Inf Manag.* 2002;16(1):46-51.

78. Poon EG, Keohane CA, Yoon CS, et al. Effect of bar-code technology on the safety of medication administration. *N Engl J Med.* 2010;362(18):1698-1707.

79. Poon EG, Cina JL, Churchill W, et al. Medication dispensing errors and potential adverse drug events before and after implementing bar code technology in the pharmacy. *Ann Intern Med.* 2006;145(6):426-434.

80. Franklin BD, O'Grady K, Donyai P, et al. The impact of a closed-loop electronic prescribing and administration system on prescribing errors, administration errors and staff time: a before-and-after study. *Qual Saf Health Care.* 2007;16(4):279-284.

81. Koppel R, Wetterneck T, Telles JL, Karsh BT. Workarounds to barcode medication administration systems: their occurrences, causes, and threats to patient safety. *J Am Med Inform Assoc.* 2008;15(4):408-423.

82. Hassink JJM, Jansen M, Helmons PJ. Effects of bar code-assisted medication administration (BCMA) on frequency, type and severity of medication administration errors: a review of the literature. *Eur J Hosp Pharm.* 2012;19(5):489-494.

83. Williams L. Ensuring pediatric safety with BCMA. *Pharmacy Purchasing and Products.* 2013;10(2). Available at: http://www.pppmag.com/article/1265/February_2013/Ensuring_Pediatric_Safety_with_BCMA/. Accessed 11.08.2013.

84. CHICA-Canada. Position statement: handling of expressed breast milk (EBM) in acute care settings. 2006. Available at: http://www.chica.org/pdf/EBM.pdf. Accessed 11.08.2013.

85. Holden RJ, Brown RL, Alper SJ, et al. That's nice, but what does IT do? Evaluating the impact of bar coded medication administration by measuring changes in the process of care. *Int J Ind Ergon.* 2011;41(4):370-379.

86. Morriss FH, Abramowitz PW, Nelson SP, et al. Effectiveness of a barcode medication administration system in reducing preventable adverse drug events in a neonatal intensive care unit: a prospective cohort study. *J Pediatr.* 2009;154(3):363-368.e361.

87. Bates DW, O'Neil AC, Boyle D, et al. Potential identifiability and preventability of adverse events using information systems. *J Am Med Inform Assoc.* 1994;1(5):404-411.

88. Bates DW, Evans RS, Murff H, et al. Detecting adverse events using information technology. *J Am Med Inform Assoc.* 2003;10(2):115-128.

89. Murff HJ, Patel VL, Hripcsak G, Bates DW. Detecting adverse events for patient safety research: a review of current methodologies. *J Biomed Inform.* 2003;36(1-2):131-143.

90. Jha AK, Kuperman GJ, Teich JM, et al. Identifying adverse drug events: development of a computer-based monitor and comparison with chart review and stimulated voluntary report. *J Am Med Inform Assoc.* 1998;5(3):305-314.

91. Classen DC, Pestotnik SL, Evans RS, Burke JP. Computerized surveillance of adverse drug events in hospital patients. *JAMA.* 1991;266(20):2847-2851.

92. Kilbridge PM, Campbell UC, Cozart HB, Mojarrad MG. Automated surveillance for adverse drug events at a community hospital and an academic medical center. *J Am Med Inform Assoc.* 2006;13(4):372-377.

93. Resar RK, Rozich JD, Classen D. Methodology and rationale for the measurement of harm with trigger tools. *Qual Saf Health Care.* 2003;12(suppl 2):ii39-ii45.

94. Rozich JD, Haraden CR, Resar RK. Adverse drug event trigger tool: a practical methodology for measuring medication related harm. *Qual Saf Health Care.* 2003;12(3): 194-200.

95. Sharek PJ, Horbar JD, Mason W, et al. Adverse events in the neonatal intensive care unit: development, testing, and findings of an NICU-focused trigger tool to identify harm in North American NICUs. *Pediatrics.* 2006;118(4):1332-1340.

96. Tham E, Calmes HM, Poppy A, et al. Sustaining and spreading the reduction of adverse drug events in a multicenter collaborative. *Pediatrics.* 2011;128(2):e438-e445.

97. Kahn MG, Ranade D. The impact of electronic medical records data sources on an adverse drug event quality measure. *J Am Med Inform Assoc.* 2010;17(2):185-191.

98. Kirkendall ES, Kloppenborg E, Papp J, et al. Measuring adverse events and levels of harm in pediatric inpatients with the global trigger tool. *Pediatrics.* 2012;130(5): e1206-e1214.

99. Dickerman MJ, Jacobs BR, Vinodrao H, Stockwell DC. Recognizing hypoglycemia in children through automated adverse-event detection. *Pediatrics.* 2011;127(4): e1035-e1041.

100. Stockwell D, Jacobs B. Automatically getting better. In: Berkowitz L, McCarthy C, eds. *Innovation with Information Technologies in Healthcare*: Springer London; 2013, p.99-109.

101. Tenner E. *Why Things Bite Back: Technology and the Revenge of Unintended Consequences.* New York, NY: Knopf; 1996.

102. Ash JS, Berg M, Coiera E. Some unintended consequences of information technology in health care: the nature of patient care information system-related errors. *J Am Med Inform Assoc.* 2004;11(2):104-112.

103. Ash JS, Sittig DF, Dykstra RH, et al. Categorizing the unintended sociotechnical consequences of computerized provider order entry. *Int J Med Inform.* 2007;76(suppl 1):S21.

104. Campbell EM, Sittig DF, Ash JS, et al. Types of unintended consequences related to computerized provider order entry. *J Am Med Inform Assoc.* 2006;13(5):547-556.

105. Ash JS, Sittig DF, Poon EG, et al. The extent and importance of unintended consequences related to computerized provider order entry. *J Am Med Inform Assoc.* 2007;14(4):415-423.

106. Berger RG, Kichak JP. Computerized physician order entry: helpful or harmful? *J Am Med Inform Assoc.* 2004;11(2):100-103.

107. Upperman JS, Staley P, Friend K, et al. The introduction of computerized physician order entry and change management in a tertiary pediatric hospital. *Pediatrics.* 2005;116(5):e634-642.

108. Sittig DF, Ash JS, Zhang J, et al. Lessons from "unexpected increased mortality after implementation of a commercially sold computerized physician order entry system." *Pediatrics.* 2006;118(2):797-801.

109. Jacobs BR, Brilli RJ, Ward Hart K. Perceived increase in mortality after process and-policy changes implemented with computerized physician order entry. *Pediatrics.* 2006;117(4):1451-1452.

110. Longhurst C, Sharek P, Hahn J, et al. Perceived increase in mortality after process and policy changes implemented with computerized physician order entry. *Pediatrics.* 2006;117(4):1450-1451.

111. Gesteland PH, Nebeker JR, Gardner RM. These are the technologies that try men's souls: common-sense health information technology. *Pediatrics.* 2006;117(1):216-217.

112. Ammenwerth E, Talmon J, Ash JS, et al. Impact of CPOE on mortality rates—contradictory findings, important messages. *Methods Inf Med.* 2006;45(6):586-593.

113. Weiner JP, Kfuri T, Chan K, Fowles JB. e-Iatrogenesis: the most critical unintended consequence of CPOE and other HIT. *J Am Med Inform Assoc.* 2007;14(3):387-388.

114. Walker JM, Carayon P, Leveson N, et al. EHR safety: the way forward to safe and effective systems. *J Am Med Inform Assoc.* 2008;15(3):272-277.

115. Singh H, Classen DC, Sittig DF. Creating an oversight infrastructure for electronic health record-related patient safety hazards. *J Patient Saf.* 2011 Dec;7(4):169-174. doi: 10.1097/PTS.0b013e31823d8df0.

116. Institute of Medicine. *Health IT and Patient Safety: Building Safer Systems for Better Care.* Washington, DC: National Academies Press; 2012.

117. Spooner SA. We are still waiting for fully supportive electronic health records in pediatrics. *Pediatrics.* 2012;130(6):e1674-e1676.

118. AAP Council on Clinical Information Technology. Health information technology and the medical home. *Pediatrics.* 2011;127(5):978-982.

119. AAP Council on Clinical Information Technology. Using personal health records to improve the quality of health care for children. *Pediatrics.* 2009;124(1):403-409.

ENGAGING PATIENTS AND FAMILIES | 8

INTRODUCTION

In the year 2001, a little girl named Josie King died from medical errors. Josie became the face behind the staggering statistic—98,000 deaths from medical errors every year, the face behind the reality that this simple five-digit numeral translates into the disturbing visual of a jumbo jet crashing every day. Perhaps it was the culmination of events that led up to her death, along with the fact that those events took place in one of our country's finest hospitals, which caused the healthcare industry to pause and take a good long hard look at itself.

Josie was admitted to the prestigious Johns Hopkins Hospital after she suffered from burns upon climbing into a hot bath. Two days before Josie was to come home, she died from severe dehydration and misused narcotics. It was not a doctor's mistake, a nurse's mistake, a misplaced decimal point, or an incorrect medication that led to her death. Josie died from a breakdown in communication, a breakdown in the system. What if the residents had noticed that her weight had dropped significantly in 24 hours? What if someone had listened to Josie's mother as she repeatedly told the staff that her daughter was really thirsty? What if there had been better communication between the doctor who changed the methadone order and the nurse who didn't realize the order had been changed? Perhaps if Josie's mother had been able to call a Rapid Response Team or if the doctors and nurses had taken their eyes off of the computer screens and clipboards and looked at the little girl, she would be alive. Maybe if someone had listened to Josie's mother as she repeatedly asked for help, none of this would have happened.

At the time of Josie's death, hospitals and healthcare providers across the country were grappling with the findings released in a November 1999 Institute of Medicine report, "To Err is Human." This report forced well-meaning, highly committed healthcare professionals to confront the fact that, despite their best efforts, every day patients are harmed and even killed in healthcare settings across the United States. The burning platform became evident, and the "patient safety movement" was launched.

Individual patient safety champions, private organizations, and the federal government began the hard work of redefining patient safety and transforming the traditional healthcare culture. Over the past decade, we have come to realize that, rather than "freedom from accidental harm," patient safety is a "discipline that utilizes a systems approach to improving healthcare processes and outcomes."[1] It has become clear that the complexity of modern healthcare has surpassed the capability of any individual provider, and patient safety requires a shift from focusing on individual performance to high-performing teams. Essential to this shift is the inclusion of patients and families as members of these teams and engaging them in all aspects of care delivery, from redesigning care processes and reimbursement models to training the next generation of providers.[2]

PATIENT ENGAGEMENT

Patient engagement has been defined in various ways, but several key elements are common across definitions. Engaged patients and families believe they have an important role to play in their care. They are willing and able to participate and have the necessary skills to manage their health and the care they receive.[3,4] The National Patient Safety Foundation describes engaged patients as informed consumers who work collaboratively with providers to share information, make decisions, and adhere to jointly agreed-upon treatments.[5] Former Centers for Medicaid and Medicare Administrator Don Berwick notes that in a truly patient-centric system, patient engagement equates with the maxim "nothing about me without me," or any component of the healthcare system that affects the patient must include the patient.[6] It extends the idea of shared decision-making to shared responsibility for processes and outcomes.

Engaging patients and family members in their care confers numerous advantages. Active patient participation has been shown to improve both patient and provider satisfaction with the care process.[7] A study of hospitalized patients found that 89.1% of those who actively participated in their care reported the quality of their experience as very good or excellent, while only 57.8% of patients who minimally participated in their care reported the same high level of quality.[8] Engaged patients also have better health outcomes, including performing more preventive (eg, annual exams, screenings) and health-promoting (eg, healthy diet, physical activity) behaviors[9] while avoiding health-damaging (eg, smoking, excessive alcohol consumption) ones. They are more likely to seek health information and self-monitor health conditions and less likely to delay care or have unmet healthcare needs. Moreover, engaged patients have up to 21% lower healthcare costs, including fewer emergency department visits and hospitalizations.[9] Finally, patient and family engagement facilitates providers' understanding and respect by incorporating the family's beliefs, needs, and preferences into decision-making, which enables the provision of services that meet each unique situation.[10]

In addition to improvements in quality, health, and cost outcomes, there is some evidence to suggest that medication errors[11] and adverse events during a hospital admission[9] decline when patients are actively involved in their care. This is in part because engaged patients tend to more closely monitor their care by seeking information and tracking their treatment.[12] Likewise, they tend to adhere better to prescribed therapies because they have explored all of their treatment options in the context of their own understanding of their condition and prognosis, as well as the potential benefits and harms of the chosen course of action.[12] However, evidence remains equivocal regarding the degree to which patient involvement results in overall improvements in patient safety.[13]

BARRIERS TO PATIENT ENGAGEMENT

A number of patient and provider barriers to patient engagement dilute the relationship between patient participation and patient safety. These barriers can be classified into three types: intrapersonal, interpersonal, and cultural.[14] Intrapersonal barriers relate to patient and provider vulnerabilities or characteristics. For patients and family members generally, the ability to assume the role of an actively engaged member of the care team is a critical barrier. First, they must be willing to accept their place as an equal contributor to the team.[15] Second, aspects of a patient's illness, such as its severity and duration, the nature and complexity of the treatment, and the healthcare setting (inpatient vs. outpatient), influence the degree to which patients and families desire to participate.[16] Third, patients and families must have the knowledge, confidence, and skills to act on their own behalf.[17] Finally, patients' and families' goals, values, religious/cultural beliefs, and life circumstances at any given point in time may enhance or inhibit their level of participation, making it difficult to predict or expect consistent engagement.[14] For providers, one main intrapersonal barrier is their level of knowledge and training in how to invite patients and families to participate in their care, including the use of understandable language and strategies for shared decision-making. A second common barrier is the degree to which providers value patient and family participation in the medical encounter versus maintaining control over the process.[15]

Interpersonal barriers concern the interactions between the provider and patients/families. When seeking care, patients and families rely on providers for information and guidance, as well as support for disease and care management.[18] However, engagement sometimes involves questioning the judgments or actions of a practitioner, which many patients and families are reluctant to do unless they perceive some benefit from these actions. Patients and families are much less likely to confront a provider if they think the stakes of the proposed outcome are low or do not believe the interaction will effect change.[18] Moreover, many patients and families fear that providers will be unreceptive to feedback, and this deters their participation.[16] In fact, without the healthcare provider's support—and even encouragement—for participation, many patients and families remain passive in their encounters.[16] Providers also experience interpersonal barriers because some patients/families want to delegate decision-making to the practitioner, even when the provider or system encourages their participation in the process.[14] How providers present options to patients and families is also an interpersonal barrier because an authoritarian stance or prefacing options with an overt or implied preference may deter asking further questions or serious consideration of other options.[14]

Cultural barriers are perhaps some of the most challenging to address, and include those that exist because of the way in which the healthcare system has been designed around medicine's traditional, paternalistic values.[14] The practice of inviting patients and families to participate in the care process conflicts with professional norms wherein the clinician makes decisions for the patient, and the patient or caregiver acts as a recipient, not a participant, in this relationship. Furthermore, despite slight increases in visit duration since 1997,[19] providers still have limited time to explain conditions and treatment options and provide health education to patients and caregivers, especially to individuals with low literacy levels.[14] Thus, efficiency goals conflict with taking the time needed to engage patients in decision-making processes. Increases in medical malpractice suits and the generally litigious nature of society in the 21st century also contribute to providers not wanting to engage patients and families for fear of litigation if a treatment selected by the patient/family does not work—especially if this choice conflicted with the provider's recommendation.[20] In inpatient settings, structures and processes theoretically designed to maximize care delivery, such as restrictions on hours and numbers of visitors, sleeping in intensive and critical care units, and participation in rounds, serve to limit patient and family engagement and retain the locus of control with the provider/provider system.[5] Several national organizations, as well as the US federal government, have been working to increase awareness of the need for a change in traditional healthcare culture to better support engagement through patient- and family-centered care. The Institute for Patient and Family Centered Care (IPFCC) has been promoting the role of patients and families as partners in care since its inception in 1992. As described by the IPFCC, patient-centeredness is "an approach to the planning, delivery, and evaluation of healthcare that is grounded in mutually beneficial partnerships among healthcare providers, patients, and families" that "redefines these relationships in healthcare."[21] The institute identifies four core concepts of patient- and family-centered care, including respect and dignity, information sharing, participation, and collaboration. The vision of IPFCC, and the focus of its educational, consulting, and technical support, is to ensure that in every patient-provider encounter, practitioners recognize and build on the strengths of patients and families to enhance their confidence, independence, and competence in decision-making. These goals are consistent with the Institute of Medicine's definition of healthcare quality, which identifies patient-centeredness as a foundational element for achieving desired health outcomes.[22]

EFFORTS TO ENHANCE PATIENT ENGAGEMENT

With a mission to "keep patients from being harmed," the Josie King Foundation was established in 2002 to develop stronger partnerships between healthcare organizations and families. In the years since its creation, the Josie King Foundation has become known throughout the country and the world for its work in preventing medical errors by aiming to change the traditional healthcare culture. The Foundation creates products and programs for hospitals, such as The Josie King Foundation Care Journal, tens of thousands of which are in the hands of patients and family members around the country. These journals provide a way to help patients and family members keep track of important information while they are in the hospital. More importantly, the journals help to bridge the disconnect that often exists between healthcare providers and the patient. As Sorrel King, mother of Josie, describes, it is quite powerful when a doctor or a nurse hands a patient a Care Journal and says to them, "this is a gift from us to you; we encourage you to keep track of information; we want you to ask questions and express your concerns; we want you to partner with us in your care."

A "Josie King DVD" was created and translated into three different languages, and is now used thoughout the healthcare industry to inspire healthcare providers to remember the importance of good communication and teamwork. An additional initiative, Condition H (Help), builds upon the success of rapid response teams (RRTs) and encourages patients and/or families to activate RRTs directly if they feel something is wrong and they can't seem to get the attention of the bedside providers. A growing number of hospitals around the country are partnering with the Josie King Foundation and other similar organizations to implement patient- and family-centered care initiatives.

Along similar lines, the National Patient Safety Foundation (NPSF) was founded in 1997 to improve the safety of care provided to patients.[23] Central to the NPSF's vision is "patient involvement in continuous learning and constant information" to advance patient safety and quality of care.

The US federal government has established a number of initiatives to promote patient and family engagement. The Agency for Healthcare Research and

Quality (AHRQ) has developed resources for consumers to learn strategies for becoming involved in their care and promoting patient safety. "Questions to Ask Your Doctor" includes pamphlets and videos with lists of questions to ask before, during, and after an appointment.[24] "Five Steps to Safer HealthCare" is a fact sheet developed by the Department of Health and Human Services in partnership with the American Hospital Association and the American Medical Association. It provides information on what patients can do to obtain safer healthcare, such as asking questions and getting test results.[25] In 2011, the Centers for Medicare and Medicaid Services launched a national "Partnership for Patients."[26] This public-private initiative has brought together over 8,000 partners, including hospitals, national organizations representing physicians, nurses, and other frontline healthcare and social service providers, patient and consumer organizations, employers, and states. The Partnership has two main goals: (1) making care safer and decreasing hospital-acquired infections by 40% over 3 years; and (2) improving care transitions and preventable complications to reduce hospital readmissions by 20% over the same 3-year period. A central feature of the Partnership is promoting best practices in patient and family engagement to improve the quality and safety of healthcare.

CREATING A STRUCTURE AND CULTURE TO SUPPORT PATIENT- AND FAMILY-CENTERED CARE

A number of healthcare organizations have begun to shift their traditional, paternalistic approach to one that is patient- and family-centered. Notable is the Dana Farber Cancer Institute (DFCI), which engaged in an organizational redesign after the death of two patients from chemotherapy overdoses. Among their key learning from the institutional overhaul was the impact of patient- and family-centered care.[27] The DFCI treats patients as "partners in care design, delivery, assessment, and improvement."[27] Through the use of patient/parent and family advisory committees (PFACs),[28] patients, parents, and family members engage in every stage of the clinical process, from Joint Commission Accreditation surveys to employee orientations and training to clinical rounds to leadership search processes. DFCI leadership has noted that they would not have been able to redesign their care system and realize the improvements in quality and safety without the active participation of their patients and families.[28]

Duke University Health System (DUHS) has also embraced patient- and family-centered care, believing that the involvement of patients and their loved ones is critical to the success of system-wide efforts to reduce harm, improve quality, and provide the ideal patient experience. DUHS's core value, "Caring for our patients, their loved ones, and each other," conveys the belief that patient safety requires teamwork, and members of the team include not only healthcare professionals but also patients and their families. Although most patient safety strategies have traditionally focused on error prevention and mitigation from a healthcare provider and system perspective, DUHS has embraced the vision of the World Health Organization's (WHO) program, "Patients for Patient Safety," where healthcare systems and providers treat patients and families as partners through honesty, openness, and transparency to prevent avoidable harms.[29]

To realize this vision, DUHS initiated Patient Advocacy/Advisory Councils (PACs), which is a group of patient volunteers who meet with Duke leadership on a routine basis. The mission of the PAC is to catalyze the transition of DUHS' culture to patient- and family-centered care by leveraging patient and family perspectives and concerns throughout every level of the health system. PACs contribute in a number of ways, including: (1) advising on policies and programs; (2) identifying system-level issues that affect patient care; (3) improving customer satisfaction; (4) providing a link between DUHS and the larger community; and (5) participating in the education of healthcare professionals. The following guiding principles provide the framework for an expanded patient advocacy presence across DUHS:

- Patients and families will be recognized and *welcomed* as important members of the healthcare team.
- Patients and families will be *engaged, educated, and empowered* to easily access information and *participate in care and decision-making* opportunities at *their level of comfort.*
- In order to provide the *best patient experience, core principles of patient- and family-centered care* (ie, respect and dignity, information sharing, participation, and collaboration) will guide the *quality and patient safety* improvement efforts and *communications.*

The PAC facilitates opportunities for patients and families to participate with DUHS leadership, voicing concerns and requesting clarification regarding processes and decision-making. Patient advocates and healthcare leaders convene in the spirit of partnership and demonstrate mutual support in their work together aimed at improving the quality and safety of care provided throughout the health system. The PAC is the foundation for this work; it serves as a "safe place" for discussions from a patient perspective, gives space for the patient voice, and supports opportunities to enhance patient engagement and promote partnership. As stated by a patient advocate leader at Duke, "Care boils down to relationships, and that's why Patient Advocacy/Advisory Councils are so important. They provide a foundation for building these relationships." (name withheld, personal communication, April 10, 2013)

Other examples of how health systems have shifted their focus to patient and family centricity is by actually measuring engagement and using this information to tailor care.[30] The Patient Activation Measure (PAM) is a standardized instrument used to assess the degree to which patients have the knowledge and confidence to act, and really perform those actions that support engagement in their health and healthcare.[30] Fairview Health Services in Minnesota, a large non-profit health system consisting of more than 40 primary practices, specialty clinics, and hospitals, collects PAM scores for all of its primary care patients, enters the score into the electronic health record, and uses the score as a "vital sign" to personalize care plans to the patient's level of activation.[31] They are also using the PAM score to reduce readmission rates by tailoring the type and amount of post-discharge support to the patient's activation level. Similarly, Peace Health Medical Group in Oregon is using PAM scores as "the new vital sign" in their patient-centered medical home.[32] Combined with the acuity of the patient's health condition, PAM scores determine the members of the healthcare team, including health coaches for those with lower activation scores. This approach has demonstrated reductions in emergency department and urgent care use, increases in the percent of patients with controlled blood pressure, and improved patient satisfaction.

ENGAGING PATIENTS AND FAMILIES

Despite the fact that many systems are not designed to support patient/family engagement in care delivery processes, the reality of medicine in the 21st century is that innovations in pharmaceuticals, medical devices, and surgical care combined with initiatives to make care more efficient mean that patients and caregivers must adhere to complex home regimens and lifestyle recommendations, make difficult care decisions, and even coordinate care among multiple providers.[33] This changing patient role not simply assumes, but indeed requires, that patients have the knowledge, skills, and confidence to act, and that they will indeed perform the necessary actions.[34] However, there exists a gap between expectations of patients and families and their actual performance.[33] For example, in the case of initiatives to promote patient safety, patients are expected to (1) assist with infection control through queries of provider hand washing; (2) choose safe providers; (3) consent and adhere to treatment; and (4) double check health records and ask questions about care processes.[35] Yet research shows that whether a patient or family member actually performs the necessary safety behaviors depends on a variety of factors. For example, the type of error they are trying to prevent, the action required, and whether that action is proactive or reactive, one-time or continuous, and involves interaction—and specifically confrontation—with a practitioner all contribute to the decision to perform safety behaviors.[35] Indeed, despite patients' and families' positive attitudes toward engaging in safety efforts, feeling comfortable about taking action and worrying about the consequences of the medical error are much better drivers of actually taking action than cognitive perceptions or explanations of a potential risk.[35]

STRATEGIES FOR ENGAGING PATIENTS

To function fully and effectively, healthcare systems must rely on patients to be engaged and perform actions to manage their health and healthcare. However, providers and healthcare systems range in their desire and capacity to engage patients in direct patient care, organizational processes, governance, and policymaking,[36] and thus limit the degree to which patients can participate. At the lowest level of engagement, patients and families serve strictly in a consultative role, such as receiving information the provider chooses to share or answering surveys of care experiences.[36] Mid-level involvement is where providers may ask about patient preferences in treatment planning or include patients and families as members of committees. At the highest level of engagement, patients and families serve in partnership or shared leadership with providers and systems, including co-developing treatment plans and co-leading key institutional committees.[36] No matter where a provider or healthcare system falls along this continuum of engagement, most individuals still need support to participate. Following are strategies to help patients and families increase their capacity for engagement, as well as their actual participation.

INCREASING PATIENT AND FAMILY CAPACITY FOR ENGAGEMENT

Improve health literacy. Health literacy is consistently a barrier to patients' ability to manage their health and exercise control over healthcare decisions.[34] Time constraints in both inpatient and outpatient settings exacerbate the problem of health literacy because clinicians must explain sometimes complicated conditions or therapies in a streamlined fashion and do not have the opportunity to expound or answer multiple detailed questions. This is where pamphlets or health information technology can increase patient knowledge and support providers in information sharing. Informational leaflets and web-based educational modules on chronic and acute illness, disease management, therapeutic options, and recommended questions to ask the provider can improve the quality and quantity of information sharing with patients and families. Patients can receive this information before and between visits or with test results, so the clinical visit can be tailored to individual patients and focus on their questions and discussions of information already received. Similarly, decision aid tools can assist patients with understanding and selecting treatment options.[34] Decision aids provide patients and families evidence-based information about all of the available options and possible outcomes, including risks and benefits.[37] Some decision aids help patients and families to consider what is important to them when considering treatment options.[38] Studies suggest that decision aids better inform patients about their options than usual care.[38] Furthermore, for conditions with stigma, such as mental health problems or HIV, decision aids can help patients and families to obtain information in a less threatening way than a face-to-face encounter with a clinician.[16]

Improve self-care and self-management. Patients play a significant role in managing their health through health behaviors, and individuals with low engagement frequently report not having the knowledge or confidence to perform the actions necessary to effectively manage their health and healthcare.[33,39] There are a number of ways that providers and healthcare systems can help patients to improve their self-management and obtain the greatest benefit from care received. Further, offering such support demonstrates to patients, caregivers, and families that the provider and the system believe they are important members of the care team and want them to assume personal responsibility to the degree possible and desired.[34] Self-care and management support can be provided at a population level, as well as one-to-one. At a population level, strategies such as health fairs and brown bag sessions for medication screenings can bring patients with various health conditions and management skills to a single venue for both general health information (eg, relationship of high LDL to heart disease) and personalized information (eg, cholesterol screen, BMI, blood pressure, onsite medication counseling with information on possible interactions).[5] At a more intensive and individualized level, patients may be offered assistance through peer mentors, patient navigators, and health coaches, who provide support and guidance, and empower patients to obtain information on their own and connect to resources for improved self-care.[40]

In a pediatric setting, parents and caregivers undertake this significant role in managing their child's illness and navigating the healthcare system.[41] Thus, educational strategies must be provided in a developmentally appropriate way, such that parents assume all or most of the control when the child is young, but this control transitions to the patient as he/she becomes capable of monitoring symptoms and taking medications independently. Furthermore, strategies to improve care and management in the pediatric setting need to consider the fact that research shows parents' and caregivers' confidence and knowledge about their *own* health directly influence their management of their child's health.[42] Parents with greater self-efficacy in managing their own conditions translated this ability to their children and reported better management of their child's health. Conversely, parents who reported low self-efficacy in managing their own health reported less confidence and knowledge to manage their child's condition. However, when parents were taught skills to better manage their child's condition, improvements in care occurred.[43] Thus, there may be benefit in understanding how parents manage their own health in order to tailor strategies for assisting them with care and management of their children.

Inform patients of their rights. Another strategy to engage patients, caregivers, and families for quality and safety improvement is to inform them of their rights within the healthcare system.[5] Many people who interact with providers and healthcare systems do not know or understand what they have a right to do and say in order to ensure they or their loved ones are receiving the highest quality and safest care available. This includes the rights to be fully informed, to ask questions, to choose among alternatives, to refuse treatment, and to delegate decision-making responsibility.[34] In a truly patient- and family-centered system, these rights extend to full transparency and a culture wherein the locus of control rests with patients, caregivers, and families to the extent they desire it, not with the provider or healthcare system.[6] The ability to exert these rights will depend in part on the degree to which providers and systems support patients and families to improve health literacy and self-management/self-care. In a fully integrated approach, educating patients and families about their rights will be incorporated into these other engagement efforts.

INCREASING PATIENT AND FAMILY INVOLVEMENT: FROM CONSULTATION TO PARTNERSHIP

In addition to implementing strategies to increase patient/family engagement in care, quality and safety will be enhanced when providers and healthcare systems move away from simply consulting with patients and families, and instead focus efforts on strategies to **partner with** them in the delivery process.[36] Some of these approaches are outlined below.

Shared Decision-Making

Partnering with patients in their treatment and inviting them to share in the decision-making process helps individuals to understand their current health status, their risks for worsening symptoms and/or events, and what to expect from the different treatment options available to them.[44] Patients and families should be as involved as they want to be in this process.[6] Involving patients in care planning and treatment decisions not only respects the patient's rights and preferences, but also aids in prevention and early identification of errors and highlights inconsistencies in protocols. For example, patients and families involved in care decisions may better recognize when treatment or its side effects deviate from what is expected, and they can alert providers more quickly and before a serious adverse event occurs.[45] Further, patients and families are more likely to adhere to treatments when they participated in deciding the course of action.[46] Shared decision-making takes several forms.

Information Sharing

For patients and families to fully participate as an equal member of the care team, they must have access to the same information as providers. This means that patients and families should be informed about any test results, treatment plans, protocols, and procedures to the degree they wish to know this information.[47] In the outpatient setting, electronic health records facilitate information sharing with limited burden on the part of the provider. Conversely, access to health records in inpatient settings is infrequent. However, a patient- and family-centered care initiative in the St. Barnabus Neonatal Intensive Care Unit (NICU) is challenging this traditional paradigm. Parents of NICU patients receive a daily update via a newsletter about their infant, "Your Baby's Daily Update (YBDU)," which is generated by the electronic health record.[48] The newsletter was developed in collaboration with parents who had children in the NICU, physicians, nurses, and informaticists, and it includes information on the baby's health status, the medical care they received, and their progress. The newsletter has helped parents be more involved in their infant's care and better contribute to medical decision-making. This model may be used in other inpatient settings to give patients and families access to the same information as providers in order to increase their capacity to participate in decision-making.

Shared Care Plans

Shared care planning involves the co-creation of a plan of care with input from both providers and patients/families.[11] The plan includes mutual goal setting about the desired health outcomes, and the treatment and self-management strategies needed to achieve those goals. In an inpatient setting, shared care planning most often occurs through conversations during critical points in the stay, including multidisciplinary bedside rounds, transitions in care, and shift changes. In outpatient settings, shared care planning may occur in a variety of ways, including online and in-person pre-visit questionnaires, conversations during the visit, in health education, coaching, or mentoring sessions with nurses or other team members, and via an electronic health record. For example, My PREVENT Plan is a personalized health and care planning tool where providers and patients can update information from test results or home monitoring. This information is shared between provider and patient via the electronic record, and it may be used to refine goals of care.[44]

Development and Review of Goals

Developing goals and associated metrics for care is critical to evaluating how patients, providers, and healthcare systems are doing. In inpatient settings, a daily goal sheet assists with this process. The daily goal sheet outlines every goal for the patient for a particular day or shift. These goals, which may address physical, emotional, or spiritual aspects of care, should be developed in collaboration with the patient and his or her family based on their preferences and discussion of the patient's clinical status and prognosis. For example, a clinical (physical) goal might be to have a patient off his or her ventilator by the end of the day. An emotional goal might be that the patient experiences less fear while weaning off the ventilator. Once the providers and patients/families agree on the daily or shift goals, they should be written on the white board in the patient's room. This way all staff associated with the patient's care, the patient, and the patient's family are on the same page as to what the patient's goals are for treatment.

Another example of goal setting is in the pediatric emergency department, where standardized tools have been used to improve parent-provider communication around the purpose of the visit and goals for treatment. A quality improvement initiative demonstrated that a one-page form asking parents about their worries, questions, and expectations for the visit improved eight domains of communication, including parents' involvement in care decisions.[49] In an outpatient setting, goals should be established collaboratively between the patient and provider in 3-, 6-, and 12-month increments and reviewed on a quarterly basis.[44] Goals should be documented in the medical record, and if the record is not electronic and accessible to the patient, they should be provided in a written form that the patient can take home, such as a calendar or goal-tracking sheet. Goals should be revised based on the patient's progress toward the goal according to self-report and clinical metrics (eg, blood pressure control, hemoglobin A1c below a desired threshold, BMI, etc.).

Coordination of Care and Care Transitions

As rates of multi-morbidity and chronic disease associated with lifestyle behaviors increase, effective care of patients requires input from various clinicians, including general and specialty providers, health educators, behaviorists, and of course, the patients themselves. Moreover, for chronically ill patients who transition between inpatient, outpatient, and skilled care facilities, communication and coordination among the various providers are critical for successful transitions. Creating and leveraging opportunities for multiple members of the care team—including patients and their families—to convene, share information, and make decisions jointly, helps to ensure that patients are actively involved in their care. In inpatient settings, conducting multidisciplinary bedside rounds that actively involve and engage the patient and family is one way to ensure patients hear from and provide their input to all members of the clinical team. As discussed in Chapter 6, these rounds are done throughout the day and at shift changes so that all team members know the treatment plan, daily goals, and progress toward meeting those goals.

Another way to ensure effective coordination and transition of care is to include patients in handovers when their care is transferred from one provider to another. During the handover, the patient is introduced to the new provider, both the patient and the new provider are updated on progress toward achieving outcomes and goals, and the patient's feelings about those goals are reassessed. Kaiser Permanente employs the Nurse Knowledge Exchange (NKE) handoff practice to involve patients in the process of nursing shift changes.[50] In the NKE practice, nurses verbally hand off patient care at the bedside using standardized tools and language. One of these tools is i-SBAR, which stands for Introduce-Situation-Background-Assessment-Recommendation. After introducing the new nursing staff, the nurses communicate with the patient regarding the status of his or her care and what to expect during the next shift. Nurses have a 60-second framing conversation before entering the patient's room to help focus the conversation and determine two to three items to keep at the forefront. Some units incorporate a whiteboard in the process so the nurse can write down what is going to happen, and patients and families can document any questions for the next exchange. Nurses finish the handoff by asking patients to "teach back" the material covered in the exchange. This is also a time to invite patient and family questions or correct information they believe is inaccurate. Similar to engaging patients in shift handovers, engaging patients and families in the discharge handover process (eg, from impatient to skilled facility or home) ensures that patients, caregivers, and families can voice any need for successfully transitioning, contribute to development of the discharge plan, and be knowledgeable of its contents, including expectations for follow-up and the metrics established to determine whether the patient is progressing or at risk for readmission.

Listen to and Learn From Patient and Family Feedback

As previously mentioned, the nuances of the care experience are not lost on patients. They are acutely aware of the efficiency (or lack thereof) of the care they receive, how well providers "get along" with each other and the system, and how well they feel on prescribed regimens or when leaving a facility. Additionally, when working across the continuum of care, patients and families are the only ones who experience and know the full journey along their illness trajectory and across sites of care. They know the "white spaces" between providers and organizations. They have knowledge that providers and health systems do not have to keep them safe in transitions. Organizations should tap into this wealth of knowledge to help identify gaps in care and areas of opportunity for improvement. Some sources for patient feedback include:

- Patient experience surveys
- Observations of the patient/family experience of care
- Focus groups
- Compliment/complaint letters

- Safety hotlines
- Staff feedback
- Community groups
- Patient and family council advisors
- Patients as members and/or co-leads of the patient safety and other committees

Information from these feedback sources should be analyzed and prioritized along with other issue identification and performance data. The patient safety officer plays a critical role in reviewing, analyzing, prioritizing, and utilizing these data in support of initiatives aimed at improvements in policies, procedures, and protocols.

Involve Patients and Their Families in Organizational and Policy Discussions and Decisions

To truly partner with patients, providers and systems must involve them in organizational policy-making. This may mean inviting them to participate on or co-lead an organization's quality or safety committee, sentinel event review panel, or other performance improvement–related committee.[36] While some organizations may balk at this idea—believing it exposes the organization to potential lawsuits or bad press—others like Duke and Dana Farber have embraced the concept, choosing to learn from patient perspectives and experiences rather than trying to deny them.

Consider this example: A patient/family advisor whose mother developed a *C. difficile* infection while hospitalized joined the safety and quality committee. As the group was setting hand hygiene improvement goals for the next year, the clinicians and staff had an extended conversation about what was an achievable goal and whether it should be 85% or 87%. The family advisor listened respectfully, and then asked "Why isn't the goal 100%?" The nature of the conversation changed dramatically to how fast the hospital could achieve 100%. Had this committee not included the patient/family representative, it is clear the goal likely would have remained below 90%, which, from this family member's perspective, was insufficient. Patient and family member participation can elevate standards, draw attention to issues that clinical and other staff do not recognize as problematic, and provide a different lens for how to frame and solve a problem. Patient and family input should also be directly involved in the design and improvement of programs that affect patients. For example, if an organization is creating a new website, they should involve patients, caregivers, and family members in the design process. Consumers can provide unique feedback on the site's ease of use and the appropriateness of the content and flow that will not only enhance the product, but also better meet the needs of those using the site.

Involve Patients in Provider Education

There is no better way to educate physicians, nurses, and other direct care providers on the importance of communicating effectively with patients than to have a patient share his or her care experiences with the team. Providers may not be aware of how their tone, affectations, and bedside manner impact patients, but listening to a patient share his or her care experience can sometimes bring new insight to clinicians. Patient/Family advisors can be highly effective in assisting with orientation of new staff and providers through sharing their stories and describing what matters to them most.

Some institutions are including patients and patient advocates as instructors in training courses for clinicians. DUHS is one of five national training sites for the Team STEPPS™ National Implementation program. Team STEPPS™ is an evidence-based, train-the-trainer curriculum that teaches effective communication and teamwork skills to participants through didactic lectures and small-group interactive sessions.[51] Duke leaders have invited members of the DUHS Patient Advocacy Council (comprised of volunteer patients and community members) to be trained as Team STEPPS™ Master Trainers, along with clinicians who complete the same training. As Master Trainers, patient advocates participate on instructor teams with clinician trainers, and teach future Team STEPPS™ courses. Patient safety leaders at Duke believe that these clinician/patient instructor teams provide a model of the institution's commitment to facilitating patient engagement and strengthening the provider/patient partnership.

Another curriculum for healthcare providers was recently created by the Josie King Foundation, in partnership with educators at Duke. The curriculum is based on the book, *Josie's Story*, written by Sorrel King to share the experience of Josie's death through her family's eyes. Over the past several years, Sorrel became aware that an increasing number of medical and nursing schools were using *Josie's Story* as a tool to educate students about the importance of patient- and family-centered care. The Josie King foundation found their mailboxes overflowing with letters and "reflection papers" from students around the country. Not only were they assigned the book to read but they were also asked to write papers on the impact the story had on them, their future careers, and their lives. In an effort to build upon this work, the Foundation reached out to educators from Duke University's School of Medicine and School of Nursing to create a more robust patient safety curriculum based on *Josie's Story*. The curriculum is centered around the notion that, while facts bring us knowledge, stories bring us wisdom. The goal of the Josie King patient safety curriculum is not only to educate the next generation of healthcare providers about the importance of patient and family engagement, but rather to inspire them to develop true partnerships with the patients and families they encounter.

Involve Family Presence Whenever Possible

Undergoing medical procedures can be intimidating, but being separated from loved ones who can provide support makes even routine procedures more stressful. This is especially so in pediatric settings, where infants and young children do not have the cognitive capacity to understand everything that is happening, and parents and children may be separated during extended stays in intensive care and neonatal units, or when parents must eat, sleep, or return to work. By necessity, parents and/or caregivers of pediatric patients will participate on behalf of or with the patient (depending upon the child's age) in discussions of diagnosis, prognosis, treatment options, and treatment decisions. The ability to participate in these discussions should be extended to other family members as well, as the patient and/or parents wish. Family members may offer a different perspective on the child, which can enhance discussions of treatment options, goals, and care plans.[9] One way to encourage parental and family involvement is to maintain open access to nursing units, intensive care units (ICUs), and the emergency department. By keeping these areas open to families 24 hours a day—even during shift changes, rounds, resuscitation events, and other emergency situations—family involvement is encouraged. Furthermore, the presence of family members who can ask questions about the care being provided and contribute information about the patient's health has the potential to decrease errors and increase patient safety. Along the same lines, those organizations that allow family members to stay during anesthesia induction, in the recovery room, in radiology, and during treatment and procedures open up the healthcare environment, increase transparency, and reduce the potential for errors. This is especially important in pediatric care, where the patient may not have the capacity to fully participate.

MEASURES OF SUCCESS

As providers and healthcare systems engage in efforts to provide patient- and family-centered care, it will be important to evaluate quality and safety metrics to determine the degree to which their efforts are making a difference. The HCAHPS (Hospital Consumer Assessment of Healthcare Providers and Systems) survey is a national, standardized, and publicly reported assessment tool that hospitals can use to assess how patients view their institution before and after implementing patient engagement strategies, as well evaluate how their ratings compare to other similar or geographically proximate entities.[52] Depending upon the changes instituted, composite scores of particular interest may include ratings of how well providers communicate with patients in general and specifically about medication, how responsive staff are to patients' needs, and whether key information is provided at discharge.

For pediatrics, individual and health system providers can obtain information about quality metrics from the CAHPS Health Plan Survey 4.0H, Child Version (CPC).[53] The CPC obtains information on parents' experience with their child's health plan, including ratings of overall health care, primary provider, specialty provider, how well doctors communicate, and shared decision-making. The Children with Chronic Conditions (CCC) measure obtains information on parents' experience with their child's health care specifically for children with chronic conditions. In addition to the above metrics, the CCC also assesses the degree to which clinicians provide family-centered care, including having a personal provider who knows the child, the parents' ability to get needed information, and how well the child's care is coordinated.[53]

The Pediatric Quality Measures Program (PQMP) is a relatively recent initiative authorized by the Children's Health Insurance Program Reauthorization Act.[54] The purpose of PQMP is to improve and strengthen the initial core set of children's health care quality measures established in February 2011 by expanding and advancing development of new and emerging, evidence-based measures. Annually the PQMP will post improved core sets of quality measures recommended by expert panels for voluntary use by state Medicaid and CHIP programs, as well as private sector insurers, providers, families, and patients. The measures identified through this process will help entities to assess quality using the most robust and cutting-edge metrics.

In addition to standardized metrics, entities also may monitor and evaluate their efforts by conducting focus groups of patients and families. Unlike quantitative surveys, focus groups can provide more in-depth information on numeric ratings, a range of opinions, and explanatory data about factors that influence opinions, behaviors, and ratings.[55] When considering possible changes or initiatives to implement, group interactions in focus groups also can stimulate new ideas and provide deeper insight into problems and solutions through in-depth discussions among people with diverse perspectives.[55] When evaluating processes and protocols, focus groups can be particularly helpful because they can elicit specific information about how well the steps work or not, and what could be done to improve them. This type of information generally cannot be obtained from standardized quantitative surveys.

CONCLUSION

Achieving a "patient-centric culture" requires significant effort on the part of institutions, their staff, their consumers, and their leaders. Institutions must invite all members to the table—from clinicians and staff to patients and families—to create a clear vision for patient-centricity, promote it among staff and patients, and invest in resources and training to build the collaborative capacity of all involved. For greatest success, system-wide change that occurs incrementally with frequent pauses for monitoring and evaluation is likely to reap the greatest benefits. However, external financial and political pressures sometimes spark swift changes for which systems may or may not be fully ready. In both cases, patient and family engagement in these processes is critical. Maintaining the presence and the voice of those whom providers and healthcare systems serve in decision-making and evaluation can help to ensure that processes, systems, and programs are as safe as possible and of the highest quality, or being modified to be so. Through the meaningful engagement and partnership of patients and families in these endeavors, true patient- and family-centered care is attainable.

IN PRACTICE

Increasing patient and family engagement in a clinical practice or institution is an iterative process that takes time. However, small steps can be taken now to begin moving toward more patient- and family-centered care. The steps below can prime the pump for true provider-health system-patient-family partnership.

INDIVIDUAL PROVIDERS

1. **Ask patients/families at least one question per visit or bedside rounds that elicits what is important to them.** Some examples include: What is one reason you want to improve your child's health? What is the best possible outcome of our time together? If we "get this right today," name one thing your child will be able to do a month from now that s/he can't do now? What do you need before you feel safe/comfortable taking your child home?

2. **Incorporate the patient's/family member's answer into your discussion of the care plan.** Patients rely on providers for information about their health and how to manage it. When you present options, link those options to what they say is important to them. For example, if the parent of a sickle cell patient says, "I would like for my child to have more pain free days, so that she can enjoy the dancing she loves," make pain management a priority of the visit.

3. **Encourage your patients to complete satisfaction surveys.** Verbally tell your patients that you – and the institution – want their feedback.

(Continued)

(*Continued*)

Remind them before they leave the office or before discharge to complete the form or web-based survey. The more you let them know you value what they have to say, the more willing they will be to participate and provide useful information.

4. **Share your HCAHP ranking.** Let clinical and non-clinical staff, as well as patients and families, know how you're doing – compare yourself to last year and to others in the region. The transparency – especially on the areas of weakness – invites patients and families into the conversation.

5. **Address your lowest HCAHP score.** Invite everyone who is involved—staff, patients, members of the community—to an open forum to discuss the score, the issues that contributed to it, and some ideas on how to raise it.

6. **Assess the state of your institution's engagement practices.** Identify if the style is based on consultation, involvement, or partnership for clinical care, processes, governance, and policy. Notice if there is alignment or mismatch in engagement practices across the different domains. Bring this information to key meetings. Bring these observations into relevant discussions.

7. **Provide patients and families with multiple ways to give feedback.** Offer comment cards, telephone numbers, web-based surveys, and mail-in surveys. Place reminders throughout the institution to complete comment cards. Making complaining as easy as—or easier—than complimenting because complaints will lead to improvements.

FAQs

1. What is the best way to provide information to patients?

   There are still limited data on the most effective forms of information delivery for patients. The best way to address this is to have at least two delivery options (eg, pamphlet and video) for any given set of information (eg, questions to ask your provider, or safety behaviors) and ask the patient/family member which they prefer.

2. How does a Patient Advisory Council (PAC) help improve patient/family engagement?

   Creation of a PAC provides structure that can facilitate efforts of healthcare organizations to treat patients and families as partners in, rather than recipients of care. Examples of PAC activities include

(1) advising on health system/hospital policies and programs; (2) identifying system-level issues that affect patient care; (3) improving customer satisfaction; (4) providing a link between the health system/ hospital and the larger community; and (5) participating in the education of healthcare professionals.

3. What practices should we implement in the clinical setting to improve patient engagement?

   Examples of evidence-based practices to enhance patient engagement include bedside rounds, daily care plan (shared care plans), and Condition H (Condition Help).

4. Where can I get help or guidance on tools and strategies to increase patient/family engagement?

   Agency for Healthcare Research and Quality (AHRQ) tool kit; Institute for Patient and Family Centered Care; National Patient Safety Foundation; Josie King Foundation.

REFERENCES

1. National Patient Safety Foundation. Patient safety imperative for health care reform. *National Patient Safety Foundation.* 2009. Available at: http://www.npsf.org/about-us/lucian-leape-institute-at-npsf/lli-reports-and-statements/the-patient-safety-imperative-for-health-care-reform/.

2. Polta. Defining patient engagement. *Health Beat: A Blog About All Things Health.* 2012. Available at: http://healthbeat.areavoices.com/2012/03/30/defining-patient-engagement/.

3. Danis M, Solomon M. Providers, payers, the community, and patients are all obliged to get patient activation and engagement ethically right. *Health Aff (Millwood).* 2013;32(2):401-407.

4. Hibbard JH, Greene J. What the evidence shows about patient activation: better health outcomes and care experiences; fewer data on costs. *Health Aff (Millwood).* 2013;32(2):207-214.

5. Awé C, Lin SJ. A patient empowerment model to prevent medication errors. *J Med Syst.* 2003;27(6):503-517.

6. Berwick DM. What 'patient-centered' should mean: confessions of an extremist. *Health Aff (Millwood).* 2009;28(4):w555-w565.

7. Haidet P, Kroll TL, Sharf BF. The complexity of patient participation: lessons learned from patients' illness narratives. *Patient Educ Couns.* 2006;62(3):323-329.

8. Weingart SN, Zhu J, Chiappetta L, et al. Hospitalized patients' participation and its impact on quality of care and patient safety. *Int J Qual Health Care.* 2011;23(3):269-277.

9. Hibbard JH, Greene J, Overton V. Patients with lower activation associated with higher costs; delivery systems should know their patients' 'scores'. *Health Aff (Millwood).* 2013;32(2):216-222.

10. An M, Palisano RJ. Family-professional collaboration in pediatric rehabilitation: a practice model. *Disabil Rehabil*. 2014;36(5):434-440.

11. Cohen M. Causes of medication errors. In: Cohen M, ed. *Medication Errors. American Pharmaceutical Association*. Washington, DC; 1999.

12. Coulter A. Paternalism or partnership. *BMJ*. 1999;319:719-720.

13. Hall J, Peat M, Birks Y, et al. Effectiveness of interventions designed to promote patient involvement to enhance safety: a systematic review. *Qual Saf Health Care*. 2010;19(5):e10.

14. Davis RE, Sevdalis N, Jacklin R, Vincent CA. An examination of opportunities for the active patient in improving patient safety. *J Patient Saf*. 2012;8(1):36-43.

15. Longtin Y, Sax H, Leape LL, et al. Patient participation: current knowledge and applicability to patient safety. *Mayo Clin Proc*. 2010;85(1):53-62.

16. Koutantji M, Davis R, Vincent C, Coulter A. The patient's role in patient safety: engaging patients, their representatives, and health professionals. *Clinical Risk*. 2005;11:99-104.

17. Hibbard JH, Peters E, Slovic P, Tusler M. Can patients be part of the solution? Views on their role in preventing medical errors. *Med Care Res Rev*. 2005;62(5):601-616.

18. Bechtel C, Ness DL. If you build it, will they come? Designing truly patient-centered health care. *Health Aff (Millwood)*. 2010;29(5):914-920.

19. Chen LM, Farwell WR, Jha AK. Primary care visit duration and quality: does good care take longer? *Arch Intern Med*. 2009;169(20):1866-1872.

20. Maurer M, Dardess P, Carman KL, et al. Guide to patient and family engagement: environmental scan report. (Prepared by American Institutes for Research under contract HHSA 290-200-600019). AHRQ Publication No. 12-0042-EF. Rockville, MD: Agency for Healthcare Research and Quality; 2012.

21. Institute for Patient- and Family-Centered Care. *Frequently Asked Questions*. 2010. Available at: http://www.ipfcc.org/faq.html.

22. Maizes V, Rakel D, Niemiec C. Integrative medicine and patient-centered care. Institute of Medicine Summit. 2009. Available at: http://www.iom.edu/~/media/Files/Activity%20Files/Quality/IntegrativeMed/Integrative%20Medicine%20and%20Patient%20Centered%20Care.pdf.

23. National Patient Safety Foundation. Available at: http://www.npsf.org.

24. AHRQ. Questions to ask your doctor. Available at: http://www.ahrq.gov/patients-consumers/patient-involvement/ask-your-doctor/index.html.

25. Five Steps to Safer Health Care: Patient Fact Sheet. 2004. Agency for Healthcare Research and Quality, Rockville, MD. Available at: http://www.ahrq.gov/patients-consumers/care-planning/errors/5steps/index.htm.

26. Partnership for Patients. Centers for Medicare and Medicaid Services. Available at http://partnershipforpatients.cms.gov/

27. Conway J, Nathan D, Benz E, et al. Key learning from the Dana-Farber Cancer Institute's 10-year patient safety journey. In: *Am Soc Clin Oncol*. 42nd Annual Meeting, Atlanta, GA; 2006:615-619.

28. Ponte PR, Conlin G, Conway JB, et al. Making patient-centered care come alive: achieving full integration of the patient's perspective. *J Nurs Adm*. 2003;33:82-90. AND Reid Ponte P, Connor M, DeMarco R, et al. Linking patient and family-centered care and patient safety: the next leap. *Nurs Econ*. 2004;22:211-213, 5.

29. World Health Organization. Patients for patient safety. Available at: http://www.who.int/patientsafety/patients_for_patient/en/.

30. Hibbard JH, Stockard J, Mahoney ER, Tusler M. Development of the patient activation measure (PAM): conceptualizing and measuring activation in patients and consumers. *Health Serv Res*. 2004;39(4 Pt 1):1005-1026.

31. Chen P. Getting patients to take charge of their health. *Well Blog - NY Times*. 2012. Available at: http://well.blogs.nytimes.com/2012/01/12/getting-patients-to-take-charge-of-their-health/?_r=0.

32. Blash L, Dower C, Chapman S. Peacehealth's team fillingame uses patient activation measure to customize the medical home. UCSF Center for the Health Professions, 2011. Available at: http://www.futurehealth.ucsf.edu/Content/11660/2011_05_PeaceHealth's_Team%20Fillingame_Uses_Patient_Activation_Measures_to_Customize_the_Medical_Home.pdf. Accessed 19.06.14.

33. Gruman J, Rovner MH, French ME, et al. From patient education to patient engagement: implications for the field of patient education. *Patient Educ Couns*. 2010;78(3):350-356.

34. Coulter A, Ellins J. Effectiveness of strategies for informing, educating, and involving patients. *BMJ*. 2007;335(7609):24-27.

35. Schwappach DL. Review: engaging patients as vigilant partners in safety: a systematic review. *Med Care Res Rev*. 2010;67(2):119-148.

36. Carman KL, Dardess P, Maurer M, et al. Patient and family engagement: a framework for understanding the elements and developing interventions and policies. *Health Aff (Millwood)*. 2013;32(2):223-231.

37. Foundation Decision Aids (Shared Decision-Making® programs). *Informed Medical Decisions Foundation*. Informed Medical Decisions Foundation. Available at: http://informedmedicaldecisions.org/shared-decision-making-in-practice/decision-aids/.

38. Patient Decision Aids. *AHRQ Effective Health Care Program*. Agency for Healthcare Research and Quality. Available at http://effectivehealthcare.ahrq.gov/index.cfm/tools-and-resources/patient-decision-aids/.

39. Barry MJ. Health decision aids to facilitate shared decision making in office practice. *Ann Intern Med*. 2002;136(2):127-135.

40. Hibbard JH, Stockard J, Mahoney ER, Tusler M. Development of the patient activation measure (PAM): conceptualizing and measuring activation in patients and consumers. *Health Serv Res*. 2004;39(4 Pt 1):1005-1026.

41. Holzmueller CG, Wu AW, Pronovost PJ. A framework for encouraging patient engagement in medical decision making. *J Patient Saf*. 2012;8(4):161-164.

42. Pennarola BW, Rodday AM, Mayer DK, et al. Factors associated with parental activation in pediatric hematopoietic stem cell transplant. *Med Care Res Rev*. 2012;69(2):194-214.

43. Warren-Findlow J, Seymour RB, Shenk D. Intergenerational transmission of chronic illness self-care: results from the caring for hypertension in African American families study. *Gerontologist*. 2010;51(1):64-75.

44. Bollinger LM, Nire KG, Rhodes MM, et al. Caregivers' perspectives on barriers to transcranial Doppler screening in children with sickle-cell disease. *Pediatr Blood Cancer*. 2011;56:99-102.

45. Burnette R, Simmons LA, Snyderman R. Personalized health care as a pathway for the adoption of genomic medicine. *J Personalized Med*. 2012;2(4):232-240.

46. Peat M, Entwistle V, Hall J, et al. Scoping review and approach to appraisal of interventions intended to involve patients in patient safety. *J Health Serv Res Policy*. 2010;15(suppl 1):17-25.

47. Martin LR, Williams SL, Haskard KB. Dimatteo MR. The challenge of patient adherence. *Ther Clin Risk Manag*. 2005;1(3):189-99.

48. Palma JP, Keller H, Godin M, et al. Impact of an EMR-based daily patient update letter on communication and parent engagement in a neonatal intensive care unit. *J Particip Med*. 2012;4:e33.

49. Porter SC, Johnston P, Parry G, at al. Improving parent-provider communication in the pediatric emergency department: results from the clear and concise communication campaign. *Pediatr Emerg Care*. 2011;27(2):75-80.

50. Nolan KM, Schalll MW. *Spreading Improvement Across Your Health Care Organization*. Oak Brook, IL: Joint Commission Resources; 2007.

51. TeamSTEPPS™. *Strategies and Tools to Enhance Performance and Patient Safety*. Avaliable at: http://teamstepps.ahrq.gov/abouttoolsmaterials.htm.

52. Center for Medicare and Medicaid Services. Hospital Consumer Assessment of Healthcare Providers and Systems. Fact Sheet, August 2013. Available at: http://www.hcahpsonline.org/files/HCAHPS%20Fact%20Sheet%20May%202012.pdf.

53. National Committee for Quality Assurance. CAHPS survey for Parents Assessment of Child Health Plans. Available at: http://www.ncqa.org/portals/0/CAHPS%20and%20CAHPS%20CC.pdf.

54. Agency for Healthcare Research and Quality. Children's Health Insurance Program Reauthorization Act. Available at: http://www.ahrq.gov/policymakers/chipra/pqmpback.html.

55. Healthcare Georgia Foundation. Available at: http://www.healthcaregeorgia.org/uploads/publications/Using_Focus_Groups_Evaluation.pdf.

SPECIAL PERSPECTIVES FOR NEONATES | 9

"The fact is that most of the biggest catastrophes we've witnessed rarely come from information that is secret or hidden. They come from information that is freely available but that we are willfully blind to because we can't handle the conflict that it provokes."

Margaret Heffernan

The history of neonatology is replete with practitioners whose lifelong focus has been to improve the lives of newborn infants. Such focus predates the existence of neonatology (or, more officially, neonatal-perinatal medicine) as a subspecialty within the field of pediatrics. Indeed, the first significant premature neonatal outcomes project dates back to the 1870s, when famed Parisian perinatologist StéphaneTarnier pioneered and publicized the use of incubators (a derivative of chicken incubators) to save premature infants from hypothermia.[1] Although incubators had also been designed by Tarnier's contemporaries in the 19th century Russia and Germany, he claimed that his implementation of incubator use at the Paris Maternité hospital resulted in a drop in mortality for infants weighing 1,200 grams to 2,000 grams from 66 to 38%[2]—an impressive quality improvement project in any era.

One may ask why neonatologists then and now are so fixated on improving the safety of newborn intensive care unit (NICU) care and improving outcomes for our NICU graduates. This chapter will begin with highlighting some of the reasons that both the NICU itself and its patients are truly different from anywhere else in a hospital. Several examples of NICU collaboratives will then be discussed—groups existing at the local, state, national, and international levels formed primarily around the goals of providing opportunities for collaboration, generating new evidence, benchmarking, and dissemination of best practices. Next, the inherently multidisciplinary process of quality improvement within the NICU will be examined through three case studies: medication safety, central-line-associated bloodstream infections, and necrotizing enterocolitis. Finally, future opportunities for improving outcomes and reducing harm in the era of "big data" will be reviewed. But first, as it is impossible to predict the future without understanding the past, further discussion of the history of achievements in neonatal quality improvement will be provided.

BACKGROUND

In the world of medicine, neonatology is a relatively young subspecialty. Both the first board exam in neonatal-perinatal medicine and the first subspecialty meeting within the American Academy of Pediatrics occurred in 1975.[3] Yet even before the field's inception, its practitioners have been tightly and jointly focused on improving the quality of newborn critical care. Over 20 years before neonatology was recognized as an official subspecialty, Virginia Apgar (an obstetric anesthesiologist) standardized delivery room management with neonatology's first "check-list"—the APGAR score.[4] Since then, efforts to reduce harm and improve neonatal outcomes have yielded many of neonatology's signature advances in the last 50 years, including:

- The development of exogenous surfactant,
- Hyperalimentation,
- Miniaturization of blood testing volumes,
- Continuous monitoring including pulse oximetry,
- Methylxanthines for apnea of prematurity,
- Therapeutic hypothermia in the setting of hypoxic ischemic encephalopathy, and more.[3]

Similarly, neonatologists' focus on the use of evidence-based medicine has also stopped us from several practices that were once canonical to the field—eg, reduced exposure to high concentrations of oxygen given association with retinopathy of prematurity,[3] more limited use of post-natal corticosteroids to prevent chronic lung disease given concerns about long-term neurodevelopmental impairment, eliminating alkalization as a therapy for persistent pulmonary hypertension, and reduced utilization of prolonged early antibiotics given their association with both necrotizing enterocolitis and death.[5]

If nearly 50 years of neonatology as an official specialty has taught us anything, it is that neonatal care in particular (and thus projects seeking to improve the quality of neonatal care) truly benefits from a multidisciplinary approach. From the earliest partnerships with colleagues in obstetrics and anesthesiology to current partnerships among NICU providers and our colleagues in pediatric surgery, cardiology, neurosurgery, and ancillary medical teams, providing care for the sick neonate must be a coordinated effort. Furthermore, new partnerships in neonatal critical care now extend well beyond medicine's traditional walls, including engineering, members of the school of divinity, and the behavioral/environmental sciences.

Such broad-reaching partnerships explain part of why it is indeed true that the NICU is "different." However, as the next section describes in detail, there is much more to answering the question: "Why?"

WHY THE NICU IS DIFFERENT?

All pediatricians remember the first time they set foot in the NICU during residency. At some point during intern year, each newly minted pediatrics resident crosses the NICU's threshold proclaiming "access restricted to official personnel only" and enters a world apart from anything they've ever experienced within medicine. It's a maxim passed from resident to resident and across generations of pediatricians: "The NICU is just different." And with good reason—the NICU is the only place in the hospital where the same providers may care for human beings 30 times different in size and many times different in age and physiologic maturity side-by-side. NICUs also have comparatively "closed" workforces wherein nurses, advanced practitioners, physicians, and ancillary staff generally spend the vast majority of their clinical time together. Also, unlike other units the NICU has relatively few "casual staff" or "floaters" assisting in the care of its patients. Finally, NICUs can vary significantly in size and acuity. Some of the biggest units in the United States top out well over 125 beds and treat the most critically ill infants in the world, while the smallest units may have fewer than 10 beds and treat mostly stable "feeders and growers."

More than staff and size though, it's the NICU's patients themselves who differentiate the unit most from the rest of the hospital when it comes to designing, implementing, and measuring quality improvement projects. These differentiating characteristics can be grouped into five major categories: population variability; rapidly changing physiology; sensitivity to error; the "starting from scratch" concept; and data richness.

POPULATION VARIABILITY

Most intensive care units in large hospitals focus on a particular disease or management process—eg, the surgical ICU, the neurological ICU, the cardiothoracic ICU, etc. Only two—the pediatric ICU and the neonatal ICU—are differentiated almost entirely by a patient's age. While the PICU certainly sees its share of variety in patients, diseases, and management needs, the spectrum of care within a NICU spans an even greater range.

Consider a day in the life of a large academic medical center NICU. In the morning, a team may focus on providing acute, critical care to newborn

24-week twins including active resuscitation in the delivery room, intubation, and urgent central venous and arterial line placement. Attention may then focus on the 2-week-old former 24-week infant on high-frequency ventilation requiring bedside surgery for ligation of a patent ductus arteriosus, or on a 3-week-old former 25-week infant undergoing bedside abdominal surgery for acute pneumoperitoneum secondary to necrotizing enterocolitis (NEC). The team may then attend a planned cesarean section delivery for an infant with a known congenital cyanotic heart lesion, and an unplanned vaginal delivery of an infant with congenital diaphragmatic hernia with birth depression requiring intubation, external cardiac massage, emergency umbilical venous access, and code-dose epinephrine to maintain circulation. Finally, the team must take care not to ignore the 70 other patients under their care in the NICU, many of whom are "stable" infants weighing less than three pounds trying to "feed and grow" their way to discharge without developing NEC, sepsis, or another complication of extreme prematurity.

While the description above likely (indeed, hopefully) does not occur every day in most NICUs, the breadth of potential clinical scenarios is not an exaggeration. Each infant in a NICU, from newborn to many months old, from extremely premature to post-term (born after 40 weeks gestation), is at a different stage in his or her own unique physiologic development. Each has different needs, limitations, restrictions, and expectations, and requires different management strategies. For example, strategies to manage hypotension while avoiding morbidity in a newborn 24-week infant are quite different from strategies needed to address the same problem in a term infant with meconium aspiration and persistent pulmonary hypertension. Such variation ultimately results in a complex array of demands on the neonatologists and their team's quest to provide the best-individualized therapies for each infant under their care.

IMMATURE PHYSIOLOGY

As has been discussed, infants within a NICU can vary significantly in their stage of development, from extremely premature to term infants, and from newborns to infants preparing to celebrate their first birthdays. Consider just the incredible changes in lung maturation that occur during gestation from 23 weeks through birth for a normal, full-term newborn. At 23 weeks, an infant's lungs are still in the "canalicular stage" of development, having barely completed branching of the bronchial tree and begun forming bronchioles.[6] At a minimum, it takes another 3 weeks before alveolar precursors begin to form, with true alveoli finally beginning to emerge around 32 weeks gestation. While 32-week lungs are orders of magnitude better prepared for ventilation than 28-week lungs, which in turn are orders of magnitude better than 23-week lungs, they still contain many millions fewer alveoli than a term infant's lungs at birth, which then still continue maturing over the first few years of life.[6]

With this in mind, it is clear why the stage of fetal lung development in which infants enter life in the NICU—23 weeks, 28 weeks, 32 weeks, etc.—dictates in large part the limits of their pulmonary physiology. However, gestational age presents only part of the challenges faced by those trying to manage ventilation for premature infants in the NICU. Antenatal steroid administration to preterm mothers is widely accepted as an effective therapy to artificially enhance lung maturity prior to delivery and improve outcomes.[3] On the other hand, "in utero" infections (eg, with *Ureaplasma* or *Mycoplasma*) may actually delay lung maturation. Finally, mechanical ventilation itself—the act of providing positive pressure ventilation either manually or via a conventional or high-frequency ventilator through an endotracheal tube—significantly alters lung development. All of these issues contribute to a developing lung physiology in premature infants that is internally changing and externally being changed throughout the maturation process.

Finally, all of that just covers the lungs—similarly lengthy stories exist for every organ system in the developing fetal body, from cardiac to gastrointestinal, immune, neurologic, even ocular development. Life in the NICU provides the neonatologist with daily reminders from early medical school coursework in embryology, physiology, and human development, all of which must be considered in the management of NICU infants' care, their safety, and ultimately their outcomes.

SENSITIVITY TO ERRORS

Several factors make infants in the NICU exquisitely sensitive to errors in patient care, most specifically around medications. First consider the size of our smallest patients, usually 350 grams to 400 grams, and the concordant volume of any medication they require. Imagine you're electively intubating a 5-day-old 400-gram infant who has failed continuous-positive airway pressure (CPAP) and you choose to use Fentanyl® as an anesthetic agent. A standard dose of 1 microgram per kilogram to 2 micrograms per kilogram for a 400-gram infant (assuming a stock Fentanyl® concentration of 50 micrograms per mL) would result in a final dose of 0.4 micrograms to 0.8 micrograms. At the high end of this dosing range, the actual drug volume is a mere 16 microliters. Recognizing the standard hub volume of a 1-mL syringe is almost 10 times that volume (generally 0.1 mL or 100 microliters), it immediately becomes clear why small errors in measuring drug doses for our smallest NICU patients can be disastrous.

Although size is a major contributor to NICU infants' risk of error, there are several other contributing factors that warrant discussion as well. NICUs are the first and foremost critical care units, a setting where caring for multiple patients on ventilators and pressors is not uncommon and bedside surgery can be a daily or weekly occurrence. Critical care units can be particularly dangerous for patients for a number of reasons[7]—many high-importance tasks are often being done simultaneously, multiple patients may have immediate simultaneous clinical needs, and almost any patient in the unit can experience respiratory or cardiac arrest and immediately become the sickest patient at a moment's notice.

Furthermore, by definition patients requiring critical care have "less reserve" than patients recovering in a regular inpatient or step-down setting. With an inherently lower tolerance for additional physiologic instability, whether caused by personal frailty or their underlying disease process, critical care patients in general and neonatal patients in particular live within a very narrow window of safety. Combine these risks with those inherent to being born 17 weeks early or having intestines in the thorax compressing the heart, lungs, and major blood vessels, and it's easy to see how the holes in James Reason's Swiss cheese model just keep getting larger.[8]

▎ OPPORTUNITY TO "START FROM SCRATCH"

Imagine caring for an average 73-year-old male patient in a medical ICU. Let's presume he's in the ICU with sepsis caused by a foot infection. He has diabetic neuropathy—which explains the foot infection—and a host of other significant co-morbidities including hypertension, congestive heart failure, chronic obstructive pulmonary disease, and hyperlipidemia. Some of his underlying conditions may have genetic underpinnings, but more likely than not much of his past medical history is defined by 73 years of living and making choices about what to eat, where and how to live, what toxic habits to engage in, and so on. Now imagine that same man 73 years ago on the day he was born—no past medical history, no chronic underlying conditions, no opportunity to have made decisions that would either positively or negatively impact his health. That's where everything begins in the NICU.

From the time of birth (in an "inborn" center, where the NICU is able to admit babies directly from the delivery service), providers in the NICU have almost 100% control of an infant's medical history from the moment he is born until the day he is discharged, transferred, or dies. An infant's genetic history, maternal contributions (eg, smoking, medicinal, or street drug use, overall health), and perinatal history (eg, perinatal infection caused by chorioamnionitis, placental abruption, umbilical cord accidents) notwithstanding, the NICU's environment of care will monitor, control, and contribute to every part of a NICU patient's developing medical history. Such practically complete ownership of a patient's outcomes is impossible to develop elsewhere in the hospital where patients enter with laundry lists of other pre-existing co-morbidities. It's an awesome responsibility but also an awesome opportunity to positively affect the trajectory of an infant's entire life as a "NICU graduate."

DATA RICHNESS

In the outpatient world, data trickles in from visit to visit – blood pressure values for chronically hypertensive patients, glucose checks for diabetics, weekly or monthly weight checks for those battling obesity. Even in the most connected, integrated health systems with the most sophisticated, interoperable electronic medical records where every visit with every provider (primary care, nurse-only visit, specialists, dietitians, etc.) is catalogued and monitored, the data available in outpatient medicine by definition are limited visit-to-visit.

In contrast, NICU providers are presented with an immense amount of data pouring in minute-to-minute from many sources at once. Blood gases, chemistries, and hematologic variables are collated and trended day-to-day and week-to-week. Repeated physical examinations over hours and days provide a picture of improving or declining health. Vital signs automatically transfer from monitors to medical record, providing opportunities not only to measure but also to analyze and act upon information and trends in a real-time manner.

Such data richness provides its own benefits and challenges. The University of Virginia published one example of potential benefits by linking trends in heart-rate variability to late-onset neonatal sepsis, adding to the real-time predictability of what is often considered an extremely unpredictable illness.[9] Such real-time data also pours into long-term storage warehouses, providing ample databases for clinical researchers to query, analyze, and tease out answers to retrospective research questions. On the other hand, such immense quantities of data can also become rapidly overwhelming, drowning out signals in a sea of noise. Ultimately, it rests on bedside clinicians' shoulders to assimilate, analyze, and act upon the rich collection of data available within the NICU to best treat their patients.

CONCLUSION

These five NICU characteristics are the primary (but by no means only) drivers of what makes the NICU "different," and must be taken into account when developing neonatal patient safety and quality improvement programs. For example, a NICU-specific program to reduce catheter-associated bloodstream infections must account for the difference in skin integrity between a

3-month-old formerly extremely premature infant and a newly born extremely premature infant, whose delicate skin could burn if exposed to the standard chlorhexidine-based cleaning solution or tear if applied with the standard surgical scrub. An effort to improve survival for extremely low birth weight infants (ELBW, weighing less than 1 kg at birth) must take into account an infant's entire hospital course beginning with the delivery room resuscitation and progressing through ventilator management, feeding strategies, fluid and blood pressure management, antibiotic use, and so on. Projects that seek to standardize medication concentrations must account for the vast differential in potential weight-based doses, balancing the overall goal of minimizing the number of potential concentrations for any one particular drug with the challenge of drawing up extremely small volumes (such as the Fentanyl* scenario described above) for extremely small patients. The list goes on.

Thankfully, such projects rarely proceed down a path that neonatologists or other NICU leaders must walk alone. Neonatology is by definition a collaborative effort, and our next section describes several efforts across the field to convene multiple sites, centers, and providers from multiple backgrounds under the banner of improving the quality of neonatal care.

COLLABORATIVE IMPROVEMENT EFFORTS

For almost 30 years, neonatologists have convened across hospitals within large multi-center collaboratives to perform clinical research, assess quality outcomes, and identify and implement best practices. The four collaboratives discussed here cover the breadth of neonatology, spanning NICUs from large to small, rural to urban, academic to private. The four groups discussed are by no means a comprehensive description of neonatal collaboratives, but are meant to serve as examples of the larger collaborative spirit generally present within neonatology as a whole, ultimately resulting in better, safer care for hospitalized neonates.

VERMONT OXFORD NETWORK

Founded in 1988 by Jerold F. Lucey, MD, Jeffrey D. Horbar, MD, and Roger F. Soll, MD, the Vermont Oxford Network (VON) began as a voluntary collective of NICUs in the United States interested in sharing both data and practices to improve neonatal outcomes.[10] Its primary goal then and now has been to improve "the quality and safety of medical care for newborn infants and their families through a coordinated program of research, education, and quality improvement."[11] From its small roots, VON today has grown to include over 900 member NICUs around the world and curates a database that already contains over one million infants and continues enrolling 50,000 new infants each year.[12]

The VON database provides a treasure trove for outcomes researchers, yielding publications around trends in neonatal mortality and premature outcomes as well as large retrospective analyses on specific clinical questions.[13,14] Membership in VON also entitles each individual NICU access to its own longitudinal outcomes data in comparison to peer institutions, allowing for invaluable benchmarking across units and identifying both best practices and targets for improvement.

VON itself has also generated new knowledge through multi-center randomized, controlled trials including seminal studies on different exogenous surfactant preparations (a substance made naturally by mature lungs but that must be exogenously delivered to premature lungs) and post-natal corticosteroid therapy.[15,16] Finally, through its "NIC/Q" and "iNICQ" collaboratives, NICU professionals can participate in hands-on quality improvement projects and education either in-person or through web-based modules.

NATIONAL INSTITUTE OF CHILD HEALTH AND HUMAN DEVELOPMENT NEONATAL RESEARCH NETWORK

In response to concerns about the lack of evidence for many "standard practices" in NICUs in the 1980s, the National Institute of Child Health and Human Development (NICHD) convened a group of academic centers in 1986 to form the Neonatal Research Network (NRN). Indeed, the NICHD itself was founded in part out of an increased national focus on neonatal health following the death of Patrick Bouvier Kennedy, a 2.11-kg infant born at 34 weeks to President John and Jackie Kennedy in August 1963. Despite his famous parents and access to the best neonatal care of the day, Patrick Kennedy died on his second day of life from "hyaline membrane disease," now known as respiratory distress syndrome, a condition resulting in large part from surfactant deficiency that today is almost always treatable if not curable.

With a focus on generating clinical evidence through large, randomized, controlled multi-center clinical trials, the NRN encompasses 20 academic centers around the United States and has been prolific in its research productivity. Led by a steering committee with representation from the National Institutes of Health (NIH), each partner NICU, and the central data coordinating center, the NRN currently has 10 actively enrolling studies at the time of this chapter's publication ranging from the Transfusion of Prematures (TOP) trial, which seeks to define the optimum transfusion thresholds for extremely premature infants, to the Optimized Cooling trial for hypoxic ischemic encephalopathy (HIE), which seeks to extend our understanding of how best to protect an infant's brain and body from long-term damage caused by an hypoxic episode using therapeutic hypothermia.

To date, the NRN has completed 37 observational and clinical trials resulting in innumerable publications in highly respected journals including *Pediatrics*, *the New England Journal of Medicine*, and *JAMA*. Many NRN studies have played a pivotal role in changing NICU practices around the country and around the world, including initiation of therapeutic hypothermia for HIE,[17] reduction in post-natal corticosteroid use,[18] and a push toward the use of non-invasive continuous positive airway pressure (CPAP) in the delivery room for extremely preterm infants.[19] Though primarily focused on clinical research, the NRN also provides opportunities for affiliated centers to benchmark their practices against each other. Within such an environment, attention has also become increasingly directed toward understanding individual practices and quality processes as "center differences in management" are consistently identified in NRN studies as a major driver of clinical outcomes.[20]

PEDIATRIX MEDICAL GROUP

Founded in 1979, the Pediatrix Medical Group employs over 900 neonatologists and 500 advanced practitioners in 34 states around the country. Part of the larger MEDNAX multi-specialty organization, Pediatrix covers over 300 NICUs ranging from smaller level 1 and level 2 units within community hospitals to large level 3 and 4 high-acuity units.

Within the framework of such a large group practice, Pediatrix maintains a Center for Research, Education and Quality that centrally coordinates efforts to improve outcomes including its own "100,000 Lives Campaign." Moreover, its enormous database including thousands of patients across 300 NICUs provides rich opportunities for clinical research and data mining to answer retrospective clinical questions. Recent papers include a description of the epidemiology of early- versus late-onset sepsis (N > 100,000 infants)[21] and a study that sought to define the reliability of cerebrospinal fluid parameters in neonatal meningitis (N > 9,000 samples).[22] The Pediatrix model demonstrates that quality partnerships to identify best practices and improve outcomes can indeed span the realm from academic to private practice.[23]

THE PERINATAL QUALITY COLLABORATIVE OF NORTH CAROLINA

Modeled on the successful experiences of the California Perinatal Care Collaborative (CPQCC) and other similar programs, the Perinatal Quality Collaborative of North Carolina (PQCNC) is a statewide collaborative that unites hospitals, family representatives, providers, payer groups, and state leaders from across North Carolina in efforts to improve the quality of perinatal care. Since 2007, PQCNC has developed and implemented several such projects including a successful central-line-associated bloodstream infection reduction program (North Carolina led the nation with the lowest in standardized infection ratios among states reporting to the CDC *National Healthcare Safety Network* from 2006-2008)[24] and the exclusive human milk for babies (EHM4B) initiative.

PQCNC also encourages partnership across the spectrum of perinatology, with a program to reduce elective deliveries prior to 39 weeks that addresses priorities important to neonatologists and maternal-fetal/high-risk obstetricians alike. Additionally, both individually and through partnership with its sister collaboratives in other states, PQCNC disseminates educational materials around developing successful NICU quality improvement programs, reliability science, and parent teaching, and provides up-to-date contact information for neonatal specialists at all partner institutions.[25] Finally, PQCNC is just one example of such state-level collaboratives in place around the United States. Other excellent examples include CPQCC, the Ohio Perinatal Quality Collaborative (OPQC), and the Tennessee Initiative for Perinatal Quality Care (TIPQC), all of whom focus on implementing statewide neonatal and perinatal quality improvement projects.

CONCLUSION

As demonstrated by these examples of NICU collaborative efforts, it is quite difficult to "stand alone" as a neonatologist in the tradition of Marcus Welby's made-for-television medical practice of yore. Within a field driven to improve outcomes for medicine's most vulnerable patients, neonatologists and their NICU teams have innumerable options to engage in quality improvement efforts at the local, state, national, and international levels. Given this breadth of opportunities for collaboration across NICUs, it is not surprising that the same level of collaboration is necessary within a NICU to ensure a quality improvement project's success. The next section will cover three case studies for improving NICU outcomes, each within a different area of both practice and process but all emphasizing the critical nature of the multidisciplinary team approach.

MULTIDISCIPLINARY CASE STUDIES

As in any aspect of quality improvement (QI), convening the right multidisciplinary team to address a problem is the first and most critical aspect of success. QI in the NICU is no different—the unique, relatively "closed" nature of NICU staffing combined with the opportunity to "own" many outcomes by caring for neonates from the very beginning of their lives on through discharge provides for a fertile QI environment.

This section will cover three cases taken from different areas of neonatal quality improvement and patient safety and focused on three specific clinical areas—medication safety, catheter-associated bloodstream infections, and necrotizing enterocolitis. Their efforts range from broad to specific and require different approaches, different measures of success, and different mechanisms to maintain improved outcomes. Taken as a whole, the three efforts described below demonstrate the possibilities for any outcomes project that emerges as the thoughtful product of a committed, multidisciplinary team in any NICU around the country.

NEONATAL MEDICATION SAFETY

According to the IOM, medication errors harm millions of patients and cost billions of dollars each year.[26] Critical care patients are known to be a high-risk population for medication errors,[7] with NICU patients specifically known to be at a higher risk than other hospitalized infants and children.[27]

With their extremely low weights, physiologic immaturity, and frequent need for off-label medication use, infants are both more vulnerable to medication errors and adverse drug events (ADEs) than older children or adults and more sensitive to them when such errors occur.[26,28] Medication error analyses performed on single drugs (eg, gentamicin or TPN) for neonatal patients report error rates >10%.[29,30] Given the number of medications our sickest NICU infants are exposed to each day, the total number of medication errors experienced by a single extremely low birth weight infant during a NICU stay remains unknown but could be staggering.

To better understand these risks, two large multi-center efforts sought to examine medication errors in NICUs using voluntarily reported, anonymous data. In the first multi-center report, investigators analyzed events reported in MEDMARX, a "voluntary, anonymous, confidential, de-identified, internet-accessible medication error-reporting program" run by the United States Pharmacopeia. In this project, investigators found 244 preventable ADEs among 6,749 medication errors within 163 NICUs over a 7-year period.[4]

In the second more detailed multi-center report, members of VON developed a multi-institutional, voluntary, anonymous, internet-based reporting system for medical errors in neonatal intensive care, evaluated its feasibility, and identified errors that affect high-risk neonates. Seven hundred thirty-nine healthcare providers (physicians, nurses, respiratory therapists, pharmacists, and others) from 54 NICUs were provided access to the error-reporting

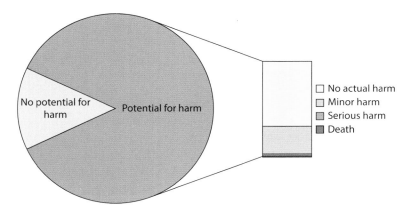

Figure 9-1 ▪ Distribution of harm related to adverse drug events in Vermont Oxford Network NICU. (Reproduced, with permission, from Suresh G, Horbar JD, Plsek P, et al. Voluntary anonymous reporting of medical errors for neonatal intensive care. *Pediatrics*. 2004;113(6):1609-1618.)

website. Phase 1 of this study included only free text reporting, while Phase 2 included specific queries including degree of harm, location, error categorization, and changes implemented to prevent recurrence.

In Phase 1, investigators determined that 581 (47%) of all reported events were related to medications, nutritional agents (breast milk, formula, and parenteral nutrition), or blood products and over half of errors occurred at either the administration or dispensing stage. In Phase 2, although only 25% of the 673 events actually caused harm, ranging from minor (eg, requirement for increased monitoring, specific treatment, other interventions) to serious harm or death, over 80% of events had the potential to cause harm (Figure 9-1). The leading identified causes of error were failure to follow policy or protocol (46.8%), communication problem (22.4%), and errors in charting or documentation (13.4%).[31]

Although our understanding of the epidemiology of neonatal medication errors remains limited, these and other early studies have led to several successful single-center efforts to reduce harm.[32-35] The first example is from the University of Iowa, whose successful implementation of bedside barcoding drastically reduced both preventable ADEs (from 15.1 per 1,000 medication doses to 4.4/1,000 doses) and near miss ADEs (0.86/1,000 doses to 0.43/1,000).[36] As described in the *Journal of Pediatrics*, Dr Frank Morriss and his colleagues assembled a multidisciplinary team including physicians, advanced care providers, nurses, respiratory therapists, and pharmacists to design and prospectively implement a bedside barcode medication administration (BCMA) system within the University of Iowa Children's Hospital NICU. By bringing together the experiences and understanding of multiple providers spanning the spectrum of neonatal care, the Iowa group was able to completely eliminate four classes of medication errors that were present prior to implementing BCMA and drastically reduce preventable harm across the board.

A similar "major-intervention" approach was implemented at Duke in 2008. In response to reports of an increased risk of ADEs for pediatric and neonatal critical care patients, Duke convened a similar multidisciplinary team to develop error-prevention strategies. The group consisted of hospital leadership including the chief executive and chief nursing officers, pharmacy leadership, NICU leadership including the division chief, as well a front-line NICU physician, pharmacist, and nurse. In its first-pass process analysis, the team identified preparation of IV medications as an area of particularly high risk, given the practical impossibility in distinguishing between two colorless, odorless liquids at the bedside. Through a failure mode effects analysis, the multidisciplinary team found several potentially error-prone processes in the medication preparation pathway that could be mitigated through barcode scanning and process simplification.

Figure 9-2 demonstrates the dramatic reduction in adverse drug events experienced after the group's recommendations were implemented in December 2008. Over the study's entire period of analysis (January 2007 to July 2010), Duke Children's Services admitted 36,811 patients who received over

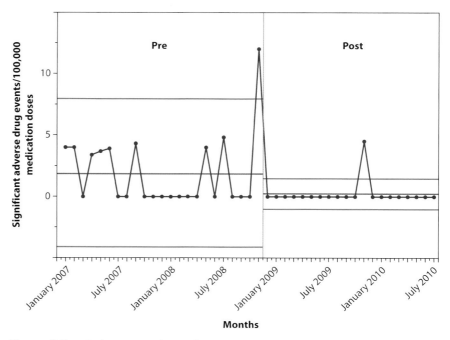

Figure 9-2 ▪ Reduction in adverse drug events requiring intervention pre/post implementation of barcoding in Duke University Hospital medication preparation room.

one million medication doses. As the figure demonstrates, adverse drug events requiring intervention dropped from 1.9/100,000 doses before the intervention to zero, resulting (in real terms) in 12 prevented adverse drug events and an estimated yearly savings of $100,000 in excess health costs.[37]

Much remains to be done in advancing neonatal medication safety, as evidence from such single-center reports becomes better understood and implemented through prospective, multi-center studies. Dabliz and Levine outlined a comprehensive approach to neonatal medication safety based on the Institute for Safe Medication Practices' Key Elements of the Medication Use System™ in early 2012[38] that may serve as a model to build such multi-center projects. Although multi-center work within medication safety will face several challenges—including creating a uniform reporting structure for ADEs, variability in voluntary reporting strategies, and overcoming institution-specific barriers in practice and process—these early single-center efforts suggest that big gains in neonatal medication safety may be possible through major, targeted interventions.

CENTRAL-LINE-ASSOCIATED BLOODSTREAM INFECTIONS

Central line access is imperative to survival in the NICU. It is simply impossible for an infant born 17 weeks before his due date to safely consume enough calories to grow just from tube feedings for days—many days—after his birth. Providing the kind of nutrition necessary to encourage growth in an extremely premature infant (well over 100 kilocalories/kilogram per day) involves concentrating protein, glucose, lipid, and solute to an osmolarity unsafe to deliver peripherally (often over 1,500 milliosmoles/liter). Even if such nutrition were possible to safety provide peripherally, multi-lumen access would be needed to give antibiotics to treat early-onset sepsis, pressors to manage hypotension, caffeine for neuroprotection and to treat apnea of prematurity, prophylactic indomethacin to prevent intraventricular hemorrhage, and so on. And if that weren't enough, imagine the struggle (for both provider and patient alike) to replace multiple peripheral IV's every day in an infant with the same mass as an average soda can.

Despite their critical contribution to saving the lives of premature infants, sick term infants, and older NICU patients with chronic medical conditions, central lines can also be deadly. Central-line-associated bloodstream infections (CLA-BSIs) have been a recognized contributor to nosocomial sepsis for decades,[39] with efforts to reduce them appearing in the literature as early as 1981.[40] Although CLA-BSIs are a scourge in any intensive care unit, infants in the NICU have long experienced challenges with CLA-BSIs and late-onset sepsis[41] with costly results in both morbidity and mortality.[42] As described earlier, infants in the NICU are inherently at a higher risk of a variety of adverse events and CLA-BSIs are no exception. On the patient side, a premature infant's poor skin integrity and immature immune system impair two of the most natural defenses against a CLA-BSI. On the unit side, that same infant may be exposed to multiple caregivers from multiple consulting services (not all of whom ascribe to the same level of hand-hygiene commitment as the core NICU staff) as well as multiple invasive procedures and that repeatedly breach his already weak skin.[43] Finally, veins capable of receiving a central line are a precious, non-renewable resource in critically ill neonates. The loss of a central venous line—either a surgically placed Broviac or bedside placed subclavian, femoral, cut-down, or peripherally inserted central venous catheter (PICC)—secondary to infection doesn't necessarily mean a new line will be easy, or even possible to place.

Early efforts seeking to understand of the epidemiology of CLA-BSIs in the NICU identified several risk factors, including extreme prematurity, time of line insertion, and colonization of the hub and insertion sites.[44,45] Furthermore, rates of NICU CLA-BSIs in the early days of analysis were reported as high 10-plus infections per thousand line days,[45] with causative organisms including the expected *Staphylococcus aureus* and virulent gram-negative species but also variable rates of both *Candida*[46] and coagulase-negative *Staphylococcus* species infections as well that are less common outside the NICU.[47-49]

Such early analyses on CLA-BSIs in the NICU and around the hospital made it clear that a single act could not and would not eliminate the problem. Indeed, as late as 2005 an article published in *Pediatrics* asked the question "Is Bloodstream Infection Preventable Among Premature Infants?" in its title![43] With these challenges in mind, efforts to reduce and later to eliminate CLA-BSIs trended early on toward a multidisciplinary, bundle-based approach.

Despite its questioning title, the article cited above describes one successful example from the George Washington University NICU. In response to a higher-than-average incidence of CLA-BSI within their NICU (as high as 16 infections per thousand line days) a team of NICU providers traveled from George Washington to Connecticut Children's Medical Center, a unit known at the time for a very low incidence of CLA-BSIs, to observe practices and develop a transferable bundle of process changes to implement back home.

During its period of observation, the group identified four major differences in practice and process between their NICU and the high-performing NICU—use of a closed medication system, limitation of line breaks, use of strict sterile-technique during central line IV tubing changes, and use of sterile technique during antiseptic dressing changes. Upon returning to their NICU, the team developed a bundle-based implementation program addressing these four major areas. Post-implementation, the George Washington NICU experienced a radical drop on CLA-BSIs from a mean of 15 infections per 1,000 line days between 1998 and 2000 to a mean of 2.1 infections/1,000 line days between 2001 and 2003.

The George Washington experience exemplifies the multidisciplinary bundle approach to reducing CLA-BSIs that has become the standard for broad, multi-center implementation both in NICUs and across the adult ICU literature.[50-53] State-wide initiatives like the pivotal Michigan Keystone ICU Project[52] have also translated to the NICU as all 19 of New York's regional perinatal centers participated in a project to reduce CLA-BSIs in the mid-2000s. The group's initial survey found significant pre-implementation variation in both process and outcomes, with CLA-BSIs ranging from 15.1 to 2.6 infections/1,000 line days across the NICUs involved.[54]Despite such variation, all 19 centers ultimately approved implementation of the study's "level-1 evidence-based central line-care bundle"[54] and maintenance checklists developed by a team of neonatologists, advanced practitioners, nursing staff, and infection control experts.[55] The adoption of both the bundle and the checklists, with optional site-by-site modifications, led to a statewide reduction in the incidence of NICU CLA-BSI by 67%. Despite such a dramatic reduction, the CLA-BSI incidence rate ratio continued to vary markedly by center (from a low of 0.04 to a high of 2.87),[55] a finding that is continually replicated in many prospective, multi-center NICU trials.

It is in the aftermath of a program like the successful New York state initiative that the recursive nature of CLA-BSI elimination becomes clear. With each new project different aspects of care can be addressed—eg, implementing a dedicated team to insert PICC lines,[56] providing either systemic or oral non-absorbed anti-fungal therapy while a central line is present,[57,58] and so on. In their 2010 article in *Clinics in Perinatology* around CLA-BSI reduction efforts in the NICU, Powers and Wirtschafter[59-61] compiled the elements of CLA-BSI bundles incorporated into eight different NICU-specific CLA-BSI reduction projects over a 9-year period.[43,62-66] Graphed in Figure 9-3, these data demonstrate the increasing complexity of bundle-based projects over time, with the most recent publications including 10 or 12 different elements.

Efforts to reduce CLA-BSIs both within the NICU and around the hospital have also benefited from a trend toward better reporting. States like Washington, Oregon, Tennessee, and Maryland have required reporting CLA-BSIs for years, while the Centers for Medicare and Medicaid Services began mandating reporting of CLA-BSI events as part of the Hospital Inpatient Quality Reporting to the National Healthcare Safety Network beginning in 2011. Such reporting processes have led to more uniform definitions of a CLA-BSI (eg, how many positive cultures with a coagulase-negative *Staphylococcus* species should be required before being considered a true infection) as well as new attention from top-level hospital administrators to CLA-BSIs as a reportable, publicly available quality measure.

The end result of a decade's worth of focus on CLA-BSIs has resulted in movable goalposts—what was once thought to be a completely unpreventable

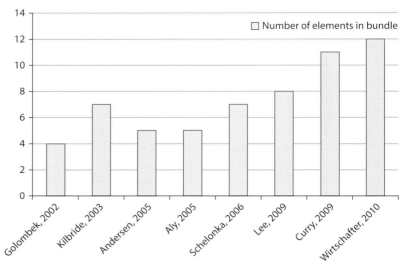

Figure 9-3 ■ Increasing complexity of NICU Bundles to prevent catheter-associated bloodstream infections. (Reproduced, with permission, from Powers RJ, Wirtschafter DW. Decreasing central line associated bloodstream infection in neonatal intensive care. *Clin Perinatol.* 2010;37(1):247-272.)

complication of NICU care is now targeted by programs actually called "getting to zero and staying there." Approaching CLA-BSIs in the NICU requires a multidisciplinary, bundle-based approach that brings providers together from every step in the line insertion, use, care, and removal pathways, ultimately leading to an almost universal focus within a NICU's entire staff on preventing these terrible infections.

NECROTIZING ENTEROCOLITIS

Necrotizing enterocolitis (NEC) is a severe, often catastrophic intestinal disease almost exclusively affecting premature infants. Of the approximately 2,000 infants born each year in the United States who develop surgical NEC, at least 50% die. Unfortunately, even those who survive have double the odds of lifelong neuro-developmental problems compared to extremely preterm infants who did not develop NEC during their NICU stay.[67,68]

Although NEC has been called "one of the most recalcitrant and entrenched fields of neonatal research,"[67] neonatal researchers have made several advances in the last 10 years in identifying factors associated with both increased and decreased risk at the patient and the unit levels. While the definitive early pathophysiologic changes that lead to NEC remain unknown and it is possible that NEC will never be entirely preventable, recent evidence does suggest that understanding and implementing changes in process and management related to these factors can help reduce the proportion of NEC cases over which we do have control.

On the increased risk side, associations ranging from confirmed and demonstrated in multi-center, prospective randomized trials to biologically plausible but untested relationships exist between NEC and all of the following:

- Prematurity (earlier gestational age at delivery = higher risk)
- Cyanotic heart disease (especially ductal-dependent lesions)
- Enteral feeding, especially aggressive feeding advancement
- Formula feeding[69]
- Long-term initial antibiotic exposure[5]
- Anemia/packed red-blood cell transfusions[68]
- H2 blocker use[70]

On the protective side, a similar collection of both proposed and confirmed associations exist, but only two have been demonstrated as safe and effective in human trials: human-milk feedings and antenatal steroids.[68] Given the myriad of potential associations, the variability in their supporting evidence, and the variability of their strength given any individual NICU's other practices (eg, fluid management,[71] PDA management, post-natal steroid use, etc.), reducing the incidence of NEC presents a useful third case study in neonatal patient safety and quality improvement.

Unlike neonatal medication safety, where a single major intervention (eg, bedside bar coding) can make a large, "one-off" difference all at once, or CLA-BSI, which more readily lends itself to a bundle-type strategy (cleaner is better), an effort to reduce NEC would need to recursively address multiple areas of safety, culture, practices, and processes across the spectrum of NICU providers, with a focus on known associations such as human milk as a primary nutrition source, antimicrobial stewardship, and avoidance of antacids as well as continued measurement and analysis to identify subsequent targets. Such a program would need to bring stakeholders together to review the breadth of evidence described above and choose targets that the unit could most effectively implement, monitor, and maintain. The Duke NICU embarked on just such an effort beginning in the early 2000s, and its efforts to reduce NEC present an interesting final multidisciplinary case study in this chapter.

As discussed in the section on collaboratives, one of the major benefits of joining a local, state, federal, or international group is the ability to benchmark a unit's outcomes in comparison to its peers. One example of such a unit is the Duke NICU, which maintains a strong, quality-focused environment with numerous outcomes among the best of the nation's largest academic medical centers. However, when Duke joined the Neonatal Research Network in 2001,

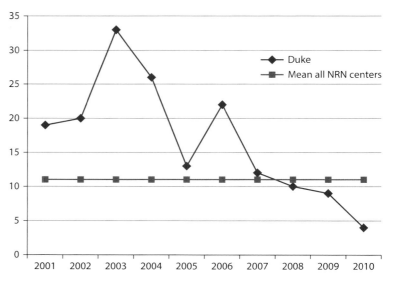

Figure 9-4 ■ Incidence of necrotizing enterocolitis, inborn extremely low birth weight infants at Duke versus cumulative incidence among 22- to 28-week infants across the Neonatal Research Network (NRN). Mean All NRN Centers = Cumulative incidence for the Neonatal Research Network for 22- to 28-week infants between 2003 and 2007 as reported by Stoll et al, 2010. (Reproduced, with permission, from Stoll BJ, Hansen NI, Bell EF, et al. Neonatal outcomes of extremely preterm infants from the NICHD Neonatal Research Network. *Pediatrics*. 2010;126(3):443-456.)

the Duke NICU leadership group noted its incidence of NEC among extremely low birth weight (ELBW) infants was higher than the overall rate across NRN centers. As shown in Figure 9-4, this trend persisted for the first few years of participation within the NRN, leading the group and its leadership to ask two questions: why, and what could be done to reduce NEC at Duke. The resulting process of introspection, analysis, and discussion resulted in a four-pronged approach that targeted each of the following:

1. Reducing prolonged (>5 day) empiric antibiotic courses,
2. Developing a robust culture around the support of human milk,
3. Reducing the routine use of reflux medications, and
4. Reconfiguring transfusion-feeding practices.

Figures 9-4 and 9-5 demonstrate the respective successes and failures of these efforts, which together resulted in an overall drop in incidence of NEC in Duke's inborn ELBW population from a high of 33% in 2003 to a low of 4% in the latest available data from 2012. At first glance, there seem to be two major drivers of success among these four projects. First, the effort among attending neonatologists to consciously focus on the length of an infant's first course of

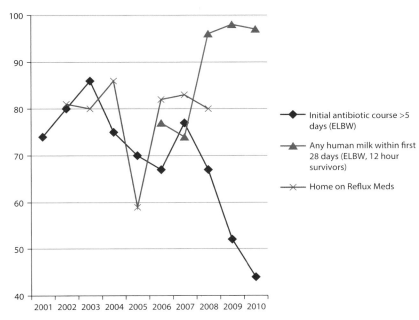

Figure 9-5 ▪ Outcomes measures for projects to reduce incidence of NEC at Duke. ELBW = Extremely low birth weight.

antibiotics was quite successful, resulting in a profound drop in the proportion of ELBW infants with an initial course longer than 5 days from a high of 86% to 44%. Second, the unit-wide focus on providing earlier feeds, early colostrum even in very small amounts for critically ill infants, and promoting human milk (either mother's milk or donor milk), which incorporated partners from obstetrics and post-partum care to provide and promote pumping resulted in a rise in human milk exposure within the most critical first 28 days of life to almost 100% by 2012.

Efforts to reduce the use of reflux medications appear to have been less successful, with a relatively similar proportion of infants discharged home on anti-reflux medications across the years measured. However, as the group's only available metric at present is medication use at discharge rather than during the timeframe infants are most susceptible to NEC within the first few weeks of life, it is possible these efforts were more successful than the data suggest. Finally, although implementing a new transfusion-feeding protocol did change practice (keeping infants NPO for 4 hours before, during, and after a packed-red blood cell transfusion), it did not change the proportion of infants who developed NEC around the time of their transfusion (data not shown, currently submitted for publication) and thus was unlikely to have affected the overall incidence of NEC.[72]

Thus, although it's safe to say that "something" changed within the Duke NICU between 2002 and 2012 that sent the incidence of NEC among ELBW infants from the roof to the basement, it's difficult to say exactly what was responsible. Given the measures of success outlined above, it's likely the combined efforts to promote human milk and reduce long-term initial courses of antibiotics—also the efforts with the strongest *a priori* evidence of potential success—are the main drivers of reduced NEC, while the focus on reflux medications and transfusion-feeding practices likely playing less of a role. However, it is hard to make a case to eliminate the changes made in any of these practices given the tremendous overall reduction in NEC, as it is impossible to actually divide the overall effort to reduce NEC into four separate QI projects. All were implemented contemporaneously in the same unit with the same staff resulting in the same changes in culture, and they likely interact in ways that aren't measurable. Furthermore, it is possible that the unit's generally increased focus on NEC overall led to other changes in practice or process that remain hidden from analysis, or that other projects (eg, a concurrent, quite successful effort to reduce late-onset sepsis) also played a role in improving and maintaining lower rates of NEC. Whatever the drivers, Duke's efforts to reduce the incidence of NEC clearly demonstrate both the challenges and potential benefits that can arise from focusing on a particular outcome, despite the difficulties inherent in changing multiple processes within the environment of care.

CONCLUSION

These three case studies offer three different views into the world of hands-on neonatal QI efforts. Each group discussed within this section has notched significant accomplishments on their scoreboard using a variety of tactics, yet all stem from the same multidisciplinary, team-based approach from the outset. Similar stories could be told for any number of neonatal quality metrics – reducing unplanned extubations, preventing admission hypothermia for ELBWs, reducing ventilator-associated pneumonias, and so on. Most would likely fall into one of the three buckets discussed here—a single large intervention, a bundle-based approach, or a recursive, multi-faceted project addressing several processes or etiologies of error at once.

Despite the immense strides made in neonatal patient safety and quality outcomes in the last century, and especially in the last few decades, there are many potentially fruitful targets for future efforts. The final section of this chapter discusses how the next generation of leaders in neonatal quality sciences can build on the successes of past generations and leverage new opportunities in data availability, computing power, and overall interconnectedness to push the boundaries of quality improvement even farther.

FUTURE TARGETS AND OPPORTUNITIES

While QI efforts in the NICU have historically focused on the types of projects we've discussed, future efforts are likely to benefit from the massive influx of clinical, administrative, and outcomes data offered by interoperable electronic medical records (EMRs). To put it bluntly, while "era of big government" may have been declared over in 1996, the "era of big data" in healthcare has only just begun.

As the healthcare providers, large and small, transition to the versions of interoperable EMRs that meet "meaningful use" requirements over the next 5 years, the amount of healthcare related data will exponentially increase. According to an estimate from SAS, one of the largest business analytics companies in the United States, healthcare data already encompassed 150 Exabytes (where one Exabyte = 1×10^{18} bytes, or one billion Gigabytes) with a single radiology-imaging provider accounting for over half that amount.[73] The last 10 years of advances in health informatics have yielded marked increases in data availability, searchability, and usability, resulting in datasets that are finally large enough, powerful enough, and coherent enough to yield meaningful results.

Examples of the power that such datasets and statistical computing packages can yield when wielded by teams of clinicians and statisticians include the NICHD's online calculator for outcomes in extreme prematurity,[74] a multivariate model that predicts a premature infant's probability of survival using gestational age, birth weight, sex, singleton status, and exposure to antenatal corticosteroids. A similar effort to provide probabilistic estimates of early-onset neonatal sepsis has also been published, incorporating gestational age, group B *Streptococcus* status, length of rupture of membranes, highest intrapartum temperature and intrapartum antibiotic therapy.[75,76] As the next generation of health services researchers learn how best to leverage these massive data sets to answer big questions, provide solutions, and create predictive modeling for continuous risk assessments at the bedside, so must the next generation of clinicians learn to think probabilistically to incorporate these findings into their practice.

Addressing cost represents a second ripe target for future efforts in neonatal quality improvement. The "Holy Grail" project within any QI program would improve both outcomes and patient safety while actually reducing overall costs; as a result, authors have increasingly begun to publish demonstrated or expected cost-savings alongside their NICU outcomes. Led by

Dr John Zupancic, the Boston Children's Hospital neonatal epidemiology group has been a leader in this arena publishing economic analyses alongside major multi-center trials including the Premature Infants in Need of Transfusion (PINT) trial, caffeine for apnea of prematurity, and inhaled nitric oxide for chronic lung disease ("NO CLD," also known as the "Ballard" protocol).[77-79] In each instance, the group demonstrated that potentially costly appearing therapies (more blood transfusions, more caffeine use, and long-term weans of inhaled nitric oxide) were actually economic "win-wins" in the long term, saving money over time by improving both short-term outcomes (eg, length of stay, number of ventilator days) and long-term outcomes (eg, survival, survival without neurodevelopmental impairment, etc.). In an environment of increasing financial pressure on the entire American healthcare system, economic analyses like these are likely to play an increasing large role in QI efforts ranging from large to small in years to come.

Finally, this section would be incomplete without a discussion of efforts to improve outcomes for neonates internationally, especially in underserved and underdeveloped nations. While neonatology in the Western Hemisphere has made immense strides since the 1960s in improving survival and other quality outcomes for premature infants, there are many places in the world today where infants like Patrick Kennedy are still dying despite the availability of proven effective therapies.

One such international effort stems from a joint program developed by the American Academy of Pediatrics, the World Health Organization (WHO), the United States Agency for International Development, Saving Newborn Lives, and the NICHD called "Helping Babies Breathe (HBB)." The program seeks to reduce the estimated one million infants worldwide who die each year from birth asphyxia, one cause of which is failure to stimulate respiration or provide assisted respiration immediately after birth. In partnership with various health organizations around the world, HBB seeks to ensure someone skilled in neonatal resuscitation is present at the birth of every baby. That "birth attendant" is tasked with ensuring that by 1 minute of age the infant is either breathing on her own or receiving assisted ventilation, a concept the group has called "the golden minute."[80]

To date, HBB has brought success in saving infants' lives to nations as diverse as Bangladesh and Guatemala, Haiti and Kenya, Mexico, and Nepal. Its curriculum is focused on providing culturally appropriate evidence-based education paired with realistic simulation and on-going mentorship to assist with implementation, measuring success, and long-term sustainment of improved outcomes. One such program in Tanzania demonstrated significant reductions in neonatal death and stillbirth, as well as increases in process measures including the use of suction and stimulation.[81] As successful international outcomes projects like HBB become increasingly well known and new programs build on previous successes, the quality obsession inherent to neonatology as a field will continue to spread, thereby improving the lives of newborns around the world.

CONCLUSION

In the larger context of a book on *Pediatric Patient Safety and Quality Improvement*, the overriding goal of this chapter has been to explain why "the NICU is different." While their population variability, relatively immature physiology, and sensitivity to error place infants in the NICU at an inherently higher risk of serious patient safety events than other children, the NICU is a data-rich environment that allows providers to "start from scratch" and own a patient's outcomes from start to finish. These dueling challenges and opportunities make the NICU unique in both its ability to understand and its ability to prevent adverse events and improve quality outcomes, engendering a spirit of cooperation and coordination that crosses professional and institutional boundaries. This spirit is exemplified by, but by no means limited to, the four groups discussed in this chapter: the Vermont Oxford Network, the NICHD Neonatal Research Network, the Pediatrix Medical Group's Center for Research, Education and Quality, and the Perinatal Quality Collaborative of North Carolina.

Highlighted in this chapter is the critical nature of multidisciplinary teams to QI efforts within the NICU, as well as reasons why the NICU's structure in particular lends itself well to cohesive team efforts. Examples have been provided to show how improvement efforts in the NICU can stem from categorical, one-time interventions, like Iowa's bar coding efforts to reduce adverse drug events. More often, however, successful efforts are more recursive in nature, like bundle-based efforts to reduce CLA-BSIs and unit-level efforts to understand and prevent NEC, where teams continually readdress remaining problems with refinements or new efforts to "get to zero." Finally, it's important to remember that no QI project happens in isolation—like most areas in healthcare, NICUs often have multiple QI projects occurring simultaneously, each of which likely impacts the other in ways that are unknown and immeasurable.

Despite these challenges, 2014 is still an exciting time to play a part in neonatal QI efforts. With the power of informatics only just beginning to be leveraged, clinicians and statisticians will be able to work together to visualize a NICU's data in ways that heretofore were unimaginable. Further, as the focus of administrative leaders at the hospital, payer, and government levels turns increasingly toward cost-savings, so have neonatologists demonstrated the cost-saving potentials even for some of our most expensive therapies. Finally, opportunities abound to improve outcomes for both premature and term infants around the world, many of whom live in nations that haven't yet experienced the benefit of inhaled nitric oxide, surfactant therapy, or even appropriate delivery room resuscitation.

In the end, the NICU faces the same challenges in preventing harm, improving outcomes, and measuring success as the rest of healthcare. With the advent of massive datasets and the computing power to put their information to use at the bedside, efforts in neonatal patient safety will continue to evolve along with the broader safety and quality movement. We as healthcare providers—physicians, nurses, students, staff, administrators, and leaders—will increasingly have the ability to understand our data in ways previous generations could only imagine. The demand is now on us to take an increasingly active role in how we put that understanding to use for our patients and their families.

> *"The truth won't set us free until we develop the skills, habit, talent, and moral courage to use it. Openness isn't the end, it's the beginning."*
> Margaret Heffernan

ACKNOWLEDGMENTS

The author would like to thank Dr David Tanaka for his mentorship during the process of drafting, revising, and final proofing of this chapter, as well as Drs Ronald Goldberg, C. Michael Cotten, P. Brian Smith, and Jeffrey Ferranti for their significant and continued contributions to his professional development. He would also like to thank Dr Karen Frush for her leadership in driving patient safety and quality outcomes within the Duke University Health System and across the nation, as well as for her long-time personal mentorship and friendship.

IN PRACTICE

- **First convene the right multidisciplinary team.** As Jim Collins would say, "getting the right people on the bus" before starting a QI endeavor is far and away the most critical step to success.[82] Having broad representation from a unit's various stakeholders will provide

(Continued)

(*Continued*)

innumerable benefits, including a greater understanding of the specific problems the group seeks to address, access to a wide range of experiences and relationships, and ultimately buy-in from those who will need to implement the team's recommendations at the bedside.

- **Identify the target as most receptive to a categorical improvement or recursive set of improvements.** Quality improvement efforts in the NICU are rarely but occasionally categorical in nature, in that one significant effort can reduce or eliminate a specific problem. More often, a process will require recursive efforts to eliminate different aspects of errors each time, ultimately resulting in a step-wise progression of bites at the QI apple.

- **Leverage cooperative efforts.** NICU professionals have a long history of focusing on QI as has been demonstrated by the four examples of multicenter/multidisciplinary collaboratives. Whatever the project your group seeks to embark upon, it is likely that other NICUs have either faced a similar problem or are actively seeking answers to the same problem right now. Explore the relationships your NICU has within and among collaboratives—even if your hospital is not a current member, many groups widely publish their projects, challenges, and successes online, and provide easily accessible educational pathways either for free or for a nominal charge.

- **Identify clear measures of success**. In each of the three areas discussed in this chapter—necrotizing enterocolitis, medication safety, and central-line-associated bloodstream infections—the outcome was clear and measurable. With the right team approaching the right problem to achieve defined measures of success, QI in the NICU has its best chances of success.

- **Lather, rinse, and repeat.** Once your project or program has demonstrated a positive effect on patient safety and outcomes in your unit, success will likely become infectious. Don't stop—build on your early successes to instill a culture of perpetual improvement and support for the QI process within your staff. When such a culture dominates among a unit's personnel, from leadership to front-line staff, it becomes incredibly difficult for other individuals with less commitment to the safety of your patients to remain around, leaving you with only the "right people on the bus" and ready to confront the next set of challenges head on!

FAQs

1. My NICU is embarking on an effort to reduce unplanned extubations but I'm struggling with how to get started—can you help?

   Absolutely! First, as with all effective QI efforts, a project around unplanned extubations needs to begin with the right team. Ask yourself "Who in my unit has any part in causing, responding to, or preventing unplanned extubations?" The team would likely involve at a minimum bedside nurses, respiratory therapists, and physicians, as well as appropriate members of unit leadership to start. Next, define the problem by leading the group through a guided process (eg, failure modes event analysis, root-cause analysis, etc.) to understand unplanned extubations—when do they occur, how frequent are they, what are the most frequency proximate causes (eg, very active infant, loose tape) as well as any issues underlying those causes (eg, sedation policies, endotracheal tube taping assessments). Identify weaknesses in any processes as well as targeted interventions to address them. Prior to implementation ensure anyone affected by each intervention understands why the issue is important, how the intervention will address it, as well as the details around each step in the new process. Finally, monitor implementation, measure results, celebrate success, and repeat the cycle as needed to address residual areas of need.

2. We recently implemented a new bundle to prevent CLA-BSIs but we're not seeing results because providers aren't following the directions. What gives?

   Implementing any new QI initiative within a unit can present many challenges, of which staff buy-in can be particularly problematic. As with any challenge, it is important to respond to pushback around QI implementation within the just culture framework. Blame and shame are rarely helpful responses—rather, ask providers their thoughts about the new bundle and any barriers they perceive to its implementation. Are supplies not readily available? Is the process thought to be too time-consuming? Were providers engaged in the bundle design process and are they involved in on-going monitoring? Often these kinds of interactions can identify specific problems with either the bundle itself or clinical support surrounding its implementation that can be easily and successfully addressed and ultimately lead to both better relationships and better outcomes.

3. We have great buy-in from staff and our catheter-associated urinary tract infection (CAUTI) program is showing fantastic results on process measures but we're not seeing the outcomes improvement we expected. What should we do?

   It is important to remember that process improvement and outcomes improvement are not always the same thing. When process measures (eg, fewer catheter days, 100% documentation of sterile insertion guidelines) show significant improvement but outcomes measures (eg, number of UTIs per catheter day) do not, there are two possible reasons. First, it's possible that not enough time has elapsed between implementation and measurement to see results. Consider a program to reduce CAUTIs that focuses on improving sterility at insertion. Such a unit may not see an improvement in actual CAUTI rates until there are no patients left in the unit with catheters inserted under the old guidelines. Second, it is possible that the intervention targeted the wrong process node—eg, despite the initial process review, insertion sterility may have actually contributed little to your unit's CAUTI rate at the outset. If you're comfortable with the length of time you've allowed for outcomes to catch up to process changes but still aren't seeing outcomes improvement, the team should reconvene around the new processes and identify a second round of targets for implementation.

4. We have completely eliminated CLA-BSIs from our unit and are incredibly excited about our results. What's next?

   First, congratulations are in order! Such success in QI should be celebrated broadly, both within your unit and across the institution. Achieving success is never easy, and it is critical to recognize every member of the team for his or her contribution to providing safer, higher-quality care for your patients. Now comes the hard part—sustaining your results in the long term. If a successful QI project has truly resulted in culture change—eg, "this is now the way we do things"—it can and often does become self-propagating as the negative, less safe behaviors are replaced. When all members of a team feel both a personal and a collective ownership of project's successful results, they become both cheerleaders and enforcers of the new processes. Ultimately new members of the team are trained in the new processes from day 1, thereby further ensuring propagation across generations of staff. However, even the most successful QI projects are subject to process drift—without continual focus on sustaining results, staff can slip back into the older, perhaps easier but less safe processes. It is just as important—and perhaps more important—to prominently display both process and outcomes results "on the wall" after achieving success as during the initial implementation process. Finally, your first success in QI will likely encourage both you and your staff to take the next steps and address other issues identified as targets for improvement within the unit. Remember to take the same thoughtful, step-wise approach each time and be mindful of how much change you ask of your staff at once. One successful project should not give rise to 12 new projects all at once—assimilating new processes into everyday care takes time, and it's important to check in with key members of the staff at every stage to ensure the whole team is ready to take on the next mountain together.

REFERENCES

1. Baker JP. The incubator and the medical discovery of the premature infant. *J Perinatol.* 2000;20(5):321-328.
2. Auvard A. De la couveuse pour enfants. *Archives de Tocologie des Maladies des Femmes et des Enfants Nouveau-nes.* 1883;10:594.
3. Philip AG. The evolution of neonatology. *Pediatr Res.* 2005;58(4):799-815.
4. Apgar V. A proposal for a new method of evaluation of the newborn infant. *Current Researches in Anesthesia & Analgesia.* 1953;32(4):260-267.
5. Cotten CM, Taylor S, Stoll B, et al. Prolonged duration of initial empirical antibiotic treatment is associated with increased rates of necrotizing enterocolitis and death for extremely low birth weight infants. *Pediatrics.* 2009;123(1):58-66.
6. Martin RJ, Fanaroff AA, Walsh MC. *Fanaroff and Martin's Neonatal-Perinatal Medicine: Diseases of the Fetus and Infant.* 9th ed. Philadelphia: Saunders/Elsevier; 2011.
7. Latif A, Rawat N, Pustavoitau A, et al. National study on the distribution, causes, and consequences of voluntarily reported medication errors between the ICU and non-ICU settings. *Crit Care Med.* 2013;41(2):389-398.
8. Reason JT. *Human Error.* Cambridge, England; New York: Cambridge University Press; 1990.
9. Griffin MP, O'Shea TM, Bissonette EA, et al. Abnormal heart rate characteristics preceding neonatal sepsis and sepsis-like illness. *Pediatr Res.* 2003;53(6):920-926.
10. Horbar JD. The Vermont Oxford Network: evidence-based quality improvement for neonatology. *Pediatrics.* 1999;103(1 suppl E):350-359.
11. Horbar JD, Soll RF, Edwards WH. The Vermont Oxford Network: a community of practice. *Clin in Perinat.* 2010;37(1):29-47.
12. Network VO. Vermont Oxford Newtork - About Us. 2013; Available at: http://www.vtoxford.org/about/about.aspx. Accessed April, 2013.
13. Horbar JD, Badger GJ, Carpenter JH, et al. Trends in mortality and morbidity for very low birth weight infants, 1991-1999. *Pediatrics.* 2002;110(1 Pt 1):143-151.

14. Walsh MC, Yao Q, Horbar JD, et al. Changes in the use of postnatal steroids for bronchopulmonary dysplasia in 3 large neonatal networks. *Pediatrics*. 2006;118(5): e1328-e1335.

15. Vermont-Oxford Neonatal Network. A multicenter, randomized trial comparing synthetic surfactant with modified bovine surfactant extract in the treatment of neonatal respiratory distress syndrome. *Pediatrics*. 1996;97(1):1-6.

16. Vermont-Oxford Network Steroid Study Group. Early postnatal dexamethasone therapy for the prevention of chronic lung disease. *Pediatrics*. 2001;108(3):741-748.

17. Shankaran S, Laptook AR, Ehrenkranz RA, et al. Whole-body hypothermia for neonates with hypoxic-ischemic encephalopathy. *N Engl J Med*. 2005;353(15):1574-1584.

18. Papile LA, Tyson JE, Stoll BJ, et al. A multicenter trial of two dexamethasone regimens in ventilator-dependent premature infants. *N Engl J Med*. 1998;338(16):1112-1118.

19. Finer NN, Carlo WA, Walsh MC, et al. Early CPAP versus surfactant in extremely preterm infants. *N Engl J Med*. 2010;362(21):1970-1979.

20. Stoll BJ, Hansen NI, Bell EF, et al. Neonatal outcomes of extremely preterm infants from the NICHD Neonatal Research Network. *Pediatrics*. 2010;126(3):443-456.

21. Cohen-Wolkowiez M, Moran C, Benjamin DK, et al. Early and late onset sepsis in late preterm infants. *Pediatr Infect Dis J*. 2009;28(12):1052-1056.

22. Garges HP, Moody MA, Cotten CM, et al. Neonatal meningitis: what is the correlation among cerebrospinal fluid cultures, blood cultures, and cerebrospinal fluid parameters? *Pediatrics*. 2006;117(4):1094-1100.

23. Pediatrix Medical Group. Home Page. 2013; Available at: http://www.pediatrix.com/. Accessed April, 2013.

24. PQCNC. North Carolina Leads States Nationally in SIR. 2013; http://www.pqcnc.org/?q=node/13026. Accessed April, 2013.

25. Carolina PQCoN. Welcome to PQCNC. 2013; Available at: http://www.pqcnc.org/. Accessed April, 2013.

26. Aspden P, Wolcott J, Bootman JL, Cronenwett LR. *Preventing Medication Errors: Quality Chasm Series*. Washington, DC: The National Academies Press; 2007.

27. Kaushal R, Bates DW, Landrigan C, et al. Medication errors and adverse drug events in pediatric inpatients. *JAMA*.2001;285(16):2114-2120.

28. Morriss FH, Jr. Adverse medical events in the NICU: epidemiology and prevention. *Neoreviews*. 2008;9(1):e8-e23.

29. Cordero L, Kuehn L, Kumar RR, Mekhjian HS. Impact of computerized physician order entry on clinical practice in a newborn intensive care unit. *J Perinatol*. 2004;24(2):88-93.

30. Lehmann CU, Conner KG, Cox JM. Preventing provider errors: online total parenteral nutrition calculator. *Pediatrics*. 2004;113(4):748-753.

31. Suresh G, Horbar JD, Plsek P, et al. Voluntary anonymous reporting of medical errors for neonatal intensive care. *Pediatrics*. 2004;113(6):1609-1618.

32. Raju TN, Kecskes S, Thornton JP, et al. Medication errors in neonatal and paediatric intensive-care units. *Lancet*. 1989;2(8659):374-376.

33. Folli HL, Poole RL, Benitz WE, Russo JC. Medication error prevention by clinical pharmacists in two children's hospitals. *Pediatrics*. 1987;79(5):718-722.

34. Simpson JH, Lynch R, Grant J, Alroomi L. Reducing medication errors in the neonatal intensive care unit. *Arch Dis Child Fetal Neonatal Ed.* 2004;89(6):F480-F482.

35. Ferranti JM, Horvath MM, Jansen J, et al. Using a computerized provider order entry system to meet the unique prescribing needs of children: description of an advanced dosing model. *BMC Med Inform Decis.* 2011;11.

36. Morriss FH, Abramowitz PW, Nelson SP, et al. Effectiveness of a barcode medication administration system in reducing preventable adverse drug events in a neonatal intensive care unit: a prospective cohort study. *J Pediatr.* 2009;154(3):363-368.

37. Ethington P. Interventions in pharmacy process reduces medication error. *PAS.* 2010.

38. Dabliz R, Levine S. Medication safety in neonates. *Am J Perinatol.* 2012;29(1):49-56.

39. Maki DG, Goldmnan DA, Rhame FS. Infection control in intravenous therapy. *Ann Intern Med.* 1973;79(6):867-887.

40. Maki DG, Band JD. A comparative study of polyantibiotic and iodophor ointments in prevention of vascular catheter-related infection. *Am J Med.* 1981;70(3):739-744.

41. Gladstone IM, Ehrenkranz RA, Edberg SC, Baltimore RS. A ten-year review of neonatal sepsis and comparison with the previous fifty-year experience. *Pediatr Infect Dis J.* 1990;9(11):819-825.

42. Leroyer A, Bedu A, Lombrail P, et al. Prolongation of hospital stay and extra costs due to hospital-acquired infection in a neonatal unit. *J Hosp Infect.* 1997;35(1):37-45.

43. Aly H, Herson V, Duncan A, et al. Is bloodstream infection preventable among premature infants? A tale of two cities. *Pediatrics.* 2005;115(6):1513-1518.

44. Mahieu LM, De Muynck AO, Ieven MM, at al. Risk factors for central vascular catheter-associated bloodstream infections among patients in a neonatal intensive care unit. *J Hosp Infect.* 2001;48(2):108-116.

45. Hruszkewycz V, Holtrop PC, Batton DG, et al. Complications associated with central venous catheters inserted in critically ill neonates. *Infect Control Hosp Epidemiol.* 1991;12(9):544-548.

46. Fridkin SK, Kaufman D, Edwards JR, Shetty S, Horan T. Changing incidence of Candida bloodstream infections among NICU patients in the United States: 1995-2004. *Pediatrics.* 2006;117(5):1680-1687.

47. Mahieu LM, De Dooy JJ, Lenaerts AE, et al. Catheter manipulations and the risk of catheter-associated bloodstream infection in neonatal intensive care unit patients. *J Hosp Infect.* 2001;48(1):20-26.

48. Stoll BJ, Hansen N, Fanaroff AA, et al. Late-onset sepsis in very low birth weight neonates: the experience of the NICHD Neonatal Research Network. *Pediatrics.* 2002;110(2 Pt 1):285-291.

49. Makhoul IR, Sujov P, Smolkin T, et al. Epidemiological, clinical, and microbiological characteristics of late-onset sepsis among very low birth weight infants in Israel: a national survey. *Pediatrics.* 2002;109(1):34-39.

50. Bizzarro MJ, Sabo B, Noonan M, et al. A quality improvement initiative to reduce central line-associated bloodstream infections in a neonatal intensive care unit. *Infect Control Hosp Epidemiol.* 2010;31(3):241-248.

51. Reduction in central line-associated bloodstream infections among patients in intensive care units—Pennsylvania, April 2001-March 2005. *MMWR. Morbidity and Mortality Weekly Report.* 2005;54(40):1013-1016.

52. Pronovost P, Needham D, Berenholtz S, et al. An intervention to decrease catheter-related bloodstream infections in the ICU. *N Engl J Med.* 2006;355(26):2725-2732.

53. Berenholtz SM, Pronovost PJ, Lipsett PA, et al. Eliminating catheter-related bloodstream infections in the intensive care unit. *Crit Care Med.* 2004;32(10):2014-2020.

54. Schulman J, Stricof RL, Stevens TP, et al. Development of a statewide collaborative to decrease NICU central line-associated bloodstream infections. *J Perinatol.* 2009;29(9):591-599.

55. Schulman J, Stricof R, Stevens TP, et al. Statewide NICU central-line-associated bloodstream infection rates decline after bundles and checklists. *Pediatrics.* 2011;127(3):436-444.

56. Taylor T, Massaro A, Williams L, et al. Effect of a dedicated percutaneously inserted central catheter team on neonatal catheter-related bloodstream infection. *Adv Neonat Care.* 2011;11(2):122-128.

57. Austin N, McGuire W. Prophylactic systemic antifungal agents to prevent mortality and morbidity in very low birth weight infants. *Cochrane Database Syst Rev.* 2013;4:CD003850.

58. Austin N, Darlow BA, McGuire W. Prophylactic oral/topical non-absorbed antifungal agents to prevent invasive fungal infection in very low birth weight infants. *Cochrane Database Syst Rev.* 2013;3:CD003478.

59. Powers RJ, Wirtschafter DW. Decreasing central line associated bloodstream infection in neonatal intensive care. *Clin Perinatol.* 2010;37(1):247-272.

60. Lee SK, Aziz K, Singhal N, et al. Improving the quality of care for infants: a cluster randomized controlled trial. *CMAJ.* 2009;181(8):469-476.

61. Curry S, Honeycutt M, Goins G, Gilliam C. Catheter-associated bloodstream infections in the NICU: getting to zero. *Neonat Network.* 2009;28(3):151-155.

62. Kilbride HW, Powers R, Wirtschafter DD, et al. Evaluation and development of potentially better practices to prevent neonatal nosocomial bacteremia. *Pediatrics.* 2003;111(4 Pt 2):e504-e518.

63. Golombek SG, Rohan AJ, Parvez B, et al. "Proactive" management of percutaneously inserted central catheters results in decreased incidence of infection in the ELBW population. *J Perinatol.* 2002;22(3):209-213.

64. Andersen C, Hart J, Vemgal P, Harrison C. Prospective evaluation of a multi-factorial prevention strategy on the impact of nosocomial infection in very-low-birthweight infants. *J Hosp Infect.* 2005;61(2):162-167.

65. Schelonka RL, Scruggs S, Nichols K, et al. Sustained reductions in neonatal nosocomial infection rates following a comprehensive infection control intervention. *J Perinatol.* 2006;26(3):176-179.

66. Wirtschafter DD, Pettit J, Kurtin P, et al. A statewide quality improvement collaborative to reduce neonatal central line-associated blood stream infections. *J Perinatol.* 2010;30(3):170-181.

67. Gordon PV. What progress looks like in NEC research. *J Perinatol.* 2011;31(3):149.

68. Neu J, Walker WA. Necrotizing enterocolitis. *N Engl J Med.* 2011;364(3):255-264.

69. McGuire W, Anthony MY. Donor human milk versus formula for preventing necrotising enterocolitis in preterm infants: systematic review. *Arch Dis Child Fetal Neonatal Ed.* 2003;88(1):F11-F14.

70. Guillet R, Stoll BJ, Cotten CM, et al. Association of H2-blocker therapy and higher incidence of necrotizing enterocolitis in very low birth weight infants. *Pediatrics.* 2006;117(2):e137-e142.

71. Uauy RD, Fanaroff AA, Korones SB, et at. Necrotizing enterocolitis in very low birth weight infants: biodemographic and clinical correlates. National Institute of Child Health and Human Development Neonatal Research Network. *J Pediatr.* 1991;119(4):630-638.

72. DeRienzo CM, Smith PB, Cotten CM, et al. Paper presented at: Pediatric Academic Societies; 2013; Washington, DC.

73. Hughes G. How big is big data in healthcare? 2011; Available at: http://blogs.sas.com/content/hls/2011/10/21/how-big-is-big-data-in-healthcare/. Accessed May 2013.

74. NICHD Neonatal Research Network. Extremely Preterm Birth Outcome Data. 2012; Available at: http://www.nichd.nih.gov/about/org/der/branches/ppb/programs/epbo/pages/epbo_case.aspx. Accessed 15.05.2013.

75. Puopolo KM, Draper D, Wi S, et al. Estimating the probability of neonatal early-onset infection on the basis of maternal risk factors. *Pediatrics.* 2011;128(5):e1155-e1163.

76. Kaiser Permanente Division of Research. Probability of neonatal early-onset sepsis based on maternal risk factors. 2011; Available at: http://www.dor.kaiser.org/external/DORExternal/research/InfectionProbabilityCalculator.aspx. Accessed 15.05.2013.

77. Kamholz KL, Dukhovny D, Kirpalani H, et al. Economic evaluation alongside the Premature Infants in Need of Transfusion randomised controlled trial. *Arch Dis Child Fetal Neonatal Ed.* 2012;97(2):F93-F98.

78. Dukhovny D, Lorch SA, Schmidt B, et al. Economic evaluation of caffeine for apnea of prematurity. *Pediatrics.* 2011;127(1):e146-e155.

79. Zupancic JA, Hibbs AM, Palermo L, et al. Economic evaluation of inhaled nitric oxide in preterm infants undergoing mechanical ventilation. *Pediatrics.* 2009;124(5):1325-1332.

80. AAP. Helping Babies Breathe. 2013; Available at: http://www.helpingbabiesbreathe.org/about.html. Accessed May, 2013.

81. Msemo G, Massawe A, Mmbando D, et al. Newborn mortality and fresh stillbirth rates in Tanzania after helping babies breathe training. *Pediatrics.* 2013;131(2):e353-e360.

82. Collins JC. *Good to Great: Why Some Companies Make the Leap—and Others Don't.* 1st ed. New York, NY: HarperBusiness; 2001.

PROFESSIONAL ACCOUNTABILITY AND PURSUIT OF A CULTURE OF SAFETY

10

You are a leader in a regional hospital or children's hospital. You walk into your office and learn that a number of "events" have occurred that need attention:

- Event 1. A representative from your Office of Patient Relations (OPR) calls and shares that she is having difficulty getting a call back from Dr Hematology to discuss a complaint filed by parents of one of her patients. Hospital policy requires OPR to contact involved physicians on an as-needed basis to assist with service recovery.
- Event 2. Dr Hospital Epidemiologist conveys a nurse's report that Dr Gastroenterology did not respond to a reminder to foam in (hand sanitize) on entering a patient's room. He stated to the nurse, "Don't need to. Just going to share test results with my patient" and proceeded to walk in.
- Event 3. Reported by Nurse X (Surgical Circulator) via the hospital's electronic event reporting system: "I attempted to call a time-out prior to the start of a neurosurgical procedure on patient Jane Doe, aged seven. Dr Neurosurgeon looked up, then continued to participate in a side conversation. I tried a second time at which point Dr Neurosurgeon interrupted, "I think we're on the same page here. Could we please just begin? I get so tired of having to waste time with this time-out nonsense."

Are the stories similar or dissimilar? Are they accurate? Which events do you address? What if you don't address each event? After all, aren't things just going to happen in a busy health system? And if you try to follow up on every event, won't you be overwhelmed?

Each event represents a behavior or performance that creates a safety risk. Each also has the potential to undermine pursuit of a "culture of safety" defined as, "The product of individual and group values, attitudes, perceptions, competencies, and patterns of behavior that determine the commitment to, and the style and proficiency of, an organization's health and safety programs. Organizations with a positive safety culture are characterized by communications founded on mutual trust, by shared perceptions of the importance of safety, and by confidence in the efficacy of preventative measures."[1]

To achieve a culture of safety requires surveillance, early reporting of events, and acting on the information to provide timely, measured feedback to team members in a highly reliable manner. Failing to act has consequences for your system and for team members' well-being.[2] The critical question is, in your leadership role, are you willing and do you have a plan to address behaviors that threaten a culture of safety?

Lack of feedback contributes to our failure to demonstrate sustained improvements in safety and quality despite the level of attention given to errors since the release of the Institute of Medicine's 1999 landmark report, *To Err is Human*.[3] Failure to have a plan and to follow the plan contributes to our inability to demonstrate sustained improvement in safety and quality.

The goals in this chapter are for the reader to understand:

- The importance of pursuing a culture of safety and reliability,
- The safety problem in healthcare stemming from our collective failure to adequately address behaviors and performance that undermine a culture of safety,[4]
- Professionalism and the key role it plays in making medicine kinder and safer,
- How infrastructure supports addressing behavior and performance through professional self- and group-regulation, and
- The skills needed to have "adult conversations" when events occur or data suggest patterns of poor performance.

PROFESSIONALISM IN THE 21ST CENTURY

Reflect back on the events reported in the beginning of this chapter, ie, lack of response to a professional colleague charged with addressing a family's concern, refusal to perform hand hygiene, and failing to observe a time-out after prompting. Do such behaviors model respect, build trust, and support team performance? If not, there arises a professional duty to address and hold colleagues accountable. Professionals have long declared they are best qualified to evaluate peers' performance,[5] but the reality is that too few organizations have effective systematized peer review or group regulation to support teams and promote safety.[6,7]

Research makes clear that medical care injures some patients[3,8–10] and faulty systems, human failures, or their interplay contributes.[11,12] The 21st-century notion of professionalism therefore requires competencies fundamental to the goal of making medicine safer. Medicine is a team activity involving the interactions of numerous parties working together. When professionals (nursing, pharmacist, physician, and others) work well together, outcomes of care are enhanced. Unprofessional behavior, in contrast, creates team dysfunction.[4,13,14]

Team member behaviors then must support team performance. "Professional" regulation needs to focus not only on cognitive and technical competencies, but also on communicating effectively, being available, and modeling respect for those who at any moment may have critical information or are in a position to prevent an error (such as wrong site surgery) if empowered to speak up. When they observe threats to safety, team members have duties to identify and report, remediate behaviors, and fix faulty systems.

In the context of the professional and the team, the professional engages in two forms of regulation: (1) self-regulation—recognizing one's limitations, referring to or seeking additional training, self-monitoring to maintain awareness of how one's behavior and performance impact others, and willingness to receive feedback, and (2) group-regulation—because one is committed to patients and his/her team members, individually or within a peer review committee, monitors, speaks up, reports, or otherwise addresses behavior or performance with the potential to undermine a culture of safety.

When professionals are willing to model respect and engage in self- and group-regulation, and are supported by a plan, Dr Hematology, Dr Gastroenterology, and Dr Neurosurgery are less likely to threaten the culture of safety.

PROFESSIONALISM AND HIGH RELIABILITY

Committed health organizations pursue high reliability, that is, right care for every patient, every time. High-reliability organizations (HROs) achieve consistent performance of high levels of safety for extended periods of time. The commercial air industry, nuclear power production, and naval carrier air operations are considered HROs because they commit to learning and change when feedback or failures suggest the need for better processes to minimize risk and increase reliability.

HROs are characterized by:

- Team members who, collectively and individually, understand the ever-present potential for injury and their crucial role in preventing harm; vigilantly monitor for any change or variation in a standard process;[15,16]

feel respected and empowered to speak up and report potential threats without fear of retaliation; and report events, "near misses" (variation in process that did not result in injury but had the potential to do so);

- Leaders who demonstrate commitment to sustaining the culture by articulating shared values and goals, providing adequate resources to create infrastructure that reinforces a culture of safety, and holding all members of the team accountable irrespective of position;

- Systematic use of tools and processes to reliably review reports and generate data that help identify gaps and deficiencies; and

- Commitment to act to remedy human behavior/performance and fix faulty systems. Remedying weaknesses promotes trust, thus reinforcing and strengthening the culture of safety to make healthcare even safer.[17,18]

Concepts of high reliability and professionalism link in that the principles that define "who I should be as a professional" are also consistent with the practices of HROs. Commitment to self- and group-regulation and infrastructure tools that support a culture of safety (described later) can transform healthcare institutions and systems into HROs.

UNPROFESSIONAL BEHAVIOR/PERFORMANCE UNDERMINES A CULTURE OF SAFETY

Healthcare professionals, like all humans, are subject to slips and lapses in behavior and performance. Everyone occasionally forgets to foam in, fails to respond to a page, or speaks in a manner perceived as disrespectful. Unfortunately, slips and lapses, whether due to carelessness, distractions, missed communications, or the stressful nature of professional practice, create risk even if they seem minor.[4,11,12,19–26] A lapse in professional performance may directly cause harm (eg, failure to sanitize hands transfers infection), or indirect harm (eg, loss of concentration when you fear another team member or incomplete communication when a physician hangs up on a nurse with a question).[4,13,25,26]

But how do we recognize unprofessional behaviors that threaten safety? Aggressive behaviors are generally easy to recognize and include "bullying, yelling, spitting, or 'cussin,'" intimidation, sexual boundary violations, and physical assault. For example, nursing professionals reported:

> Dr Infectious Disease came in, cursing loudly and screaming how stupid I was. It was witnessed by many people, not only patients and families, but also staff who reported to me.[27]

The fellow told her to come out of the room. She asked if she could give the pain med first and he said "No, come out now." She stepped to the door … He started yelling at her and said he would not follow the rules for contact precautions on his patients because "the rule is stupid" … After approximately two minutes, he told her she was completely inappropriate for asking him to gown and glove and walked off.

Passive-aggressive and passive behaviors, however, may be equally destructive to the pursuit of safety.[4] Jousting[13,14,28,29] (gratuitous negative comments about a professional, practice, or healthcare institution), condescension, and modeling disrespect for safety systems impair relationships and undermine trust:

After the therapist left the room, my husband's nurse made his opinion of the therapist's actions clear to everyone: "stupid…stupid…stupid…" and a few other choice words

We had just installed a new order entry system. Dr Internist walked by a terminal, picked up a paper towel, wrote orders on it, and gave it to me.

Dr Surgeon was entering a patient's room, and I noticed she did not foam in. She did not respond to my verbal prompt so I offered her a pair of gloves. She took the gloves, turned, held the gloves over a trash pail, let go, and proceeded to the bedside, ungloved.

Passive behavior, too, threatens patient care when professionals fail to respond to calls or emails (Event 1), arrive late to meetings, rounds, or the operating room, ignore others, or fail to communicate with team members. Such behaviors make it more difficult to provide appropriate medical attention and for patients to fully understand what they need to do or what to expect.

Dr Oncologist and I followed a patient together. He's the primary oncologist, and I am the child's stem cell transplant physician. While I was reviewing the child's scans, so we could present the information to the family together, Dr Oncologist discussed the future care with the parents. Dr Oncologist left without discussing these plans with me and never paged to communicate with me before I walked in to see the family.

I [patient] kept trying to ask Dr Oncologist questions, but he just kept texting and wouldn't answer. He suddenly said, "excuse me" and walked out of the room.

Because a wide range of behaviors threaten safety, we define unprofessional (disruptive) behavior as any behavior **or** performance that interferes, or has the potential to interfere, with the medical team's ability to achieve intended outcomes.[3,30] We define unprofessional behavior more broadly than bullying, physical violence, boundary violations, or discrimination, because of the critical importance of team performance within a culture of safety. The inclusive definition allows professionals greater latitude (and ability) to address issues of conduct and performance, for example, when Dr Neurosurgeon continues to engage in a side conversation and then announces, "Can we move along…?" or when someone fails to practice good hand hygiene.

As we think about professional accountability, reflect on those moments when any one of us does not perform at our best. Professionals pledge to one another willingness to give and receive feedback, to help prevent pattern development, and where patterns appear to exist, to fairly address with the individual. Whether an unprofessional act is intentional or not, failure to follow best practices threatens care. The patient who acquires a central-line-associated bloodstream infection (CLABSI) because a physician forgot or chose not to follow best practices is just as ill. Further, when co-workers observe others not following important safety procedures, they may feel exempt or conclude that the practice must not really be that important.

The critical question that remains is, are chair, chief medical officer, chief nursing officer, director, division chief, chief of service, vice-president of medical affairs, and others prepared to support professionals trying to do good work? For healthcare organizations to become HROs, executive officers and leaders at the bedside must understand the linkage between attributes of professionalism, teamwork, reliability, and safety.[31]

WHY DO PROFESSIONALS FAIL TO BE PROFESSIONAL?

Understanding the definition of unprofessional behavior is important. We must also ask why it is that a medical professional behaves or performs in a way that undermines a culture of safety. Many factors contribute.

To begin with, the interaction between professionals and their health systems is challenging. Being a healthcare professional is inherently stressful, and many practice in dysfunctional systems. Increasing demand for services, declining reimbursement, and efforts to increase production take their toll. Perhaps, for example, the neurosurgeon does not want to pause for a time-out because of pressure to shorten operating room (OR) turnaround time to accommodate case volume. Professionals get conflicting messages from hospital leadership, eg, conduct timeouts *and* shorten OR turnaround times. Other stressors include concerns or fear that another professional or system failure has harmed or placed their patient in danger of harm. Although occasional passive, testy, or aggressive behavior may be understandable, it still needs to be addressed.

In addition, a host of human conditions may impair one's ability to "play well" with others, including substance use/abuse, psychiatric, including personality (narcissism) disorders, medical illness, or cognitive impairment.[32,33] Family/home problems spill over into a professional's life and vice versa.

Some behaviors reflect long-standing dysfunctional habits or patterns. As examples, professionals may continue to wrestle with "family of origin" (the family into which they were born)[34] issues such as alcoholism and co-dependency, or demonstrate a history of unprofessional behaviors stretching from when they were in medical school to state medical board sanctioning decades later.[35]

Stressors or personality/behavioral factors, however, are "*antecedents,*" that is to say, triggers or predispositions to unprofessional acts. They are not the reason that patterns develop. What perpetuates unprofessional behavior are the types of consequences that follow.[36,37]

Imagine a 4-year-old and the parent at a store. The child makes a request for a treat. The parent decides that fulfilling the request is not in the child's best interest and simply but kindly says, "no." The child immediately escalates, turning up both verbal and non-verbal communication. The parent weighs his/her options: repeat "no," provide an explanation, attempt to distract, promise something later, or in the face of the child's persistence, just give in.

How often is it that when a particular team member makes a demand, especially someone with "special value," others jump to respond because of conditioning, fear, or both? How often do team members create workarounds because Dr Interventional Radiologist does not want to enter orders into the electronic ordering system or engage in time-outs? Have they come to recognize that if they attempt a second request, Dr Interventional Radiologist will only escalate resistance? How often does the parent rationalize, "Just this one time." The child learns a "valuable" lesson.

When team members fail to do something important for patient care, do we look the other way? Consider the ophthalmologist who, for whatever reason, does not want to come in to the emergency department (ED) to evaluate a child with trauma to the eye. The ophthalmologist might model passive behavior (and just not seem to have his/her pager on), passive-aggressive behavior ("I'll come in, but you guys really should learn to do a proper slit lamp exam"), or become aggressive ("Another ED physician called me earlier and like I said before, I don't want you calling me to come in unless the child needs surgery. They can come to my office on Monday," then slams down the phone). Regardless of the form of unprofessional behavior, is the ophthalmologist's "inner 4-year-old" in command?

Thus, most professionals who fail to wash their hands, ignore insertion bundles, prescribe non-indicated antibiotics, fail to respect time-outs or accumulate incomplete operative notes and discharge summaries do so because there are no negative consequences. In other words, for some reason, the offending professionals are not motivated to self-regulate, and observers neither report nor act to support group regulation. Pediatricians, above all disciplines, should understand this principle that it is not about punishment when someone fails—we're all human—but rather about using appropriate and measured feedback to re-point people in the direction of safety.

BARRIERS TO ADDRESSING BEHAVIORS THAT UNDERMINE A CULTURE OF SAFETY

If Dr Surgeon has behaved "that way" for years, many are likely to assume "(s)he will not change." Perhaps not, but by not addressing, team members may normalize behaviors and undermine efforts to move the safety agenda forward. Further, consider if it is professional or even fair to Dr Surgeon that colleagues and co-workers continue to talk *about* but not *to* him?

What barriers keep concerned professionals from acting? Barriers may be systemic, personal, or a combination of the two. Leaders must be able to articulate the barriers in order to develop effective plan to support reporting and acting.

Team Member Barriers

Among the more common systems obstacles that should be addressed in order for team members to more fully participate in sustaining safety are:

- *Inadequate policies.* When you review your current professionalism policy, do you (really) understand it? Non-existent, weak, confusing, or difficult-to-understand professional conduct policies written in "legalese" hinder pursuit of a culture of safety. Policies should clearly define the types of behaviors and performance that should be reported or acted upon, outline options for reporting and action, and prohibit retaliatory behavior for good faith reporting; and
- *Lack of user-friendly reporting systems.* If you have a surveillance system for event reporting, is it easy to use? If not, do team members understand their chain of command and how to use it? Your health system, regardless of size, must provide reminders that a responsible healthcare professional is alert to and reports variation from standardized processes, unprofessional behavior, apparent conflicts of interest, or compliance concerns. Implementing accessible (eg, present on all workstations), easy-to-use electronic reporting surveillance systems help well-intentioned, busy people report.

Team members also face *personal* barriers to reporting. These include:

■ *Fear of backlash* if a report is not kept confidential and/or creates tension within the team:

A surgeon in our facility routinely "hazes" nurses publicly, which results in disruption of care if the nurse is overwhelmed by the attack. I [nurse] try to ignore the behavior and not throw gasoline on the fire.

Some professionals, however, exhibit personal courage and do the right thing anyway:

The patient was not getting appropriate care. I found it difficult to speak out because I feared asserting myself would cause difficulty working with them in the future. My actions did cause some hurt feelings. I had to "smooth over" the situation with the nurses involved even though their inaction caused potential harm to the patient.

■ *Experience of previous intimidation* that makes one too fearful to report.

After it was reported, the physician is still in the clinic and I refuse to put anything else in writing for fear of retaliation. I cannot sleep the night before and suffer anxiety when he is in the clinic.
 They "hung me out to dry" to save their neck. I was afraid to tell anyone above the director. I felt gun-shy after that experience.

■ *Rationalization* that a colleague or co-worker's "bark is worse than his/her bite; or "I can (*or should be able to*) handle it;"
■ *Decision that a "workaround"* is easier than interacting with a potential offender:

Dr Surgeon hates to be called when she's on rounds … most times I just order tests for her patients that I think she'll want.
 Every time I need to send a patient to the ED for a surgical consult, I check first to make sure Dr Surgeon is not on call. If it is Dr Surgeon, I casually ask the page operator which surgeon will be on call when the switch occurs, hoping I can wait before sending the patient over;

■ *Lack of awareness* that evidence-based best practices for hand hygiene or line insertion bundles can achieve meaningful differences in outcome.[38,39,40] (Think of Dr Neurosurgery scoffing at "this time-out nonsense");
■ *Misperception of the downstream effects of unprofessional conduct.* A professional may shrug off as inconsequential an encounter in which a family felt disrespected. Failure to respond to the episode perpetuates an ongoing threat to safety that can lead to serious consequences should

the family hesitate to call when their child's illness does not follow the expected pathway to recovery; and

■ *Belief it is futile to speak up*, ie, "Nothing will be done if I report." Lack of confidence that leadership will intervene is a reasonable conclusion when "Dr Cardiologist still behaves that way even after all of our reports." Certain professionals with "special" value always seem to get a pass:

He should have been written up this time but the CEO chose to let it go.

Leader Barriers

Although aware that unprofessional conduct occurs, is under-reported, and poses threat to safety,[4,41] two-thirds of executives believe they do not deal with these issues effectively.[27]

Some of the systemic barriers include:

■ *Uncertainty of authority to act* or fear that those higher up the chain might not support their efforts or overtly oppose;

■ *Lack of training* to know how to create infrastructure that supports a safety culture;

■ *Incomplete understanding of the costs of not acting* (more later) and so choose to allocate resources to other priority needs; and

■ *Lack of awareness* that failure to impose negative consequences for unprofessional behavior is the primary reason the behavior persists.

Leaders' personal barriers to addressing unprofessional behavior include:

■ *Aversion to conflict* even among "C-suite" officers (eg, chief executive/ nursing/medical officers);

■ *Treating certain professionals as "special,"* eg, high-revenue generators, difficult-to-recruit skill set, robust research grant support or tenure (academic centers), or personal relationships with Board members or high-ranking officers, erodes trust that team members' reports are dealt with fairly and consistently.[27] When leaders declare a goal to eliminate "wrong site" surgery and establish policy mandating universal time-out protocols and Team Stepps[42] training, they may yet permit key figures to not attend training (passive) or to ignore time-outs (passive-aggressive); and

■ *Self-assigned special status* whereby some high-level administrators themselves behave unprofessionally at times (and with impunity):

Our organization was acquired by another. The new CEO, who is now my boss, screams, curses, and gets physically aggressive whenever he disagrees with any member of the former leadership team. This has prevented me

from providing to our team's members the type of support that formerly was part of my role. I find myself "holding back."

If healthcare leaders articulate the barriers to addressing non-professional behavior in their group or system, they can develop effective plans to remedy. There is no role for either the coward or the zealot on a self-righteous mission. What it takes are leaders at all levels—unit/team leaders, division chiefs, chairs/ chiefs of service, chief executive/medical/nursing officers, and members of the Board—willing to develop a thoughtful plan and act in a fair and measured way:

Dr Neurosurgeon raged at me [charge nurse] … I reported him … because I would never be able to look my nurses in the eye when I recommend they report unprofessional behavior … This episode was … a personal watershed moment for me—I have resolved to NEVER stand by and let someone in my facility get by with harmful behavior … I admit it's stressful to struggle against bad behavior and worry about who will stand with me, but this is a better, healthier stress. I can sleep with the stress that comes from working on progress … We teach other people how to treat us, and for too long this physician and others like him have been trained that abominable behavior is all right because of who they are and what they do … An elementary school teacher told me that to change the bullies, we have to change the bystanders. If bystanders let it be known they won't tolerate bullies attacking victims, things change.

MAKING THE CASE FOR ADDRESSING UNPROFESSIONAL CONDUCT

Despite barriers to act, the case for action is strong. Safety and organizational behavior science tells us that unprofessional behavior threatens trust, creates team dysfunction, and diverts attention from the task on hand, contributing to slips, lapses, and errors.[11-13] Human costs of unprofessional behavior and performance therefore include patient harm and team member distress.[13,43-45] As will be seen, financial impacts include costs associated with high staff turnover and recruitment, treating preventable patient harm, and medical malpractice claims.

FAILURE TO ACHIEVE INTENDED OUTCOMES

Suppose you are a nursing professional performing a complex task when Dr Intensivist walks into the intensive care unit (ICU). Aware of her reputation as one who may suddenly lash out and belittle, at least some of your attention shifts from your task to focus on her movements, increasing risk for a slip or lapse in performance.[46] Furthermore, because any barrier to team communication places patients at increased risk of harm, efforts to avoid interacting with Dr Intensivist or failures on her part to listen to other members are maladaptive. In "fishbone"[47] analyses of adverse outcomes in emergency medicine, women's health, pediatrics, and trauma care, impaired communication was identified as a major contributor to adverse events in up to two-thirds of cases:[19–21,23,24]

> *Dr Intensivist … [is] argumentative, demeaning, and rude, not just to nurses but to [physician] colleagues. We are all a team but, unfortunately, patient care, and morale [suffer]. Nurses are afraid … to talk to Dr Intensivist and delay … as long as possible, sometimes avoiding Dr Intensivist altogether.[25]*
>
> *No one wants to get report from this nurse due to her curt responses as well as the "interrogation" as to why thing were done this way, etc. She creates tension and anxiety in the workplace … affects my ability to concentrate on the work at hand is a huge distraction. It is easy to see how this could become a patient safety issue.*
>
> *I [resident] was asked to assist Dr Intensivist with a chest tube insertion. Dr Intensivist took a cellphone call and motioned to me to take over the procedure. I felt uncomfortable and tried to let Dr Intensivist know that I've not yet done this procedure although I've seen it done a couple of times. Dr Intensivist waved at me to go back to the procedure and continued talking on the phone.*

Furthermore, in a study that also looked at patient and family complaints,[19] in half of the cases with communication failures, the physician was described by complainants as having demonstrated other unprofessional behaviors. One patient, for example, noted:

> *It was difficult observing one person humiliating another. It made me feel unsafe myself.*

Patient outcomes also suffer when patients and families who witness or experience disrespect firsthand decide to not adhere to medical recommendations, fail to follow up, or drop out from the practice:[48–53]

> *I do not want to come back … Dr Intensivist was loud and rude to his staff during the visit and I am not comfortable with him.*

COSTS OF DISRESPECT

Perceived mistreatment and disrespect for team members lowers trust and reliability, and contributes to poor team morale and burnout.[54] Those who feel unvalued or repeatedly targeted find little joy and meaning in their work:[55-57]

> *Dr Otolaryngologist dismisses my comments and plans ... speaks in a condescending manner in reports to senior management who assume the physician is correct. This promotes lack of initiative, giving up, burn-out, and/or inhibits professional development.*
>
> *Working with a pathologic bully for 10 years ... I am frightened. It clearly affects my ability to concentrate and is a huge distraction. It is easy to see how this could become a patient safety issue.*
>
> *[Nursing colleague] makes me dread coming to a job I used to love and look forward to.*

Many unhappy professionals leave their jobs.[58] In a 2009 study by the Center for Patient and Professional Advocacy at Vanderbilt and the Studer group, two-thirds of nurses interviewed considered leaving because of unprofessional conduct in the workplace; 41% said they had left a position at some point for this reason.[27]

To assess the magnitude of associated costs, consider a hypothetical organization with 2,000 staff nurses and an annual turnover rate of 13%; 260 nurses depart each year. Of these, suppose as few as 6%-12% (n = 16-31) leave for reasons related to failures of the health system to reliably address unprofessional conduct, such as:

> *The DoN [Director of Nursing] won't do anything about ... verbal abuse by surgeons and anesthesiologists in public areas and in front of patients and peers ... makes it challenging to do your job or even want to come to work.*

Costs incurred when nurses depart include advertising, recruiting, hiring temporary staff, overtime pay for some, loss of productivity from increased stress, and orienting and training new team members. In FY 2007, such costs ranged from $82,000 to $88,000 per new recruit.[59] Thus, our hypothetical organization could incur expenses on the order of $1.3-$2.8 million annually to replace nurses who leave because of others' unprofessional behavior. Harassment claims impose further financial burdens, and the reputation of the health system as a bad place to work interferes with staff retention and recruitment.[60] Furthermore, nursing turnover impacts patient safety as turnover rates over 12% are associated with higher risk-adjusted mortality rates and length of stay.[61]

COSTS OF PATIENT HARM

Unprofessional behaviors cost health systems in other ways. Failure to adhere to common evidence-based practices, including hand hygiene or use of bundles to perform common procedures, places patients at risk for nosocomial infections, surgical occurrences and other adverse outcomes, as well as the attendant costs of treatment. Billions of dollars are wasted annually in the United States caring for preventable healthcare-associated infections (HAIs) such as central-line-associated bloodstream infections (CLABSI), catheter-associated urinary tract infection (CAUTI), or ventilator-associated pneumonia (VAP).[62] Increasingly, the costs to care for these infections are often uncompensated if payers deem them avoidable.[63] In contrast, compliance with surgical sign-in, time-out, and sign-out checklist procedures helps prevent complications and generates cost savings.[64,65]

From an economic point of view, it is not hard to make a case for addressing single episodes in which physicians, nurses, and other professionals fail to follow best practices in order to prevent pattern development.

IMPACT ON REPUTATION

The professional's and health system's reputations suffer when patients leave a practice or refuse to return to a hospital because of their dissatisfaction with care and/or how they were treated. While only a fraction of unhappy patients voice concerns directly to the organization (estimates range from 1 of 3 to fewer than 1 in 50),[66–69] most share their poor experience with an average of 10 to 20 friends and neighbors.[70,71] When patients and others in their circles leave, so do their dollars.

MEDICAL MALPRACTICE CLAIMS COSTS

Medical malpractice claims risk and unprofessional behaviors are linked. Studies of medical malpractice claims demonstrate non-random distribution of claims even within disciplines where overall annual claims rates reach close to 20%.[72,73] A small subset of physicians (3%–8%) within any discipline account for almost half of all malpractice claims and 75%–85% of all indemnity payouts.[74]

Researchers investigating why some physicians are associated with high numbers of suits relative to their peers found little difference between the practices of high and low claims physicians in terms of patient mix, acuity, and documented medical care. Where groups differed, however, was in how patients reported their experiences with these professionals. Patients of high claims physicians expressed more dissatisfaction with their physicians:[75,76]

As soon as the doctor walked into the room his first comment was, "This is so typical of you people" … disrespectful, hurtful.

Dr Pulmonologist told her that his word is final in that clinic because he is the boss and it doesn't matter what Dr Pediatrician says about the patient. Mother is very upset by this because she really likes Dr Pediatrician and feels like he's the only doctor who is trying to figure out what is wrong with her son.

Patient's father states he has left multiple messages with the unit and at the MD's office … the doctor still hasn't called back.

Patients of high claims physicians were three times as likely to report such behaviors to the research team compared with patients seen by low claims physicians.[76] Subsequent studies confirmed the association of claims risk with patient and family reports of their observations or experiences of professionals' behaviors that undermine safety.[77–82]

You, a leader or team member, undoubtedly, observe or experience behaviors that undermine a culture of safety. Invariably you weigh the pros and cons of reporting or acting. Competing priorities, lack of training, belief that certain individuals can never change, or fear of antagonizing a "special" person within the organization or their protector may deter you. These barriers, however, must be weighed against the costs of failing to act: damage to staff morale, retention issues, the institution's reputation, liability and risk management costs, and most importantly, the contribution to unsafe conditions and poor outcomes of care for the patients we collectively serve.[83] For leaders and team members to attain the level of commitment needed to take on the challenge of addressing unprofessional behavior and performance requires an understanding of consequences of failing to act. There are no spectators in a culture of safety; real professionals observe and are willing to act.

Pause and reflect on the last three unprofessional events you witnessed or were reported to you in your official role. Did these episodes place patients at risk? Did they impact (or could have impacted) members of your team? How did you weigh the pros and cons as you decided whether to report or act? Did you act within your capacity to address or report, or did you rationalize that it was okay to look the other way just this time?

INFRASTRUCTURE ELEMENTS FOR PROMOTING PROFESSIONAL ACCOUNTABILITY

Reliably addressing behaviors (single acts or patterns) that undermine a safety culture requires more than just good intentions. Professionals and organizations need a plan supported by leadership commitment. Eight key elements

Table 10-1	INFRASTRUCTURE ELEMENTS FOR PROMOTING PROCESS RELIABILITY AND PROFESSIONAL ACCOUNTABILITY

1. Leadership commitment
2. Mission, goals, core values, and supportive policies
3. Surveillance tools to capture observations and reports
4. Processes for reviewing observations and reports
5. Model to guide graduated interventions
6. Multi-level professional/leader training (on infrastructure and communication skills)
7. Resources to help address the causes of unnecessary variation in performance (both system and individual)
8. Resources to help those affected

support self- and group-regulation by promoting process reliability and professional accountability.[18,84] (Table 10-1)

As you review this subsection, think about your practice/group/health system. Which elements exist and which need further development or better support?

LEADERSHIP COMMITMENT

It is reasonable to assume that "C-suite" executives (including chief executive/medical/nursing officers, chairs/chiefs of service, and members of the Board of Directors) do not want "never" events, including wrong site, wrong procedure, or wrong patient surgery to occur. This desire, however, is not sufficient. Leaders signal real commitment to a culture of safety by:

- Establishing and supporting an infrastructure to reliably address professional accountability;
- Encouraging and supporting team members to report or act. At any time, a nursing professional who observes someone not sanitizing his/her hands or honoring a time-out process has a moment to be a safety leader. Recognizing, however, that not all prompts are received in a professional manner, leaders support personnel who are threatened or assaulted, verbally or otherwise, for doing the right thing;
- Making clear that reporters' observations are reviewed and acted upon in a fair and measured way with progressive messages that support professional accountability;
- Not "blinking," ie, using their authority to act in a fair and consistent manner and not looking the other way. The Joint Commission emphasizes in a safety culture, all team members should be held "accountable

for modeling desirable behaviors" and the code of conduct enforced "consistently and equitably among staff regardless of seniority or clinical discipline."[4] Doing so sets the stage for self-reinforcing culture change;[85] and

■ Embracing the principles of professionalism and high reliability and incorporating them as core organizational values.

To assess commitment, ask each leader to declare "I recognize the importance of and will ...":

■ Enforce policies and processes that support a culture of safety, including evidence-based practices such as time-outs, hand hygiene, and use of line insertion bundles;

■ Use my authority to act in a fair and consistent manner when a resister invokes his/her "special" status as a reason for exemption from a safety practice or behavioral norm; and

■ Be prepared to terminate individuals who, after receiving measured feedback, continue to demonstrate unwillingness or inability to model behaviors/performance consistent with professional standards.

As a leader or future leader in your health system, reflect on the three events reported to you earlier. Would you be willing to provide feedback to those involved in each (or support a designee)? Would others within your organization be willing to do the same? It is important to consider the answers to these questions because without shared commitment, the ability to reinforce process regularity and continual vigilance is hampered. Knowing the answers also means that when you are ready to act, you do not belatedly discover there is no one standing with you. As Benjamin Franklin wisely reflected at the signing of the Declaration of Independence, "We must all hang together or, assuredly, we shall all hang separately."[86]

MISSION, GOALS, CORE VALUES, AND SUPPORTIVE POLICIES

Establishing an organizational mission, goals, and core values (credo), and developing supportive policies models leadership and promotes accountability. Adopting and promulgating throughout the system common principles, expectations, language, and a defined process promotes accountability and fairness.

Most successful teams develop goals and share with team members (eg, win the Superbowl, grow to qualify for trading on the New York Stock Exchange, train the next generation of medical leaders). Isn't it reasonable for your practice or system to have articulated goals such as "eliminating central-line-associated bloodstream infections" aligned with the group's mission? Small groups to large health systems need to articulate their mission (vision) and define and share performance goals so that team members understand. An example of a health system's mission statement, for example, might be "to serve our local, national, and world communities through innovative research and education, and delivery of high quality, safe, compassionate health care." Pursuing reliability requires team members to understand why they come to work and how their duties are aligned with the organization's mission. Alignment further supports joy and meaning in the workplace.[2]

Establishing a yearly set of operational goals across the organization focused on the well-being of team members, quality and safety, innovation, and financial performance is important as is interconnectedness among the goals. One example of an operational goal might be "to eliminate catheter associated bloodstream infections." Senior and mid-level management should always ask whether any new or existing initiative aligns with the organization's goals and mission (vision). Too often, quality and safety initiatives fail because they are not prioritized at a high enough leadership level within the organization nor sufficiently recognized as critical to the success of other operational goals.

Medical groups and systems also need to define who they are. Credo, a set of core values developed through an iterative, collaborative process, can help with this identity. Credos should align with standards of professionalism to which team members ascribe. As an example, development of the Vanderbilt University Medical Center (VUMC)'s credo began in 1995, involving 900 high-performing team members (including nursing, physicians, reception, transport, medical staff, dietary services, pharmacy) working in focus groups. The participants were asked to draw "what professionalism looks like," using paper and markers. Thousands of illustrations were ultimately distilled into six core principles and transformed into VMUC's statement of "who we are," ie, "our credo[87]":

- I make those I serve my highest priority.
- I respect privacy and confidentiality.
- I communicate effectively.
- I conduct myself professionally.
- I have a sense of ownership.
- I am committed to my colleagues.

Note that each statement begins with "I" and not "we." Personalizing each declaration aligns with the concept of reliability, ie, that these behaviors are normative, habitual, and predictable. VUMC team members sign the credo in public and wear it on their identification badges. The credo is discussed in staff and faculty meetings and leaders present "credo awards" to team members with distinguished performances. Significantly, credo principles are part of team members' performance evaluations. As will be seen, credo principles serve as one of the bases for having some of the challenging conversations in support of high reliability.

Written policies should specifically articulate the organization's mission and its safety and quality goals. Policies serve to outline process regularity and establish expectations for behavior and performance. They incorporate important concepts—event reporting, mandated reviews, protection of and non-retaliation against reporters, addressing patient complaints, defining egregious behavior—and convey that reporting and action are about doing the right thing (supporting a culture of safety). Professional conduct policies should expressly link attributes of professionalism to effective teamwork and charge each team member to take lapses in basic safety practices seriously and address (report or act) lapses promptly and in a reliable manner.

Policies need to be written in language that is understandable to the healthcare professional, not just those schooled in the law, and enforceable as written. Opaque language that drives healthcare professionals to seek legal interpretation also impairs the ability of individuals, leaders, and/or organizations to respond as rapidly as is needed within an HRO. Well-written policies serve a key role in administering a practice/group/health system in that they establish a shared approach to addressing issues. Leaders new to their role should review the organization's policies; familiarity with policies avoids needing to "study up" from scratch after a problem is identified. Leaders should also review policies again for clarification before approaching a problem.

Written goals, credos, and policies that support a culture of safety serve as reference points and the basis for human conversation when events occur that do not appear to conform to self-regulation. Credo, for example, helps clarify and communicate expectations when there appears to be performance inconsistent with the organization's quality and safety goals. A team member's failure to follow an evidence-based insertion bundle when placing a central line, for example, represents not only a technical failing but also a behavior inconsistent with a credo that makes "those we serve our highest priority."

Onboarding new team members to a group practice or hospital staff includes making sure they know the organization's mission, goals, core credo values, and policies. This helps set expectations for standards of behavior and performance right from the start. If these expectations are a routine part of onboarding, and documented, then even if a team member asserts "I didn't know," you proceed. Furthermore, properly trained team members should be more willing to act when they observe, for example, inappropriate work-related material posted by a fellow team member on social media.

Explicit discussion of the organization's defined values declares the importance of respect for other team members' contributions and how respect builds trust and supports reliability and favorable outcomes of care. Orienting new affiliates to learn how to use the chain of command communicates that you are not only permitted but encouraged to go up the chain to promote patient safety. The group's values and the mechanics of "how to" are best learned during onboarding, before you are in a situation where you need to make rapid decisions about handling delicate situations.

Organizations that declare their overarching mission and goals, adopt core credo values, write and articulate understandable policies, and seek to assure that all team members, new and existing, understand their duty to uphold all are able to use this shared language in two important ways. First, the concepts facilitate recognition of behaviors that undermine a culture of safety. Second, having common language helps team members efficiently, and in a readily understandable way, articulate feedback to colleagues regarding specific behavior "that does not appear consistent with our shared values." Significantly, the ability to use common language in a shared approach promotes a reliable response when an event occurs. When organizations use processes that are consistent, regular, and predictable, they deal with humans fairly.

Pause and reflect. Do you know your organization's mission statement and goals? Do you have a credo? Have you read and do you understand your policies (really?), and do they specifically refer to safety?

▌SURVEILLANCE TOOLS

Consider the three events described at the beginning of the chapter. In your practice or organization, is there a system that enables patients to file complaints and patient relations professionals to provide service recovery?[88] Is there a system for observing and reporting hand hygiene compliance issues or reporting team member resistance to time-outs? Exactly how does a professional concerned about a lapse in a safety practice share his/her observations with those authorized to take action?

Surveillance tools enable leaders to know what is going on within the practice or health system. Organizations routinely collect many types of data—administrative data, claims file extracts, direct observations to assess hand hygiene,[38] safety culture surveys,[89–91] patient satisfaction surveys,[92] and employee satisfaction community surveys[93,94]—to name but a few.

Contemporaneous co-worker reporting occupies a particularly crucial role in pursuing and sustaining a safety culture. Because the reports they file often identify behavior and performance that pose threats, healthcare personnel need ready access to an electronic event reporting system or their chain of command. Best practices are for those designated within the organization to receive and review the reports to thank the reporters, confirm that there is a process for review, and remind the reporter of the organization's non-retaliation policy. As team members develop trust, their confidence in the culture strengthens.

Patient and family ("patient") reports, too, are critical in support of a culture of safety. Patients assess how well team members communicate, model respect, and take the time to listen and explain. Sometimes patients witness or are the target of unprofessional behaviors and practices that other members of the team no longer "see" or long ago gave up trying to change. For example, a healthcare professional may have behaved unprofessionally all too often for 20 years, but a patient seeing the behavior for the first time may recognize it to be unreasonable and declare it unacceptable. In that regard, patients' observations cast fresh eyes on what sometimes are old problems. Patient feedback can help practices and institutions identify areas of unsafe behavior and practices, including threats to team function. The following are sample patient and family reports:

> *Dr Anesthesiologist was awful … talked down to his staff in front of us … disrespectful and condescending.*
>
> *The anesthesiologist and resident brought my son to the recovery room. The anesthesiologist started to reprimand the resident right in front of us. She was rude and unprofessional. The resident seemed embarrassed, and I felt uncomfortable.*

Patient complaints also alert the organization of problems with care. For example, patient admissions with surgical complications are associated with more complaints than surgical admissions without complications.[95] Furthermore, at times the only notice the group or institution has of an error or sentinel event is a patient's unsolicited complaint report.[81] Patients and staff should be told that their input is important and taken seriously whenever they see something that just doesn't seem right.

PROCESSES FOR REVIEWING REPORTED OBSERVATIONS

Making families and team members aware of reporting systems is essential but must be associated with an established process for review. Consider the following report filed by a nursing professional:

> *Dr Trauma Surgeon was screaming, pounding his fists in the air and throwing his glasses off of his head … the patient and family was visibly confused and upset at what he said and how he said it … The staff*

were at the desk talking about how he never changes and no one does anything about his aggression.

The reporter makes the institution aware of Dr Trauma Surgeon's behavior, the fact that patients and families bear witness and are affected, and that other team members do not trust leadership to act. By virtue of filing, only the author appears to recognize his/her professional duty to report or has already decided to depart and say something on the way out. When professionals fail to take action and address or report observations, they contribute to the development of patterns that undermine a safety culture.

To positively reinforce reporting behavior, organizations should make clear that reports are reliably and promptly reviewed. If your organization collects reports, why do it unless they are screened for immediate and emerging threats in order to avert or mitigate harm? As defined by policy, reports of unprofessional behavior should be referred to designated personnel within the health system who are then expected to share and provide feedback to involved professionals. Similarly, reports regarding faulty systems are referred to appropriate managers, oversight committees, and other designated leaders to work on improving. In all circumstances, leaders must maintain awareness of how behavior, performance, and systems interplay.

As reports accumulate, they begin to suggest patterns. Organizations have a responsibility to code, aggregate, and analyze for persistent or recurrent signals, patterns, or themes in order to identify faulty systems and hold professionals who stand out from comparative and peer groups accountable. Data help professionals fulfill their duty of promoting professional and group accountability by providing opportunities to intervene. Practice and unit leaders are able to reflect on and address low performance or system failures.

A MODEL TO GUIDE GRADUATED INTERVENTIONS: THE PROMOTING PROFESSIONALISM PYRAMID

Beyond reviewing data, practices and health systems need a model to address individual events and apparent patterns. Depending on the data source(s), leaders have the ability to share the data with involved professionals (or managers/directors for units with lagging performance), allow time for self-correction, and then escalate to a higher tier in the model if performance does not change. Leaders should also share results of periodic culture of safety surveys and community surveys with team members.[96]

Supporting professional accountability requires patience. Although there are circumstances that require immediate action (more later), in most cases, one should be willing to allow events/data sufficient time to accumulate to

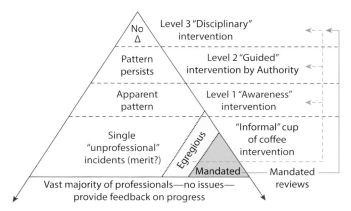

Figure 10-1 ■ Promoting professionalism pyramid. (Adapted, with permission, from Hickson GB et al. A complementary approach to promoting professionalism: Identifying, measuring, and addressing unprofessional behaviors. *Acad Med.* 2007;82:1040-1048.)

reveal any larger picture, accept incremental successes in the direction of safety, and persistently keep the process moving forward. A leader can afford to be patient as long as there is ongoing surveillance to identify outlier behavior or performance.

Using a predictable process and model well understood throughout the practice or health system builds trust and dissipates fear. Figure 10-1 illustrates one validated model for delivering graduated interventions, the Promoting Professionalism Pyramid (Pyramid).[84,38,97] Universal and consistent use of the model provides a fair process in those cases where individuals appear unable or unwilling to respond. The model can also be applied to support unit/clinic performance, as will be shown later through the example of a feedback and intervention program for increasing hand hygiene rates.

The following subsections further examine this model. Each level of the model is associated with a suggested conversation.

SINGLE UNPROFESSIONAL INCIDENT

As you view the Pyramid, notice its base. You know that the vast majority of professionals with whom you work are outstanding and treat others with respect, wash their hands, and regularly engage in self-reflection. However, within any environment, "stuff" can happen, and when it does, team members need a respectful and measured way to share with each other.

Single "events" related to observed or reported behavior need to be addressed early and as often as they occur to help the individual recognize that (s)he is part of a culture pursuing high reliability in which all commit to helping one another self-regulate. The first tier of the model involves feedback after such an event, using what we refer to as a "Cup of Coffee conversation" ("CoC"). A collegial conversation between two people, the individual whose behavior is observed and the person who observes or receives a report, CoC is predicated on the notion that professionals should be willing to deliver and receive feedback.

CoC discussions have three goals: (1) share about a single event (the organization has eyes and ears), (2) share that such behavior/performance does not seem consistent with "the professional I know you to be" (or "our credo"), and (3) "get out of dodge."

When sharing about single events, we suggest the following principles:

- A CoC is not authority-based. Any two co-workers can engage in a CoC, irrespective of job title;
- Consider how you would want information delivered to you;
- Discuss privately and with minimum distraction (same principles as delivering bad news to a patient or family);
- Seek to maintain respect and trust. A CoC is non-judgmental;
- Be clear about your intent. All you want is for the recipient to hear you. The conversation is not about control;
- Avoid the use of the "you" word, a word that tends to promote conflict. Focus instead on using "I" statements—I heard, I saw, I received a report;
- Balance empathy and objectivity;
- Allow the recipient to express his/her view. This models respect and may facilitate insight;
- Recognize that your colleague may "push back" and explain why the report is not true or the behavior justified. You acknowledge but you stay on message: "but what I saw/reviewed … did not seem consistent with …"
- CoC conversations are non-directive. Resist your natural inclination to diagnose your colleague's problem or to share what you think they ought to do. You do not have the right or duty, even if (s)he asks. You are not trying to fix the person. You reinforce an expectation that the individual receiving the message is a problem-solver who will do the right thing (even if you have doubts); and
- Do not expect thanks or even acknowledgement.

Remember that CoC conversations may seem "unsatisfying." You do not demand that the professional acknowledge the event is true or declare "I'll never do it again." If the professional denies the event, you repeat that you brought the observation to his/her attention because it is professional for each of us to share. You acknowledge that while perceptions sometimes differ, you felt it was important to make him/her aware.

Always keep in mind that the observation or report you received could be wrong. Investigation of single reported events is almost always absent from the process except in cases mandated for review or allegations of "egregious" events (Table 10-2). CoCs do not require confirmation of reported "facts" before proceeding; in fact, the information contained in the event report is delivered with

---

Table 10-2   **MANDATED REVIEWS AND "EGREGIOUS EVENTS"**

The **RED** triangle in the lower right hand corner of the Pyramid represents those events that require "Mandated Reviews," ie, prompt formal review by designated offices or authority. These alleged events, once raised, must never be handled in an informal way, even if "I've known Dr XX for years, and I find the story/event impossible to believe." A formal approach allows protection of those alleging harm and future potential victims, and also protects the rights of the professional who may be falsely accused.

Allegations that require Mandated Reviews (and the office/authority to which they are referred) include those pertaining to:

- Acts that, if true, would be criminal or otherwise illegal (law enforcement).
"Dr XX came back very angry and threw the chair against the wall ..."You just shut up."... He then smacked me on the left side of my face."

- Discrimination (Equal Opportunity, Affirmative Action, and Disability Office).
"I was in shock when she called me a [?@#/%]."*

- "HIPAA" violations[a] (Privacy Office).
"Dr XX called my ex-husband and shared the results of my herpes culture."

- Fraud (Compliance Office).
Dr XX billed for a week of procedures where he supposedly was supervising residents. He was on vacation in Hawaii. He states, "Well, I was a phone call away if needed."

The **YELLOW** triangle represents additional issues that The Joint Commission allows hospitals to designate as "egregious." Egregious behavior generally will require involvement of that individual's authority figure/supervisor, Employee/Physician Wellness, or other resources to address and/or undertake corrective/disciplinary action.

Note the YELLOW and RED arrows that point to various levels of the Pyramid. These arrows indicate the types of interventions that leaders may determine are appropriate for a mandated or egregious event. Mandated events, for example, always require, at a minimum, intervention by an authority. An egregious event is never addressed with a cup of coffee conversation but requires, at a minimum, an awareness conversation. Leaders should have latitude to address behavior in ways commensurate with the issues presented. Thus, for example, how a leader addresses a professional with an excessive number of incomplete hospital discharge summaries for the first time likely will differ from how (s)he addresses an individual who threatened another team member.

---

[a]Health Insurance Portability and Accountability Act of 1996 (HIPAA). Pub. L. 104-191 (1996); 45 CFR §§ 164.502, 164.508.

an understanding that the report could be wrong. Investigations can constitute a fatal flaw to the process of promoting professional self-and group-regulation. Investigating each complaint is likely to result in a "he said/she said" situation and creates "analysis paralysis." It delays timely delivery of a simple message: "I received a report … I observed an event … does not seem consistent … I value you as a fellow professional." The unspoken concept is self-regulation.

Pause and reflect on a past experience where a colleague shared an observation about your behavior with you. How did you feel? Did your reaction change through the course of the conversation? Did you reflect? Did you adjust your behavior? Simple sharing is effective.

THE ESPRESSO CONVERSATION

Sometimes with "single" events you, as supervisor or leader, need a bit more leverage to expedite self-reflection and self-correction or to place the individual on notice. Specifically, an event may represent an imminent safety risk or a repeat of a previous behavior for which the individual was provided with a CoC. We refer to such a conversation as an Espresso. This conversation is a sub-type of a CoC with three differences.

The Espresso conversation is also respectful and confidential. Similar to a CoC in most ways ("I saw/ heard/ received a report which seemed inconsistent with the professional I know you to be. I am confident you will reflect on the information and consider what you might do"), three features of this conversation profoundly change the dynamic. In the Espresso conversation, you make clear that:

- You are coming to the professional in your leadership role within the organization;
- You want to know if the event as reported is factually true; and
- You will write a note documenting that the conversation occurred:

I am coming today as your [leader] to share a report I received. The reported event did not seem consistent with who I know you to be and inconsistent with our commitment to (universal hand hygiene, professional behavior, time-out protocols, etc.). [You briefly review the story you received.] Is the report factually true? [Allow response]

You will likely hear one (or more) of several possible responses—Yes; No; I don't know what you're talking about; It wasn't me; It's the system. If you note denial or deflection, do not argue and do not dial up the heat. Just simply respond:

You know, I just couldn't believe such a report knowing who you are.

The point of the conversation is to signal that the organization has eyes and ears and that there may be consequences. Someone is watching.

> *In this circumstance, I will document the fact that I have shared the story with you and trust we will not need to have a similar conversation again. You are appreciated as a member of this team. There are certain standards, however, to which we are committed.*

If at all possible, this conversation should take place in the recipient's office. Once more, there is no expectation of acknowledgment or confession, but also no question that, in a measured and deliberate way, the professional has been made aware that his/her behavior/performance is noted and the sharing documented.

Leaders can face the challenge of either seeming to be too focused on "gotcha" or too permissive. As leaders gain more experience in addressing the performance and behavior of their team members, however, they develop a better sense of norms. Most individuals are never associated with patient or staff complaints, while some are heard about on a regular basis.[77,78] It is important to provide every opportunity for professionals to self-regulate; this requires willingness to deliver messages (data) in a timely manner, not only the first, but the second and third reports as well.

AN APPARENT PATTERN

While there always are some unreasonable observers, once a professional accumulates more reports than his/her peers, the likelihood that all are misreported becomes exceedingly small. In your leadership role, you receive a third report involving Dr Neurosurgeon and his apparent resistance to the time-out process:

> *The team attempted to perform a time-out prior to a shunt revision on a two year old. Dr. Neurosurgeon asked everyone to listen carefully and then, as the process started, he began whistling a tune. "We believe it was the Mickey Mouse Club theme song."*

You review the Pyramid (Figure 10-1)[97,98] to determine where you are. You recognize that there is a professional duty to address this third event. The behavior as reported appears intentional and to suggest a pattern. Your organization's infrastructure for reliable surveillance, report review, and data analysis to assess distribution across the population of professionals gives you confidence that Dr Neurosurgeon's future behavior will continue to be monitored. You decide it is time to make Dr Neurosurgeon "aware" of what appears to represent a pattern. You still hope he develops insight and, as a professional, self-regulates.

The "awareness" conversation takes place at a scheduled meeting where a leader within the professional's chain of command or a trained peer messenger within the organization's peer review function is charged with delivering the message.[7] The awareness discussion is intended to:

- Make the party aware that there "appears" to be a pattern,
- Remind that a pattern is not consistent with the group's collective commitment to professionalism and "who we are,"
- Reinforce that there is surveillance (and it will continue),
- Make clear that the process may escalate if there is no improvement, and
- Demonstrate respect for the individual and trust them to self-regulate.

To prepare for an awareness conversation, we suggest that the leader or peer messenger:

- Send a letter to the professional prefacing with the organization's commitment to professionalism and pursuit of safety, and requesting to meet to share the reports and data with which Dr Neurosurgeon has been associated;
- Prior to the meeting, review all reports and know the data;
- Know the goals for the meeting;
- Schedule adequate time and do not allow the recipient to torpedo the conversation. If told, "I'm sort of busy today. How long will this take?" reveal no disappointment or irritation but agree and immediately reschedule a time "that works better for you." This sends the clear message that the process is not going away.
- Follow a similar structure to the previously described CoC conversation:
  - Thank the professional for his/her time;
  - Ask, "Did you get the letter?";
  - Explain the reason for the meeting ("The data suggest a pattern of reports and/or data inconsistent with ...");
  - Present colleague with his/her aggregated data (even if just a collection of three stories);
  - Invite colleagues to take time after the meeting to reflect on ways to address whatever the issue/performance issue is;
  - Express appreciation for the individual's contributions to the organization followed by "however, the reports/data do not appear consistent with our professional standards."
  - Express confidence that "I know you will reflect on the data and problem-solve"
  - Confirm that follow-up data will be provided as available.
- All "awareness" conversations are documented.

Again, the messenger and message are not judgmental. The meeting is non-directive, and the messenger resists telling someone what to do. Avoid defaulting to your problem-solving nature, training, and desire to be a "fixer." There are too many problems for you to fix them all. Furthermore, if your colleague (subordinate) does not respond, there will be an opportunity to be more directive.

"Awareness" conversations are effective.[38,97,99] The conversation and data from your surveillance system separate out those who are able to respond because they develop insight and change versus those who do not and, therefore, require direction.

A PERSISTENT PATTERN

Although research reveals that most professionals respond to interventions delivered by peer colleagues, some will not. Generally, an individual is provided two chances to respond, based on policy and the rate at which meaningful data can accrue, unless risk is imminent. Giving professionals the opportunity for self-correction protects the integrity of the process and is fair. At some point, however, you have to escalate to guided intervention under authority. The authority figure moves from appealing to self-regulate to an "accountability action plan" designed to facilitate improvement.

Despite the awareness intervention, Dr Neurosurgeon continues to demonstrate disrespect for universal time-out protocols. You receive additional reports. The following is representative:

> Dr Neurosurgeon arrived, announced the need to answer calls during the time-out process, and declared, "Come get me when all this 'stuff' is done. I've got work to do …"

You (the authority figure in this case) prepare for the meeting by reviewing the organization's by-laws and relevant policies (including "Professional Conduct"). You commit to seeing the process through to the resolution, with the professional improving or failing to do so and escalating to a higher tier in the Pyramid, including the possibility of limitation of privileges or separation (termination). You review the data and reports and anticipate what resources might be necessary to address the professional's performance.

You send a letter in advance to the professional declaring the need to meet. You arrange for the discussion to take place in your office (not the professional's office) and make clear, as you did in the Espresso conversation, that this meeting is different:

> I am meeting with you as your [leader] for the purpose of developing an accountability plan aimed at addressing a pattern of behavior/

performance … in this case, accumulating staff complaints which reflect disregard for an important and endorsed safety practice.

We suggest use of the acronym, EDICTS, to serve as a guide to elements that should be considered for delivery in the meeting and documented:

E: "These are our group's **expectations**." Ground your expectations in policy, such as a professional conduct policy, practice and safety policies, faculty handbook, institutional credo, mission statement, contract, and/or medical staff bylaws.

D: "These are the ways in which your behavior/performance is **deficient**, ie, inconsistent with our expectations. Note that you no longer use "appears to be." With accumulation of data and previous sharing, there is now reasonable certainty that a pattern exists.

I: "We are here to develop an accountability action plan," ie, the **intervention**. Asking the professional to participate in developing the plan may increase his/her ownership. You also make clear that you hold authority to approve or modify the plan. Possible plan elements include obtaining skills training or continuing education, bringing in a coach to observe the professional's interactions with patients and staff, conducting a practice survey, making changes to the practice such as adding a partner or re-training staff, improving the phone/scheduling systems, and/or referring the professional for medical and mental health evaluations.

C: The leader again expresses confidence that reports will cease, but also makes clear that there *may* be **consequences** if substantial improvement is not seen within a stated period. The reason we suggest the use of the word "may" instead of "will" is that leaders sometimes find themselves trapped if they use the "will" word, draw a line in the sand, and then a minor or ambiguous infraction occurs. Leaders should never abdicate their authority role in deference to a rule that, under certain circumstances, may not seem to apply or would appear unjust. Decision-making and judgment comes with the leadership role. Deliberation and fairness, not rationalizing or drawing lines in the sand, mark leadership.

T: The leader should provide the professional with a defined **timeframe** within which (s)he will follow up.

S: The leader advises the professional that there will be ongoing **surveillance** for reports (or whatever data supported the progressive intervention).

Leaders who undertake an authority-guided intervention need to follow through and adhere to stated timelines, share follow-up data, and administer consequences as outlined if there is lack of improvement.

Table 10-3 **SUMMARY OF PROGRESSION OF TIERED INTERVENTIONS**			
Type of Conversation/Intervention	Who Conducts?	Times Occurring Before Escalating?	Documented?
Cup of coffee	Collegial; may be peer, co-worker, or supervisor clarifying "non-supervisor hat"	1-3 based on timeframe and imminence of safety risk	No
Mandated review	Designated office or authority	N/A (immediate review)	Yes
Espresso	Supervisor within professional's chain of command clarifying "supervisor hat"	1-2 based on timeframe and imminence of safety risk	Yes
Awareness	Member of peer review committee or supervisor within professional's chain of command	1-2 based on timeframe and evidence of self-correction	Yes
Authority	Supervisor and subordinate	1-3 based on professional's response to accountability action plan	Yes
Corrective/disciplinary	Executive committee constituted to limit privileges or terminate	N/A	Yes

CORRECTIVE/DISCIPLINARY ACTION

In rare cases, the professional's pattern will persist or review for a "mandated" issue or alleged egregious act demonstrates that the asserted facts are true. In such circumstances, organizational leaders must be prepared to advance to corrective/disciplinary action, which may lead to restrictions on the individual's practice or a required departure from the organization (Table 10-3).

MULTI-LEVEL PROFESSIONAL/LEADER TRAINING

For any accountability methodology and process to work, team members and leaders should seek to acquire the skills needed so they are comfortable having conversations that fall within their authority. Training should include an experiential component. The organization should also maintain local experts who can provide refresher training when needed, including just-in-time executive coaching to reinforce and debrief.

The importance of training in every level of conversation and intervention in which you might be called upon to participate cannot be overstated. Recall the first time you took a history from a patient? How long did it take?

How long does it take now? Training, practice, reflection, practice, reflection—achieve expert status.

RESOURCES TO HELP ADDRESS UNNECESSARY VARIATION

As leaders develop accountability action plans within the authority-guided intervention, or are approached by professionals for help or information, they soon recognize that no plan is "one size fits all." Each professional will need appropriate targeted remedies.[100]

Although a full discussion of available resources is outside the scope of this chapter, some resource options were presented earlier in the discussion of Intervention under EDICTS. It is our experience that improvement often occurs after coaching or by addressing dysfunction within the practice. Physical and mental evaluations sometimes reveal serious health issues, such as cancer, heart disease, cognitive impairment, or psychiatric disorders, and/or substance abuse problem.[83,101,102] In the rare instances where individuals are not able to return to their usual professional duties due to illness or cognitive impairment, they are able to retire with dignity.

RESOURCES TO HELP THOSE AFFECTED

Co-workers and colleagues who observe or experience the consequences of behaviors that undermine a safety culture may also need support in the aftermath, whether they are the primary victim, ie, the target of unprofessional behavior, or the second victim, a professional whose care was somehow related to a patient's adverse outcome.[103]

PROFESSIONALS AND STAFF AS THE TARGET OF UNPROFESSIONAL BEHAVIOR

Team members humiliated or embarrassed by other team members, especially when the abuse is recurrent, may need psychological and emotional support resources. For this reason, leaders should routinely ask team members how they are doing after a reported event and be familiar with community resources that can provide help. Many organizations, for example, encourage referral to their Employee Assistance or Wellness program.

Event reporting systems in some respects are a resource to assist traumatized professionals and staff because, by reporting, the individual is able to take defined action to (1) hold parties accountable and make the system better, which, for many, are part of the healing process, and (2) ensure appropriate follow-up in circumstances where the reporter describes behavior suggestive of discrimination or boundary violation, and designated offices or authorities (such as the Equal Opportunity, Affirmative Action, Disability Office (EAD) or law enforcement) are mandated to investigate.

Care teams also need systems support to lessen environmental triggers of unprofessional behavior. This is not to say that faulty systems are ever the excuse for, or give a "pass" to, someone who emotionally "floods" or lashes out. As previously seen, defective systems are only antecedents to, but not the reason for behavior. Nonetheless, failing systems should be fixed; experts who redesign flow and process can support safety and professionalism by, example, placing foam containers for hand hygiene in convenient locations. Thus, holding professionals accountable and fixing defective systems are both part of our professional duty.

PROFESSIONALS AND STAFF AS THE "SECOND VICTIM"

When behavior or performance contributes to harm or death of a patient, a modern approach is to support all impacted parties.[104] Tending to the patient's immediate medical needs and providing emotional support to the family are paramount. So, too, is addressing the needs of the "second victim,"[103] ie, the professional(s) who cared for the patient. Healthcare professionals involved in harm-causing error often bear a heavy emotional burden, which may include feelings of sadness, embarrassment, or guilt for not having done all they could to help avert, or fear they will be sued or looked at differently by their peers and patients.[103,105–108] A patient's bad outcome may be particularly distressing to a professional who had recognized an emerging problem but whose concerns were dismissed or calls for help were ignored by another professional, especially when the professional realizes that his/her failure to attempt to re-engage or use the chain of command to get help may have contributed to the outcome. Professionals often experience grief after such events.[103]

Risk managers and leaders should make involved professionals aware that when error is suspected or confirmed, they may experience these intense emotions, including anger at other team members for their performance or contributory behaviors, and/or disorientation due to an altered sense of one's abilities.[103,105–107] Because strong emotions affect judgment, team members should be encouraged to obtain professional help during a crisis when appropriate.

Structured review of an event to understand what happened not only helps prevent future occurrences, but also serves as a reality check to those who were involved to step back and see the larger picture. Therefore, it is important that professionals: (1) report adverse events promptly to expedite review; and (2) participate in root causes analyses and multidisciplinary morbidity and mortality conferences that can help identify causal human behaviors and systems factors that need to be addressed.[18,109,110]

Healthcare professionals should also engage with the patient and family to disclose information and keep channels of communication open. Disclosure is a process over time that involves sharing what is known about the event, what is not yet clear, what will be done to try to get answers, and offering an apology if medical error contributed to the harm.[108] Understanding that failures to communicate are the trigger for many lawsuits[111,112] reinforces the importance of taking steps to increase understanding and reduce tension within the professional–patient relationship.

Paying for out-of-pocket expenses or temporary housing while a patient undergoes treatment for medical injury, and/or offers of early settlement in appropriate cases can help maintain the relationship and, in many cases, avoid litigation.[113–117] Doing the right thing by the patient and family may also help bring closure to the healthcare professional(s) who were involved in the genesis of the adverse event.

On a last note, consider the many circumstances where patients were not physically injured by care experience dissatisfaction and unprofessional behavior. Every practice and health system needs a way for patients to complain and for trained patient relations professionals to utilize best practices in service recovery to help make right what patients and families perceive as wrong.[88] By facilitating communication, patient relations personnel help defuse situations in which clinical professionals come under verbal assault from angry family members.

EFFECTIVENESS OF THE PYRAMID MODEL

But does any of this really work? Once a practice or health system's infrastructure successfully implements a model for reporting, reviewing, and addressing unprofessional behavior and performance through graduated interventions, will change follow?

ADDRESSING MEDICAL MALPRACTICE CLAIMS RISK

The evidence-based literature about physicians' malpractice claims experience reveals that only a small group of physicians within any medical discipline account for the majority of medical malpractice claims.[7,77,78] The non-random association between complaints and claims is also well established.[77–82] While specialty type and productivity also predict risk (gender as a predictor is an

Table 10-4 **INCURRED EXPENSE BY RISK CATEGORY**				
Predicted Risk Category	Number of Physicians (%)	Relative Expense (multiples of lowest risk group)	% of Total Expense	Risk Score
1 (low)	318 (49)	1	4%	0
2	147 (23)	6	13%	1–20
3	76 (12)	4	4%	21–40
4	52 (8)	42	29%	41–50
5 (high)	51 (8)	73	50%	>50
Total	644 (100)		100%	

Data from Moore IN, Pichert JW, Hickson G, Federspiel C, Blackford JU. Rethinking peer review: detecting and addressing medical malpractice claims risk. *Vanderbilt Law Rev.* 2006;59:1175-1206.

Predicted Risk Category: Five (5) empirically determined risk categories into which physicians were grouped based on a regression analysis involving type of practice (Medicine or Surgery), service volume, and number of unsolicited patient complaints as predictors of risk management activity risk.

Relative Expense: Ratios of grouped physicians' risk management-related expenses where the lowest risk category's expense equals one.

Risk Score: Weighted sum algorithm over 4 years in which more recent complaints have greater impact on the score than remote complaints. Column presents the observed ranges of Risk Scores corresponding to related Predictive Risk Category.

inconsistent finding), their effect is modest when compared with the unique ability of a physician and his or her practice to create patient dissatisfaction as measured by coded and aggregated unsolicited patient and family complaint reports.[77,78] For example, in a study of a large academic medical group's claims experience, physicians with no patient complaints during a 6-year audit accounted for less than 4% of the group's risk management-related costs while 8% of the physician group with the highest numbers of complaints (risk score >50%[118,119]) accounted for 50%.[77] (Table 10-4) Study findings were replicated at a regional medical center.[78]

Simply describing the relationship between patient complaints and malpractice claims, however, does not lower a physician's risk. If there is no intervention, high-risk physicians remain at a high risk.[120] The Pyramid model was conceptualized 20 years ago to help physicians become aware of concerns, develop insight, change behavior and performance, and reduce excess medical malpractice claims risk.[84,98,100] Using patient complaint reports filed within VUMC's Office of Patient Relations, the Vanderbilt research team developed a coding system, analytic methodology, and ability to generate graphic individualized and comparative peer group data.[121]

Data alone, however, are not sufficient to promote change unless they are delivered. Recognizing studies that demonstrate the effectiveness of peer-based sharing,[122–124] the team included within the model peer professional "messenger" colleagues to deliver the data. Professionals are recruited to serve as members of a peer review committee and trained to deliver "awareness" interventions through role play exercises, including how to handle "push-back." Messengers are then assigned to deliver data to colleagues with high risk scores and at increased risk for claims.[84,96–99] Leaders who do not "blink" further support the process by assuming responsibility for authority-guided interventions and beyond.

A study has analyzed response to the tiered intervention process for the years 2004–2009 at Vanderbilt and 15 community and academic health systems. Ongoing surveillance of 25,000 physicians' patient complaint profiles revealed 373 physicians at high risk for medical malpractice claims. Overall, 64% of these high-risk physicians responded to the peer-based intervention model with an 80% average reduction in complaints and concomitant reduction in risk score.[97,99] Extending the results of the previous study for the years 2000 through 2013, surveillance of patient complaint profiles of over 45,000 physicians based at more than 75 sites resulted in interventions for 912 physicians. Of these, 77% demonstrated reduced complaints, 17% did not improve, and 6% departed from their institutions.[97]

Review of claims experience at two academic centers utilizing the Pyramid for intervening with high-risk physicians demonstrates a significant downward slope in malpractice suits.[98]Vanderbilt's malpractice claims experience additionally compares favorably with that of non-Vanderbilt physicians in middle Tennessee.[125] With the understanding that other risk prevention initiatives were introduced at Vanderbilt, particularly over the last decade, conservative estimates of the impact of the Pyramid model suggest return on investment of greater than 25:1.[125]

In sum, the process for promoting professionalism—surveillance, capturing reports, coding and aggregating data, and addressing high claims risk via graduated data-based, peer-delivered interventions for those professionals who demonstrate outlier results—effectively supports change.

IMPROVING HAND HYGIENE COMPLIANCE

Can the intervention process based on the Pyramid be adapted to address other safety and quality concerns? Between 2004 and 2009, VUMC, like many healthcare organizations, had attempted to increase compliance with hand hygiene (HH) best practices through training, awareness events, and a direct observation methodology, with similar limited success. Concerned about healthcare acquired infections, coupled with surveillance data suggesting continued low adherence with HH, a hospital epidemiologist (also a member of the peer committee charged with delivering data to high claims risk Vanderbilt physicians) suggested that the tiered intervention strategy used to address high claims risk might help the group attain "professional" levels of hand hygiene.

A team was assembled to steer the project, create a comprehensive plan using a "new project bundle"[18] tool designed to help launch safety and quality initiatives and support sustainability, and track success. The foundation of the project was an agreement that not practicing appropriate hand HH is an unprofessional act. Therefore, addressing compliance became a matter of promoting individual and group regulation, consistent with professionalism and high reliability.

To assess leadership commitment, several scenarios were posed to the system's CEO, COOs, CNOs, CMOs, and chairs, and included the following:

- If a professional team member failed to practice appropriate HH and it came to your attention, would you support sharing in a CoC conversation?
- If observations of the team member failing to foam in continued, would you escalate and share in an Espresso conversation?
- If the behavior/performance persisted, would you take action based upon your authority within the institution?
- In support of professional self- and group-regulation, would you support progressive interventions ("awareness" on up) with the leadership of units with persistently low HH rates?

VUMC leaders publicly declared their willingness to support the plan, their expectation that team members would appropriately self-regulate, and affirmation that they would address any team member who displayed unprofessional behavior following a reminder to foam in. Leaders furthermore declared they would support tiered unit interventions with the leaders of those units. The project leadership team also identified a methodology for measurement. Acknowledging that no measurement system is perfect, VUMC leaders collectively agreed to use the methodology and not attack or discredit data when an individual unit leader did not like his/her results.

Prior to launch, observers were trained to prompt team members observed to not foam in through a CoC conversation. Once HH observations commenced, did all team members conduct themselves as professionals in response to prompts? Not surprisingly, there were some who did not. In one instance, an observer was told:

> *This is so stupid! We're busy, we have sick patients to care for, and you're just standing around … why don't you do some real work?*

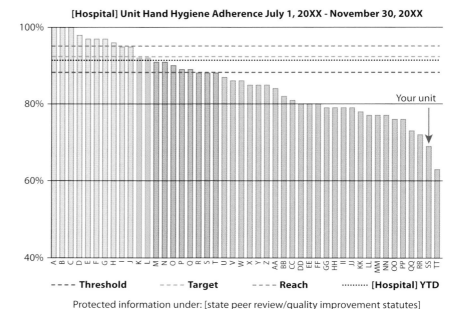

Figure 10-2 ■ "You are here" chart example. (Reproduced, with permission, from Vanderbilt University Medical Center.)

Nonetheless, the team was prepared with a plan to address such occurrences, commencing with observers reporting through the organization's event reporting system or up the chain of command, and members of the Hand Hygiene Executive Committee (HHEC) acting in accordance with the Pyramid to address behaviors.

As observation data were collected and aggregated, the interdisciplinary HHEC regularly reviewed and identified variation in unit performance. Representatives of the HHEC conducted "awareness" interventions with the dual leadership (nurse manager and medical director) of units with low HH compliance rates, presenting comparative data, including a "You Are Here" chart. (Figure 10-2)

If a unit did not improve HH compliance, intervention escalated up the Pyramid to guided intervention under authority.

The HHEC established Threshold, Target, and Reach levels of compliance for each year of the project and offered a financial incentive. Rebates on a portion of the malpractice premium for all departments depended on the level of compliance achieved for the medical center; all units had a stake in the success of all other units. Threshold/Target/Reach goals were raised as compliance increased.

Of the 179 discrete Vanderbilt units and clinics, 31% required awareness interventions. Seventy percent (70%) of units receiving awareness intervention achieved institutional goals. The remainder escalated to guided intervention under authority. Overall HH compliance rates went from a baseline of 58% (July 2009) to 85% (August 2012).[38] HH compliance rates are now over 92% (unpublished data). Although not a single factor attribution, improvement in HH was inversely correlated with a decline in device-associated (CLABSI, CAUTI, and VAP) standardized infection ratios (SIRs).[38]

In sum, VUMC increased HH compliance by adapting the method and process previously used successfully to reduce medical malpractice claims risk. The project succeeded largely due to two important principles:

1. Embedding the practice of appropriate HH within the concept of professionalism and in the pursuit of safety called upon people to be professional and self-regulate; and

2. Using the tiered intervention infrastructure of the Pyramid promoted individual and unit accountability. Observers were empowered to prompt and engage in CoC conversations when appropriate. In addition, leaders from the HHEC were committed to sharing with local leaders to hold them accountable for getting their units in order. Throughout the 3-year project, institutional leaders did "not blink" when certain units failed to exceed expected performance. In addition, the system regularly celebrated successes.

Consider for a moment the state of your HH efforts within your practice or health systems. Do you collectively consider foaming in a professional act? What other potential areas of behavior or performance could be addressed using the Pyramid and progressive accountability?

PRINCIPLES UNDERLYING GRADUATED INTERVENTIONS

Leaders sometimes hesitate to take steps that might lead to someone losing their job, in part, because they are aware loss of income impacts a person's life and family. Many leaders are concerned that they could be sued. Fear of litigation, however, should not paralyze leaders, groups, or health systems from doing the right thing. The key is to have a supported, defined process, and to pause and reflect before you move forward, especially where taking action is not comfortable and the next step might have consequences for the professional's ability to practice within your organization.

We find that a principled approach to decision-making and action diminishes legal concerns and allows leaders to be more comfortable doing what is right for patients, the clinical team, and the organization.[100] The potential for liability usually arises out of a failure to maintain process regularity. Therefore, act early and as often as indicated, and follow your own defined process in support of professional accountability.

As you begin to administer a stepwise, measured, and consistent approach to addressing unprofessional behavior and performance, keep in mind the underlying principles:

- Focus on doing what is right. This promotes justice and is the professional thing to do;
- Assiduously avoid conflicts of interest or the appearance of a conflict.
- Gather observations and analyze data in a fair and consistent way to promote reasonable certainty of behavior and/or performance issue(s).
- Administer feedback, corrective action, and disciplinary measures in ways that maximize opportunity for your professional colleague to gain personal insight so (s)he may self-regulate to return to responsible performance and behavior;
- If your colleague fails to self-regulate, deal fairly in separating those unwilling or unable to change from the organization.

We will discuss each underlying principle in greater detail.

Promoting justice in the context of addressing unprofessional behavior means that all individuals are treated in accordance with organizational policies and other applicable governing documents. Each organization's policies should put forth the uniform expectation that professionals will behave professionally and that deficiencies in professionalism are addressed early and consistently.

Note that the specific relationship of the professional to the organization (eg, employee, faculty-independent contractor, *locum tenens*), and other internal sources of authority, such as terms of affiliation contracts, medical staff bylaws, the faculty handbook, and credentialing and privileging requirements, may affect specifics of the process or actions that can be taken. Nonetheless, even when there are differences in how variation from expected performance is addressed because of the relationship, the fact remains that measured and escalating intervention occurs for any affiliate whose behavior or performance falls outside accepted norms. No one, irrespective of status within the organization, is granted a pass because "I am special and the policy, therefore, does not apply to me." Thus, organizations must also affirmatively consider how they will approach follow-up to events if the professional involved is a leader. Our hope is that professionals within the organization would seek to support leaders' professionalism as well.

As previously discussed, providing timely, measured feedback helps change behavior in most cases. Therefore, justice requires addressing the disruptor's behavior to lessen the chance of recurrence. By doing so, professionals and leaders also acknowledge the needs of team members whose work was disrupted and support joy and meaning in the workplace.

Avoiding conflicts of interest means that you ask yourself, "Do I (or the committee I represent) have authority to act? Am I the right person to be doing this review or inquiry?" Conflicts of interest may be evident or subtle. Before an authority guides an intervention or refers for a hearing that could result in corrective/disciplinary action, s/he stops and self-examines for any negative motivator that could influence a decision either for or against.

Even if a participant in a review or intervention process has no subjective conflict of interest, consider whether an objective assessment suggests the appearance of one. Before evaluating data about a practice, group, or colleague, ask yourself if the person to be reviewed is a competitor or if there is "bad blood" between the two of you. Will you be able to fairly consider the data?

The appearance or existence of a conflict may not necessarily preclude the leader from delivering the data, guiding an intervention, or referring to an executive board for further action, but you must declare. All potential conflicts of interest must be out in the open so others may determine if it is surmountable, or whether someone else within the organizational structure without a conflict should take charge of the matter.

Reasonable certainty means that the data are sufficient to serve as a basis for decision-making. You are aware that every story has at least two sides, and leaders and committees with responsibility for determining reasonable certainty do not rush to judgment. One does not need a significance level of <0.05% in order to act at any level on the Pyramid. For the first two levels, it is part of the culture to provide feedback. However, by the very nature of the process, as events continue to accumulate, the "certainty" increases. The more data you have, the greater the confidence you have in the information that emerges.

Experienced leaders can make reasonable judgments that the data are sufficiently convincing to allow moving forward when patterns are discernible from one or more sources of information, for example, patient and/or co-worker complaints, formal event analyses, performance evaluations, medical records, and risk management files. The ability to accumulate data over time and compare patterns of behavior and performance of the individual against peer groups is also helpful. Leaders often are able to sense, "How often do I receive reports or data about Dr Surgeon compared with how often I hear about the vast majority of the professionals in this practice/group/department/health system?"

Providing multiple opportunities to acquire insight means that professionals with patterns of noncompliance with important safety practices who do not respond at first to attempts at intervention are given more opportunities. The reason is that they might yet change. Some professionals take longer to respond than others but, as consequences increase, eventually gain genuine insight. Therefore, processes that build in opportunities at every level of intervention to acquire insight are fair and support professionalism. In one study, half of physicians who did not respond to initial "awareness" interventions, eventually significantly reduced patient complaints and claims risk after accountability action plans were implemented and enforced through authority-guided intervention.[98]

Unfortunately, some who prove unable to change are found to suffer from physical or mental health problems, but is it not professional to identify and support peers who need compassion and further care?

Dealing fairly in separating means that if disciplined data analysis and step-wise intervention (including directing the individual toward professional evaluation and treatment if behaviors or poor performance persist) do not result in restoring the professional to organizational norms, they will need to separate. Organizations that commit to pursuit of a culture of safety almost invariably find that some will need to voluntarily or involuntarily depart. Multiple sources of data that demonstrate consistent patterns and failure to respond are persuasive evidence that corrective/disciplinary action is appropriate.

If the professional does not leave to pursue other practice opportunities, leaders must carefully follow the medical staff bylaws and provide notice to the professional of his/her due process hearing rights and adhere to all deadlines. If leaders have evenhandedly and fairly applied the stepwise process, and the individual chooses to litigate, a court is likely to find that the move to separate was neither arbitrary nor motivated by ill-will or other unacceptable reasons for termination.[126,127]

In sum, considering legal ramifications is important, but concern that "Dr Surgeon will sue us," should not trump potential harm to patients and team members when unprofessional behavior is allowed to persist. Consider within your own practice, group, or health system how many colleagues, right now, are not following hand hygiene best practices (and increasing infection rates), failing to respond to pages (delaying necessary care), and refusing to follow universal time-out protocols (resulting in risk for wrong site, wrong patient, wrong procedure surgery). Is acknowledging and acting to address not the most professional response? Speculating that colleagues will resent or be antagonistic to feedback should not be used as an excuse to ignore behavior/performance and undermine a culture of safety. Seek assistance from your legal counsel as needed, but do not allow fear of litigation paralyze you from attending to your duty to promote kinder and more reliable care, and to exercise the personal courage of a professional.

❙ CONCLUSION

Promoting professionalism and professional accountability supports quality team-oriented care, high reliability, and pursuit of a culture of safety. In the 21st century, professionals engage in self- and group-regulation as part of their professional duty and commitment to respect and protect patients from harm, and support other team members in their professionalism. Professionals are supported by an infrastructure with the following elements: committed leadership; alignment of safety initiatives with the organization's mission and goals; understandable and supportive policies; ongoing surveillance; safety for reporters; timely review of reports; and graduated, tiered interventions in accordance with a model for addressing unprofessional behavior and performance.

IN PRACTICE

- Model professionalism in your practice: wash your hands, communicate effectively, accept feedback, and routinely pause and reflect about how your behavior influences the performance of other team members.
- When you observe slips and lapses in professionals' performance, in a respectful and professional way, share. Over the next several months, practice sharing "cups of coffee." Then pause and self-reflect on the ways in which you supported professional accountability.
- Recognize that other team members, including patients and families, make important observations about the performance of your practice. Take patient observations seriously. Be sure that the practice or system in which you practice has a mechanism to make patients aware that their voice is important. Review any observations related to you and your practice.
- Work with others within your practice to ensure that you have an articulated mission and that it is supported by a set of core values.
- If you are positioned as a leader in any capacity, do self-assessment. The next time you are presented with an event or data that suggest(s) unprofessional behavior by a colleague or subordinate, ask yourself if you are spending more time ruminating about it, or sharing. If you do not share, consider "why" in this case or this one time. Do you decide, "The issue is really not that serious?"

FAQs

1. I want to implement a "professional accountability" program. How do I get started? Implementing a robust program that promotes process reliability and professional accountability in order to pursue a culture of safety takes resources. You can start by evaluating the status

of the eight elements that promote process reliability and professional accountability. Do a gap analysis:

a. Leadership commitment:
   i. Are your practice, hospital, and health system leaders committed to taking action to reduce medical error?
   ii. Do they understand the need for surveillance in order to identify risk?
   iii. Are they willing to routinely and reliably review event reports and respond?
   iv. Will they commit the necessary resources to support the infrastructure?
   v. Do they publicly declare their commitment and incorporate their declarations into the organization's goals?

b. Mission, goals, core values, and supportive policies:
   i. Do they exist? If so, review to see areas of alignment and areas of conflict. If not, develop. As a starting point, see what peer institutions have developed, then modify to conform with your vision and organizational structure.
   ii. Do they reflect current intentions of the organization? You must know what leaders, including members of the Board of Directors, are committed to.
   iii. Are policies as written understandable and enforceable? Create interdisciplinary focus groups to review policies and provide feedback.
   iv. Are you willing to hold all members of the healthcare team accountable for behavior and performance, ie, no one has "special status" that allows him/her a "pass?"

c. Surveillance tools to capture observations and reports:
   i. Do you have an electronic event reporting system? If not, find out what reporting systems are currently available and their capabilities. Consider contacting peer organizations to see what system they use and evaluate each for strengths and weaknesses.

d. Processes for reviewing observations and reports
   i. Do you have a designated team for reviewing reports and sharing information with those with a "need to know," ie, those empowered to address?
   ii. Are you willing to aggregate and analyze data in order to identify trends and patterns?

e. Model to guide graduated interventions
   i. Are you willing to allow professionals an opportunity to self-correct? Most will.
   ii. Are leaders willing to work with professionals who may take longer to correct and to provide specific guidance and follow-up?

   iii. If the individual has not improved behavior and/or performance after appropriate opportunities to do so, will the institution "blink," or will the institution follow through on consequences outlined in policy?

  f. Multi-level professional/leader training (on infrastructure and communication skills)

   i. Are leaders willing to invest resources for training? Without adequate training, the program may be "dead on arrival."

   ii. "Train-the-trainer" training supports a sustainable process.

   iii. Are you committed to training all personnel in "Cup of coffee" conversations, how to report events or observations of potential unsafe conditions or behavior, and how to use the chain of command?

   iv. Are you committed to training all local leaders and higher-level leaders in guided intervention under authority?

  g. Resources to help address the causes of unnecessary variation in performance (both system and individual):

   i. Can you identify referral resources to support guided intervention? These may include your Employee Assistance or Wellness program, programs for distressed professionals, CME programs, additional training, coaching, mentoring/proctoring, and practice review.

   ii. Do you have internal expertise to conduct root causes analyses, multidisciplinary morbidity and mortality conferences, risk management file review?

   iii. Do you have a plan for addressing faulty systems and holding professionals accountable?

  h. Resources to help those affected:

   i. The first step is awareness that some professionals who, in some way, may have contributed to or witnessed medical injury are impacted emotionally and/or professionally.

   ii. Can you identify resources that can support these professionals?

2. What if our leaders are hesitant to address "rainmakers"?

  a. Create ongoing dialog about the true costs of allowing professionals who behave or perform unprofessionally to continue unabated.

  b. If your mission/goals/credo/policies are aligned, unprofessional behavior and performance is more readily identifiable and easier to address.

3. What can my hospital do about conflict-averse group or institutional leaders?

  a. Training is helpful.

  b. Aligned mission/goals/credo/policies are a resource for framing the message and guiding stepwise action.

4. Is it really possible to change culture at a hospital? It takes time to promote culture change in an environment where consistent modeling of professionalism has not been the norm.
   a. Steadily gain allies and be persistent.
   b. Do not give up when things do not go well. Even with an infrastructure in place and skills in having progressive conversations, things do not always go well.
   c. Do not allow single anecdotes to paralyze group commitment to doing the right thing. The goal is to get it right in the aggregate, but it will never occur in every single circumstance.

REFERENCES

1. The Advisory Committee on the Safety of Nuclear Installations, as adopted by the UK Health and Safety Commission; 1993.
2. Leape L, Berwick D, Clancy, et al. Transforming healthcare: a safety imperative. *Qual Saf Health Care*. 2009;18:424-428.
3. Kohn L, Corrigan J, Donaldson M, eds. *To Err Is Human: Building a Safer Health System. Report of the Institute of Medicine.* Washington, DC: National Academy Press; 1999.
4. The Joint Commission's Sentinel Event Alert #40 (July 2008), Behaviors that undermine a culture of safety. Available at: http://www.jointcommission.org/assets/1/18/SEA_40.PDF. Accessed 26.02.2013.
5. Cruess SR, Johnston S, Cruess RL. "Profession:" a working definition for medical educators. *Teach Learn Med*. 2004;16(1):74-76.
6. Scheutzow SO. State medical peer review: high cost but no benefit-is it time for a change? *Am J L Med*. 1999;25(7):7-60.
7. Moore IN, Pichert JW, Hickson GB, et al. Rethinking peer review: detecting and addressing medical malpractice claims risk. *Vanderbilt Law Rev*. 2006;59:1175-1206.
8. Brennan TA, Leape LL, Laird NM, et al. Incidence of adverse events and negligence in hospitalized patients: results of the Harvard Medical practice study I. *New Engl J Med*. 1991;324:371-376.
9. Mills DH. Medical insurance feasibility study. A technical summary. *West J Med*. 1978;128:360-365.
10. Thomas EJ, Studdert DM, Burstin HR, et al. Incidence and types of adverse events and negligent care in Utah and Colorado. *Med Car*. 2000;38(3):261-271.
11. Reason J. Human error: models and management. *Brit Med J*. 2000;320:768-770.
12. Gluck PA. Medical error theory. *Obstet Gyn Clin N Am*. 2008;35:11-17.
13. Felps W, Mitchell TR, Bylington E. How, when, and why bad apples spoil the barrel: negative group members and dysfunctional groups. *Res Organ Behav*. 2006;27:175-222.
14. Hickson GB, Entman SS. Physician practice behavior and litigation risk: evidence and opportunity. *Clin Obstet Gynecol*. 2008;51(4):688-699.
15. McPherson K, Wennberg JE, Hovind OB, Clifford P. Small-area variations in the use of common surgical procedures: an international comparison of New England, England, and Norway. *N Eng J Med*. 1982;307:1310-1314.

16. Wennberg JE. Dealing with medical practice variations: a proposal for action. *Health Affair*. 1984;3(2):6-32

17. Kozlowski SW, Ilgen DR. Enhancing the effectiveness of work groups and teams. *PSPI*. 2006;7:77-124

18. Hickson GB, Moore IN, Pichert JW, Benegas MJr. Balancing systems and individual accountability in a safety culture. In: Berman S, ed. *From Front Office to Front Line*. 2nd ed. Oakbrook Terrace, IL: Joint Commission Resources; 2012:1-36.

19. Hain PD, Pichert JW, Hickson GB, et al. Using risk management files to identify and address causative factors associated with adverse events in pediatrics. *Ther Clin Risk Manag*. 2007;3(4):625-631.

20. Morris JA, Carrillo YM, Jenkins JM, et al. Surgical adverse events, risk management and malpractice outcome: Morbidity and mortality review is not enough. *Ann Surg*. 2003;237(6):844-851

21. Pichert JW, Hickson GB, Bledsoe S, et al. Understanding the etiology of serious medical events involving children: implications for pediatricians and their risk managers. *Pediatr Ann*. 1997;26(3):160-172.

22. Wachter RM, Shojania KG. *Internal Bleeding: The Truth Behind America's Terrifying Epidemic of Medical Mistakes*. New York, NY: Rugged Land, LLC; 2004.

23. White AA, Pichert JW, Bledsoe SH, et al. Cause-and-effect analysis of closed claims in obstetrics and gynecology. *Obstet Gynecol*. 2005;105:1031-1038.

24. White AA, Wright S, Blanco R, et al. Cause-and-effect analysis of risk management files to assess patient care in the emergency department. *Acad Emerg Med*. 2004;11:1035-1041.

25. Rosenstein AH, O'Daniel M. Disruptive behavior and clinical outcomes: perceptions of nurses and physicians. *Am J Nurs*. 2005;105(1):54-64.

26. Rosenstein AH, O'Daniel M. Impact and implications of disruptive behavior in the perioperative arena. *J Am Coll Surg*. 2006;203(1):96-105.

27. Center for Patient and Professional Advocacy at Vanderbilt (CPPA) and Studer Group. Creating great places to work by eliminating disruptive behaviors. *Mod Healthc*. 2009.

28. Donn SM. Medical liability, risk management, and the quality of health care. *Semin Fetal Neonat M*. 2005;10:3-9.

29. Hickson GB, Entman SS. Physicians influence and the malpractice problem. *Obstetr Gynecol*. 2010;115(4):682-686.

30. Reason J. *Human Error*. Cambridge, UK: Cambridge University Press; 1990.

31. Hickson GB, Moore IN. Risk prevention, risk management, and professional liability. In: Rock JA, Jones HW III, eds. *TeLinde's Operative Gynecology*. 11th ed. Philadelphia, PA: Lippincott Williams & Wilkins; Forthcoming [chapter 4].

32. Williams BW, Williams MV. The disruptive physician: a conceptual organization. *J Med Lic Disc*. 2008;94(3):12-20.

33. Banja J. Empathy in the physician's pain practice: benefits, barriers, and recommendations. *Pain Med*. 2006;7(3):265-275.

34. Samenow CP, Swiggart W, Spickard A. A CME course aimed at addressing disruptive physician behavior. *Physician Exec*. 2008:32-40.

35. Pappadakus MA, Hodgson CS, Teherani A, Kohatsu ND. Unprofessional behavior in medical school is associated with subsequent disciplinary action by a state medical board. *Acad Med*. 2004;79:244-249.

36. Krause TR. How senior leadership behavior influences world-class safety. Available at http://www.efcog.org/wg/ism_pmi/docs/Safety_Culture/How_Senior_Leadership_Behavior_Influences_World-Class_Safety.pdf.

37. OSHA. Introduction to practical behavior-based safety. Available at: http://www.osha-train.org/pdf/otn717w.pdf.

38. Talbot TR, Johnson JG, Fergus C, et al. Sustained improvement in hand hygiene adherence: utilizing shared accountability and financial incentives. *Infect Control Hosp Epidemiol.* 2013; 34(11):1129-1136.

39. Pronovost PJ, Goeschel CA, Colantuoni E, et al. Sustaining reductions in catheter related bloodstream infections in Michigan intensive care units: observational study. 2010. *BMJ.* 340:c309.

40. Lipitz-Snyderman A, Steinwachs D, Needham DM, et al. Impact of a statewide intensive care unit quality improvement initiative on hospital mortality and length of stay: Retrospective comparative analysis. *BMJ.* 2011;342:d219.

41. Weber DO. Poll results: Doctors' disruptive behavior disturbs physician leaders. *Physician Exec.* 2004;30(5):6-14.

42. AHRQ. TeamSTEPPs: National Implementation. Available at: http://teamstepps.ahrq.gov/.

43. Leape LL, Shore MF, Dienstag JL, et al. A culture of respect, Part 1: The nature and causes of disrespectful behavior by physicians. *Acad Med.* 2012;87(7):845-852.

44. Leape LL, Shore MF, Dienstag JL, et al. A culture of respect, Part 2: The nature and causes of disrespectful behavior by physicians. *Acad Med.* 2012;87(7):853-858.

45. Pearson CM, Porath CL. On the nature, consequences, and remedies of workplace incivility: no time for "nice". Think again. *Acad Manage Perspect.* 2005;19(1):7-28.

46. Lewick RJ, Bunker BB. Developing and maintaining trust in work relationships. In: *Trust in Organizations: Frontiers of Theory and Research;* 1996:114-139.

47. Ishikawa K. *Guide to Quality Control.* 2nd ed, revised. Tokyo: Asian Productivity Organization; 1986:226.

48. Düsing R, Weisser B, Mengden T, Vetter H. Changes in antihypertensive therapy: the role of adverse effects and compliance. *Blood Press.* 1998;7:313-315.

49. Ware JE, Davies AR. Behavioral consequences of consumer dissatisfaction with medical care. *Eval Program Plann.* 1983;6(3-4):291-297.

50. Kravitz RL, Cope DW, Bhrany V, Leake B. Internal medicine patients' expectations for care during office visits. *J Gen Intern Med.* 1994;9:75-81.

51. Jackson JL, Kroenke K. The effect of unmet expectations among adults presenting with physical symptoms. *Ann Intern Med.* 2001;134:889-897.

52. Jayadevappa R, Schwartz JS, Chhatre S, et al. Satisfaction with care: a measure of quality of care in prostate cancer patients. *Med Decis Making.* 2010;30:234-245.

53. Borras JM, Sanchez-Hernandez A, Navarro M, et al. Compliance, satisfaction and quality of life of patients with colorectal cancer receiving home chemotherapy or outpatient treatment: a randomised controlled trial. *BMJ.* 2001;322:1-5.

54. Spickard A, Gabbe SG, Christensen JF. Mid-career burnout in generalist and specialist physicians. *JAMA.* 2002;288:1447-1450.

55. Leape L, Berwick D, Clancy C, et al. Transforming healthcare: a safety imperative. *BMJ.* 2009;18:424-428.

56. Mkary MA, Sexton JB, Freischlag JA, et al. Patient safety in surgery. *Ann Surg.* 2006; 243(5):628-635.

57. Nahrgang JD, Morgeson FP, Hofmann DA. Safety at work: a meta-analytic investigation of the link between job demands, job resources, burnout, engagement, and safety outcomes. *J Appl Psychol.* 2011;96(1):71-94.

58. Pearson CM, Porath CL. On the nature, consequences and remedies of workplace incivility: no time for "nice"? Think again. *Acad Manag Exec.* 2005;19(1):7-18.

59. Jones CB. Revisiting nurse turnover costs. *JONA.* 2008;38(1):11-18.

60. Kramer M, Schmalenberg C, Maguire P. Nine structures and leadership practices essential for a magnetic (healthy) work environment. *Nurs Admin Q.* 2010;34(1):4-17.

61. Kiel JM. An analysis of restructuring orientation to enhance nurse retention. *The Health Care Manager.* 2012;31(4):302-307.

62. Scott RD. The direct medical costs of healthcare-associated infections in U.S. hospitals and the benefits of prevention. Division of Healthcare Quality Promotion, National Center for Preparedness, Detection, and Control of Infectious Diseases, Coordinating Center for Infectious Diseases, Centers for Disease Control and Prevention. March 2009. Available at: http://stacks.cdc.gov/view/cdc/11550/. Accessed 14.08.2013.

63. Miller A. Hospital reporting and "never" events. *Medicare Pat Management.* 2009;4(3):20-22.

64. Haynes AB, Weiser TG, Berry WR. A surgical safety checklist to reduce morbidity and mortality in a global population. *N Engl J Med.* 2009;360:491-499.

65. Semel ME, Resch S, Haynes AB, et al. Adopting a surgical safety checklist could save money and improve the quality of care in U.S. hospitals. *Health Affair.* 2010;29(9):1593-1599.

66. Allsop J, Mulcahy L. Adverse events, complaints, and clinical negligence claims: what do we know? Chief Medical Officer's Advisory Group on Complaints and Clinical Negligence, Department of Health, London, UK. 2002;14.

67. Annandale E, Hunt K. Accounts of disagreements with doctors. *Soc Sci Med.* 1998;46:119-129.

68. Mulcahy L, Tritter JQ. Pathways, pyramids and icebergs? Mapping the links between dissatisfaction and complaints. *Sociol Health Ill.* 1998;20(6):825-847.

69. Schlesinger M, Mitchell S, Elbel B. Voices unheard: barriers to expressing dissatisfaction to health plans. *Milbank Q.* 2002;80:709-755.

70. Jennings ME. Utilization of patient satisfaction-patient retention strategies in the primary care healthcare setting. *GARJMBS.* 2012;1(1):1-5.

71. TARP. *Consumer Complaint Handling in America: An Update Study Part II.* Washington, DC: United States Office of Consumer Affairs; 1986.

72. Kane CK. Medical liability claim frequency: a 2007-2008 snapshot of physicians. *Policy Research Perspectives No. 2010-1.* Chicago, IL: American Medical Association; 2010. http://www.ama-assn.org/resources/doc/health-policy/prp-201001-claim-freq.pdf.

73. Jena AB, Chandra A, Lakdawalla D, Seabury D. Malpractice risk according to physician specialty. *N Engl J Med.* 2011;365:629-636.

74. Sloan FA, Mergenhagen PM, Burfield WB, et al. Medical malpractice experience of physicians. Predictable or haphazard? *JAMA.* 1989;262(23):3291-3297.

75. Entman SS, Glass CA, Hickson GB, et al. The relationship between malpractice claims history and subsequent obstetric care. *JAMA*. 1994;272(20):1588-1591.

76. Hickson GB, Clayton EW, Entman SS, et al. Obstetricians' prior malpractice experience and patients' satisfaction with care. *JAMA*. 1994;272(20):1583-1587.

77. Hickson GB, Federspiel CF, Pichert JW, et al. Patient complaints and malpractice risk. *JAMA*. 2002;287:2951-2957.

78. Hickson GB, Federspiel CF, Blackford JU, et al. Patient complaints and malpractice risk in a regional healthcare center. *South Med J*. 2007;100(8):791-796.

79. Cydulka RK, Tamayo-Sarver J, Gage A. Association of patient satisfaction with complaints and risk management among emergency physicians. *J Emerg Med*. 2011;41(4):405-411.

80. Fullam F, Garman AN, Johnson TJ, Hedberg EC. The use of patient satisfaction surveys and alternative coding procedures to predict malpractice risk. *Med Care*. 2009;47(5):553-559.

81. Levtzion-Korach O, Frankel A, Alcalai H, et al. Integrating incident data from five reporting systems to assess patient safety: making sense of the elephant. *Jt Comm J Qual Patient Saf*. 2010;36(9):402-410.

82. Stelfox HT, Gandhi TK, Orav EJ, Gustafson ML. The relation of patient satisfaction with complaints against physicians and malpractice lawsuits. *Am J Med*. Oct;118(10):1126-1133.

83. Rawson JV, Thompson N, Sostre G, Deitte L. The cost of disruptive and unprofessional behaviors in health care. *Acad Radiol*. 2013;20(9):1074-1076.

84. Hickson GB, Pichert JW, Webb LE, Gabbe SG. A complementary approach to promoting professionalism: identifying, measuring and addressing unprofessional behaviors. *Acad Med*. 2007;82(11):1040-1048.

85. DuPree E, Anderson R, McEvoy MD, Brodman M. Professionalism: a necessary ingredient in a culture of safety. *Jt Comm J Qual Patient Saf*. 2011;37(10):447-455.

86. Houldin AD, Naylor MD, Haller DG. Physician-nurse collaboration in research in the 21st century. *J Clin Oncol*. 2004;22(5):774-776.

87. Vanderbilt Medical Center. elevate credo. Available at: http://biostat.mc.vanderbilt.edu/wiki/pub/Main/RecognizeReward/vumc-credo.pdf.

88. Hayden AC, Pichert JW, Fawcett J, et al. Best practices for basic and advanced skills in health care service recovery: a case study of a re-admitted patient. *Jt Comm J Qual Pat Saf*. 2010;36(7):310-318.

89. Surveys on patient safety culture. Available at http://www.ahrq.gov/professionals/quality-patient-safety/patientsafetyculture/index.html.

90. AHRQ. The Safety Attitudes Questionnaire. Available at: http://psnet.ahrq.gov/resource.aspx?resourceID=3601.

91. Sexton JB, Berenholtz SM, Goeschel CA, et al. Assessing and improving safety climate in a large cohort of intensive care units. *Crit Care Med*. 2011;39:934-939.

92. Fowler L, Saucier A, Coffin J. Consumer assessment of healthcare providers and systems survey: implications for the primary care physician. *Osteopathic Fam Phys*. 2013;5(4):153-157.

93. Studer Q. *Hardwiring Excellence: Purpose, Worthwhile Work, Making a Difference*. Gulf Breeze, FL: Fire Starter Publishing; 2003.

94. Das S, Chen MH, Warren N, Hodgson M. Do associations between employee self-reported organizational assessments and attitudinal outcomes change over time? An

analysis of four Veterans Health Administration surveys using structural equation modeling. *Health Econ.* 2011;20:1507-1522.

95. Murff HJ, France DJ, Blackford JU, et al. Relationship between patient complaints and surgical complications. *Qual Saf Health Care.* 2006;15:13-16.

96. Colla JB, Bracken AC, Kinney LM, Weeks WB. Measuring patient safety climate: a review of surveys. *Qual Saf Health Care.* 2005;14:364-366.

97. Pichert JW, Moore IN, Karrass J, et al. An intervention model that promotes professional accountability: peer messengers and patient/family complaints. *Jt Comm J Qual Patient Saf.* 2013;39(10):435-446.

98. Hickson GB, Pichert JW. Identifying and addressing physicians at high risk for medical malpractice claims. In: Youngberg B, ed. *Patient Safety Handbook,* 2nd ed. Sudbury, MA: Jones and Bartlett; 2013.

99. Pichert JW, Hickson GB, Moore IN. Using patient complaints to promote patient safety: the patient advocacy reporting system (PARS). In: Henriksen K, Battles JB, Keyes MA, Grady ML, eds. *Advances in Patient Safety: New Directions and Alternative Approaches.* Bethesda, MD: Agency for Healthcare Research and Quality (AHRQ); 2008;2:421-430.

100. Reiter CE, Hickson GB, Pichert JW. Addressing behavior and performance issues that threaten quality and patient safety: what your attorneys want you to know. *Prog Pediatr Cardiol.* 2012;33(1):37-45.

101. Oreskovich MR, Kaups KL, Balch CM. Prevalence of alcohol use disorder among American surgeons. *Arch Surg.* 2012;147(2):168-174.

102. Leape LL, Fromson JA. Problem doctors: is there a system-level solution? *Ann Intern Med.* 2006;144(2);107-115.

103. Wu A. Medical error: the second victim: the doctor who makes the mistake needs help too. *Brit Med J.* 2000;320:726-727.

104. Hickson GB, Moore IN. Risk prevention, risk management, and professional liability. In: Rock JA, Jones HW III, eds. *TeLinde's Operative Gynecology.* 11th ed. Philadelphia, PA: Lippincott Williams & Wilkins; in press.

105. Christensen JF. The heat of darkness: the impact of perceived mistakes on physicians. *J Gen Int Med.* 1992;7:424-31.

106. Schwappach DLB, Boluarte TA. The emotional impact of medical error involvement on physicians: a call for leadership and organisational accountability. *Swiss Med Wkly.* 2008;138(1-2):9-15.

107. Waterman AD, Garbutt J, Hazel E, et al. The emotional impact of medical errors on practicing physicians in the United States and Canada. *Jt Comm J Qual Patient Saf.* 2007;3(8):467-476.

108. Pichert JW, Hickson GB, Pinto A, Vincent C. Communicating about unexpected outcomes, and adverse events, and errors. In: Carayon P. *Human Factors and Ergonomics in Health Care and Patient Safety.* 2nd ed. Boca Raton, FL: CRC Press; 2012:401-421.

109. Deis JN, Smith KM, Warren MD, et al. Transforming the morbidity and mortality conference into an instrument for system-wide improvement. In: Henricksen K, Battles JB, Keyes MA, Grady ML, eds. *Advances in Patient Safety: New Directions and Alternative Approaches.* Vol. 2. Rockville, MD: US Agency for Healthcare Research and Quality; 2008.

110. Percarpio KB, Watts BV. A cross-sectional study on the relationship between utilization of root cause analysis and patient safety at 139 department of veterans affairs medical centers. *Jt Comm J Qual Patient Saf*. 2013;39(1):32-37.

111. Vincent C, Phillips A, Young M. Why do people sue doctors? A study of patients and relatives taking legal action. *Lancet*. 1994;343:1609-1613.

112. Hickson GB, Clayton EW, Githens PB, Sloan FA. Factors that prompted families to file medical malpractice claims following perinatal injuries. *JAMA*. 1992;267(10):1359-1363.

113. Kraman SS, Cranfill L, Hamm G, Woodard T. Advocacy: the Lexington veterans affairs medical center. *J Comm J Qual Imp*. 2002:646-650.

114. Kachalia A, Kaufman SR, Boothman R, et al. Liability claims and costs before and after implementation of a medical error disclosure program. *Ann Intern Med*. 2010;153:213-221.

115. Gallagher T, Studdert D. Disclosing harmful medical errors to patients. *N Engl J Med*. 2007;356:2713-2719.

116. Boothman RC, Blackwell AC, Campbell DA, et al. A better approach to medical malpractice claims? The University of Michigan experience. *J Health Life Sci Law*. 2009;2(2):125-159.

117. Lembitz A. Litigation alternative: COPIC's 3Rs program. Available at: http://www.aaos.org/news/aaosnow/sep10/managing7.asp Accessed 13.08.2013.

118. Stimson et al. Medical malpractice claims risk in urology: an empirical analysis of patient complaint data. *J Urol*. 2010;183:1971-1976.

119. Mukherjee K, Pichert JW, Cornett MB, et al. All trauma surgeons are not created equal: asymmetric distribution of malpractice claims risk. *J Traum*. 2010;69(3):549-556.

120. Bovbjerg RR, Petronis KR. The relationship between physicians' malpractice claims history and later claims. Does the past predict the future? *JAMA*. 1994;272:1421-1426.

121. Hickson GB, Pichert JW, Federspiel CF, Clayton EW. Development of an early identification and response model of malpractice prevention. *Law Contemp Probs*. 1997;60(1):7-29.

122. Ray WA, Federspiel CF, Schaffner W. Prescribing of tetracycline to children less than 8 years old: a two-year epidemiologic study among ambulatory Tennessee Medicaid recipients. *JAMA*. 1977;237:2069-2074.

123. Ray WA, Federspiel CF, Schaffner W. Prescribing of chloramphenicol in ambulatory practice: an epidemiologic study among Tennessee Medicaid recipients. *Ann Intern Med*. 1976;84:266-270.

124. Schaffner W, Way WA, Federspiel CF, Miller WO. Improving antibiotic prescribing in office practice: a controlled trial of three educational methods. *JAMA*.1983; 250(13):1728-1732.

125. Pichert JW, Hoffman WW, Danielson D, et al. Application of a project bundle to planning implementation of the Patient Advocacy Reporting System throughout the Sanford Health System. In: Battles JB, Reback KA, Azam I, eds. *Advances in Patient Safety and Medical Liability*. Bethesda, MD: Center for Quality Improvement and Patient Safety, Agency for Healthcare Research and Quality (AHRQ); in press.

126. Merkel PL. Physicians policing physicians: the development of peer review law at California hospitals. *USF L Rev*. 2004;38:301-330.

127. Grogan MJ, Knechtges P. The disruptive physician: a legal perspective. *Acad Radiol*. 2013;20(9):1069-1073.

Index

Note: Page numbers followed by *f* denote figures; page numbers followed by *t* denote tables.

A

Accountability, 117, 147*f*, 270
    action plans, 267, 268, 270, 280
    algorithm for assigning, 115
    appropriate (*See* Appropriate
        accountability)
    development of, 147
    for high-alert medications, 84
    lack of, 129
    methodology, 269
    professional, 260 (*See also*
        Professionalism)
        and pursuit of culture of safety,
            230–284
Ad hominum process, 110
Adverse drug events (ADEs), 73, 79,
        157, 216
    automated surveillance of,
        166–169
    background, 47–50
    challenge of keeping patients safe,
        55–56
    complexity of care, 52–55, 53*f*
    complex systems, accident causation in,
        64–66
        Swiss-cheese model, 66*f*
    error reduction principles, 66–69
    errors in medicine
        systems flaws, not character flaws
            production of, 60*f*
    incidence of, 74
    measures of, 161
    no data without story, no story without
        data, 50–51
    problem in, 51–52
    reduction in, 218*f*
    risk of, 218
    safe practice
        violations of, 63–64
    structure for, 219
Adverse events (AEs), 54
Agency for Healthcare Research and
        Quality (AHRQ), 185

Agency for Healthcare Research and
        Quality, and Health Level Seven
        (HL7), 159
Alert fatigue, 164–165
Ambulatory care, 74, 80
American Academy of Pediatrics, 206, 228
American Recovery and Reinvesting Act
        (ARRA), 158
Ann & Robert H. Lurie Children's
        Hospital of Chicago, 78, 86
Annotated control chart
    example of, 46*f*
APGAR score, 206
Appropriate accountability
    definition of, 106
    safe and reliable pediatric care,
        115–118
Assignable variation, 19
Automated dispensing device (ADD),
        84, 96
Automated trigger tools
    use of, 169
Awareness
    discussion, 266
    preparation for, 266

B

"Ballard" protocol, 228
Barcode medication administration
        (BCMA) system, 165–166, 217
    implementation of, 166
    pediatric considerations for, 166
Barcoding systems, 96
Baseline data
    example of, 42*f*–43*f*
Behaviors
    of teams in pediatric care, 113*f*
    unprofessional
        professionals and staff, 270–271
Body mass index (BMI), 11
Brainstorming, 16
Bulletin boards, 120, 123
    types of, 124

C

California Perinatal Care Collaborative (CPQCC), 214
Care delivery processes, 188
Catheter-associated bloodstream infections, 216
Catheter-associated urinary tract infection (CAUTI), 252
Center for Patient and Professional Advocacy, 251
Center for Research, Education and Quality, 214
Centers for Disease Control and Prevention (CDC) national healthcare safety network, 215
Centers for Medicare and Medicaid Services, 159, 186
Central-line-associated bloodstream infections (CLA-BSIs), 219–221, 244, 252
   epidemiology of, 220
Change concepts, 6
   categories of, 6
      change the work environment, 8
      design systems to avoid mistakes, 8–9
      eliminate waste, 6
      enhance the provider/customer relationship, 8
      focus on the product or service, 9
      improve workflow, 8
      manage time, 8
      manage variation, 8
      optimize inventory, 8
Chemotherapy Safety Committee, 88–89
   responsible for, 88–89
Children with chronic conditions (CCC), 197
CHIP programs, 198
Clinical decision support (CDS), 75, 78, 161–165
   alert fatigue, 164–165
   definition of, 161
   medication-specific functionality, 162t
   medication with computerized physician order entry, 161–163
   pediatric systems, 163–164
Closed-loop communication, 144
Coagulase-negative *Staphylococcus* species, 221

Code response simulation, 93
Common cause variation. *See* Random variation
Communication. *See also* Debriefing
   development of, 68
   errors, 129
   exchange, 139
   in learning systems, 111–113
   of medical information, 79
   to primary care provider, 32, 36f, 37f
   rate of, 32
   structured, 111, 138
   teamwork and, 66, 112–113, 129–152
      achieving high-functioning teams, 146–148
      emergency department discussion, 133–136
         learning points, 136
      learning from errors, 147f
      pediatrician's office, 130, 144–145
         discussion, 131–132, 145–146
         learning points, 132, 146
      pediatric intensive care unit, daily rounds, 140
         discussion, 140–142
         learning points, 142
      pediatric intensive care unit, next day, 142–143
         discussion, 143–144
         learning points, 144
      pediatric intensive care unit, patient handoff from operating room, 136–137
         discussion, 136–137, 137–139
         learning points, 139–140
      TeamSTEPPS™ framework, 148f
Complexity of care
   factors in, 54
Computed tomography (CT) scan, 132
Computerized physician order entry (CPOE), 56, 74, 77, 78, 80, 95, 159–161
   advantages of, 159
   design of, 160
   evaluation tool, 163
   FMEA, 90
   implementation of, 170, 171
   pediatric specific functionality, 160t
   potential of, 169

Congenital diaphragmatic hernia, 208
Connecticut Children's Medical
        Center, 220
Continuous learning, 106, 107, 120
    definition of, 119
Continuous-positive airway pressure
        (CPAP), 209
Conversation
    point of, 265
Costs
    of disrespect in professionalism, 251
    medical malpractice claims, 252
    of patient harm, 252
"C-suite" executives, 254
Culture. *See* Safety culture
Cup of coffee conversation (CoC), 262
    goals for, 262
    principles of, 262
    sub-type of, 264

D
Dana Farber Cancer Institute (DFCI), 186
Data collection process, 10, 33, 42
    instruments, 38, 40
Debriefing, 119, 120
    defects identified from, 124
    by ED team, 135
    participate in, 135
    process of, 124, 136
    results of, 124
Decision-making processes, 183, 191
Define, measure, analyze, improve, control
        (DMAIC) framework, 14–15
Deming's theory of profound
        knowledge, 2
    components of, 2
Department of Health and Human
        Services, 186
Discharge handover process, 194
Discharge progress, 39, 45
Disclosure, 272
Dispensing, 82–84
    administration, 83
    formulations and dosage forms,
        82–83
    high alert and look-alike-sound-alike
        medications, 83–84
    measures for, 82–83
Dosing errors, 81

Down syndrome, 57
Duke University Health System (DUHS),
        186, 196
    Patient Advocacy Council, 196

E
Education
    for end-users and monitoring
            compliance with, 87
    evidence-based, 228
    on handoff techniques, 138
    important aspect of, 142
    involve patients in provider, 196
    to patients and caregivers, 184
    staff, 88
    targeted for, 145
    team disassociation and, 141
Edwards, W.
    system of knowledge, 1
Effective leaders, 115
Electronic health records (EHRs)/
        Electronic medical records
        (EMR), 227. *See also* Health
        information technology
    CPOE system, 165
    definition of, 158
    programmer, 29
    types of, 169
Electronic medication administration
        record (eMAR), 165
Electronic prescribing systems, 78
Electronic trigger tool, 168
    strategies for implementing, 168
Emergency departments (EDs), 75, 245
    case study, 20, 132, 151*t*
    pediatric, 193
Emergency medical services (EMS), 75
Endogenous factors, 62
Equal Opportunity, Affirmative Action,
        Disability Office (EAD), 271
Error-prone processes, 218
Error-reduction principles, 67
Errors
    human, 56
    juxtaposition, 170
    medical (*See* Medical errors)
    types, 170
Evidence-based medicine
    use of, 206

Exclusive human milk for babies
    (EHM4B), 215
Exogenous factors, 62
Experienced leaders, 279
Extremely low birth weight (ELBW)
    infants, 212, 224

F
Failure modes effects analyses (FMEAs),
    16–18, 90
Fatigue, 62–63
Fentanyl® scenario, 212
First-pass process analysis, 218
Fishbone diagrams, 16
10-Fold errors, 77
Food and Drug Administration (FDA), 172
Four-pronged approach, 224

G
Goal-directed therapy, 20
Good Health Center Clinic System, 33

H
Hand hygiene (HH) best practices, 274
Hand Hygiene Executive Committee
    (HHEC), 276
Handoff
    from operating room, pediatric
        intensive care unit, 136–137
        discussion, 137–139
        learning points, 139–140
    techniques, 138
Harvard Medical Practice Study, 49, 50
Healthcare-associated infections (HAIs), 251
Healthcare Finance Administration
    (HCFA), 182
Healthcare industry, 2, 49
Healthcare office
    characteristics of, 131
Healthcare organizations, 81
Healthcare professionals, 242, 271, 272
Healthcare providers, 58, 141, 216, 227
Healthcare systems, 18, 52, 189, 191
Healthcare team, 129
Health information technology
    (HIT), 157, 172. *See also*
    Electronic health records
    (EHRs)/Electronic medical
    records (EMR)

importance of, 158
unintended consequences of, 169–172
    EHR harm mitigation, 171–172
    Pittsburgh CPOE case, 170–171
Health Information Technology for
    Economic and Clinical Health
    (HITECH) Act, 158
key hallmarks of, 158
Health IT and patient safety, 172
Health literacy, 189
Helping babies breathe (HBB), 228
Hemophilia, 52
High-alert medications, 85f
High-frequency ventilator, 209
High-functioning healthcare teams,
    143, 146
High-reliability organizations (HROs), 59,
    65, 241
    characterized by, 241–242
"Holy Grail" project, 227
Hospital-acquired infections, 186
Hospital Consumer Assessment of
    Healthcare Providers and
    Systems (HCAHPS) survey, 197
    health plan survey, 197
    score, 200
Human errors, 56. *See also* Errors
    performance, 61–63, 61f
    "swamp" of, 58–59
Human factors, 59–60
    background, 47–50
    challenge of keeping patients safe,
        55–56
    complexity of care, 52–55, 53f
    complex systems, accident causation in,
        64–66
        Swiss-cheese model, 66f
    component tasks, 59
    error reduction principles, 66–69
    human error
        performance, 61–63, 61f
        "swamp" of, 58–59
    infractions, 61
    no data without story, no story without
        data, 50–51
    problem in, 51–52
    safe practice
        violations of, 63–64
    understanding of, 66

Human factors engineers (HFEs), 60
Human papilloma virus (HPV) vaccine, 164
Hypoxic ischemic encephalopathy (HIE)
    Cooling trial for, 213
    therapeutic hypothermia, 214

I

Illegal drugs
    use of, 117
Improvement process, 2
    definition of, 107
Information systems
    improve access to, 68
    use of, 166
Information technology
    electronic trigger tool examples, 167*t*
    importance in pediatric patient safety,
        157–173
        adverse events, automated
            surveillance of, 166–169
        barcode medication administration
            (BCMA), 165–166
        clinical decision support (CDS)
            medication-specific
            functionality, 162*t*
        computerized physician order entry
            (CPOE), 159–161
            pediatric specific functionality, 160*t*
        health information technology,
            unintended consequences of,
            169–172
Institute for Healthcare Improvement
        (IHI), 167
    improvement model, 37
Institute for Patient and Family Centered
        Care (IPFCC), 184
    vision of, 185
Institute for Safe Medication Practices
        (ISMP), 77, 94, 219
Institute of Medicine (IOM), 74, 94,
        157, 172
    To Err is Human, 52, 157, 181, 240
    Health IT and patient safety, 172
    report, 27
Integrated health systems, 211
Intensive care units (ICUs), 84, 88,
        93, 197, 249
Interpersonal barriers, 183
Intervention process, 279

"In utero" infections, 209
Ishikawa diagrams, 16

J

James Reason's Incident Decision Tree, 115
Joint Commission, 63
    accreditation, 186
    list of high-alert medications, 93
    medication reconciliation in, 79
Joint Commission National Patient Safety
        Goal (NPSG), 79
Josie King Foundation, 185
Just culture, 106, 115
Just culture algorithm, 117

K

Kaiser Permanente, 194
Key driver diagrams, 16, 36–37
    example of, 36*f*–37*f*
    for interventions, 17*f*
Keystone ICU Project, Michigan, 221
Knowledge, skills, and
            attitudes (KSAs), 147

L

Langley, G.
    change concepts, 6
        categories of, 6
Language
    common, 258
    critical, 113, 114
    opaque, 257
Leaders
    challenge of, 265
    commitment to, 254–255
    definition of, 105
    effective, 125–126
    feedback for, 111
    impact of, 126
    power of, 118
    psychological safety and, 110–111
    responsibilities of, 108–109
    role in safe and reliable pediatric care,
        108–111
Leadership
    barriers, 248–249
        personal barriers, 248–249
        systemic barriers in, 248
    component of, 103

Lean principles, 12–14
   create flow by eliminating waste, 13–14
   identify customers and specify value, 12
   identify the value stream, 12–13
   let the customer pull value, 14
   pursue perfection, 14
   wastes in healthcare, 13t
Leape, Lucian, 49
Leapfrog Group for Patient Safety, 163
Learning
   boards, 124
   components of, 103
Learning systems, 103, 106, 111,
      118–120, 125
   building of, 126
   communication in, 111–113
      teamwork and, 112–113
   comprised of, 119
   continuous learning, 119
   effective teams, 112–113
Lesch–Nyhan syndrome, 52
Leveraging automation, 96
Licensed independent
      practitioner (LIP), 84
Look-alike-sound-alike (LASA)
      medications, 83

M
"Major-intervention" approach, 218
Massachusetts Institute of Technology, 12
Measurement
   definition of, 107
   types of
      balance, 5
      outcome, 5
      process, 5
Medical errors, 49, 73
   Alyssa Shinn, case study, 51
   background, 49–50
   challenge of keeping patients safe,
      55–56
   complexity of care, 52–55, 53f
   complex systems, accident
      causation in, 64–66
      Swiss-cheese model, 66f
   error reduction principles, 66–69
   no data without story, no story without
      data, 50–51
   problem in, 51–52

   rates of, 76
   safe practice
      violations of, 63–64
   Sheridan Cal, case study, 50
   systems flaws, not character flaws,
      56–57
Medication administration
   definition of, 83
Medication administration
      record (MAR), 85
Medication decision support systems
   types of, 163
Medication reconciliation process, 96
   obtain a medication history, 79
   reconcile again upon transfer and
      discharge, 80
   reconcile and resolve discrepancies and
      prescribe the medications, 79
   share the list, 80
Medication-related errors. See Medical
      errors
Medication Safety and Pharmacy and
      Therapeutics Committees, 84
Medication Safety Committee, 85
Medication use process, 77–81, 95
   computerized provider order entry and
      clinical decision support, 78–79
   medication reconciliation, 79–80
   prescribing, 77
   processing/verifying, 80–81
Memory
   avoid reliance on, 67
Metrics, 31–33
Michigan Keystone ICU Project, 221
Model for Improvement
   components of, 10
   focus of, 5
   key elements, 27
   questions of, 27
   steps in
      attainable, 4
      measurable, 4
      relevant, 4
      specific aims, 3
      time bound, 4
   types of measures
      balance, 5
      outcome, 5
      process, 5

N

National Asthma Education Prevention Program, 164
National Center for Health Statistics, 75
National Coordination Council for Medication Errors Reporting and Prevention (NCC MERP), 83, 89
National Institute of Child Health and Human Development (NICHD), 213
National Institutes of Health (NIH), 213
National Patient Safety Foundation (NPSF), 182, 185
National pediatric database, 168
National Transitions of Care Collaborative, 29
Necrotizing enterocolitis (NEC), 208, 222
    incidence of, 224f, 225f, 226
    proportion of, 223
Negotiation
    definition of, 106
    goal of, 114
Neonatal intensive care unit (NICU), 54, 92, 192
Neonatal medication errors, 217
Neonatal medication safety, 223
Neonatal research network (NRN), 213, 223
Neonates
    background, 206–207
    central-line-associated bloodstream infections, 219–222
    collaborative improvement efforts, 212
    conclusion, 211–212, 215, 226–227
    data richness, 211
    future targets and opportunities, 227–229
    immature physiology, 208–209
    multidisciplinary case studies, 215–216
    National Institute Of Child Health And Human Development Neonatal Research Network, 213–214
    necrotizing enterocolitis (NEC), 222–226
    neonatal medication safety, 216–219
    NICU, 207
    opportunity to "start from scratch," 210–211
    Pediatrix Medical Group, 214
    perinatal quality collaborative of North Carolina, 214–215
    population variability, 207–208
    sensitivity to errors, 209–210
    special perspectives for, 205–234
    Vermont Oxford Network, 212–213
Neonatology
    history of, 205
Neurosurgical procedure, 239
Newborn intensive care unit (NICU), 119, 205, 207, 210, 230
    bundles
        complexity of, 222
    characteristics, 211
    medication errors in, 216
Nitric oxide for chronic lung disease (NO CLD), 228.
    See also "Ballard" protocol
Nolan, Tom
    model for improvement, 3
Normal Gaussian distribution model, 61, 61f
Nurse knowledge exchange (NKE), 194

O

Office of Patient Relations (OPR)
    calls, 239
Ohio Perinatal Quality Collaborative (OPQC), 215
On-line event reporting system
    use of, 89
Opaque language, 257
Operating room (OR), 133, 136, 244
Organizational excellence framework, 104f, 107–108
Organizational fairness
    algorithm
        logic of, 117
    definition of, 106
Outcomes
    adverse, 63, 65
        creation of preventable, 66
        production of, 60f
    patient-relevant, 31
    quality, 161
    suboptimal, 119
    treasure trove for, 213
Ovals mark, 33

P

Pareto principle, 18
Patient activation measure (PAM), 187
    scores, 188
Patient Advocacy/Advisory Councils
        (PACs), 187
    contribute in, 187
    framework for, 187
Patient engagement
    barriers to, 183–185
    creating structure and culture to
        support patient/family-centered
        care, 186–188
    efforts to enhance, 185–186
    engaging patients and families, 188
    increasing patient and family capacity
        for, 189–191
        improve health literacy, 189–190
        improve self-care and self-
            management, 190
        inform patients of their rights,
            190–191
    increasing patient and family
        involvement, 191–197
        coordination of care and care
            transitions, 193–194
        development and review of goals,
            192–193
        information sharing, 191–192
        involve family presence whenever
            possible, 197
        involve patients and their families
            in organizational and policy
            discussions and decisions, 195
        involve patients in provider
            education, 196
        listen to and learn from patient and
            family feedback, 194–195
        shared care plans, 192
        shared decision-making, 191
    measures of success, 197–198
    strategies for, 189
Patient/parent and family
        advisory committees
        (PFACs), 186
Patient safety experts, 58
Pediatric care
    lifecycle of, 53–55, 54f
    risk of harm in, 55

Pediatric care, safe and reliable
    aims, tests of change, and strategy and
        actions, 121f
    appropriate accountability, 115–118
    communication in learning systems,
        111–113
    department or unit is made up of
        culture and learning, 103–107
    essential behaviors of teams, 113f
    fair evaluation and response chart, 116f
    improvement and measurement,
        120–122
    increasing insights, 109f
    leaders, role of, 108–111
    learning systems, 118–120
    management of, 123f
    negotiation, an intrinsic part of team
        function, 114–115
    role in leadership, 103–127
    safe & reliable healthcare, 108f
    socio-technical framework and
        organizational excellence,
        107–108
    transparency and visibility, 123–125
Pediatric Emergency Care Applied Research
        Network (PECARN), 75
Pediatric emergency department, 193
Pediatric health information systems
        (PHIS), 168
Pediatric intensive care unit (PICU), 136,
        159, 207
Pediatric medication safety
    automated dispensing device
        drawers, organization and
        labeling of, 87f
    Chemotherapy Safety Committee,
        88–89
    children at greater risk, 76–77
    definitions and epidemiology of, 73–76
    dispensing, 82–84
    establishing an event review
        structure, 89
    high-alert medications, 85f
    improvement of, 90–92
    LASA medication list and
        precautions, 86f
    medication administration
        oversight, 86–88
    medication use process, 77–81

NCC MERP safety event category
impact scale
percent of doses dispensed, 91*f*–94*f*
planning in new hospital, 92–94
role of pharmacist, 81–82
safety event reporting and learning
from mistakes, 89–90
sequence for implementation of
technology, 95*f*
starting point of, 94–95
technology utilization to enhance
medication dispensing and
administration safety, 84–86
Pediatric patients, 146
risk for, 76
*Pediatric Patient Safety and Quality
Improvement,* 228
Pediatric Pharmacy Advocacy Group
(PPAG), 77
Pediatric Quality Measures Program
(PQMP), 198
Pediatrix Medical Group, 214
Peer-based intervention model, 274
Perinatal Quality Collaborative of North
Carolina (PQCNC), 214
Peripherally inserted central venous
catheter (PICC), 220
Pharmacist, role of, 81–82
Pharmacy system, 165
Planning, Doing, Studying, and Acting
(PDSA) cycle, 6, 10–11, 21–23,
37, 40, 45, 120–122
example of, 42*f*–43*f*
impact of implementation, 12
test cycles, 12
Post-natal corticosteroid therapy, 213
Premature Infants in Need of Transfusion
(PINT) trial, 228
Premature neonatal outcomes project, 205
Process mapping, 33, 34
constructing, 36
definition of, 15
Professional accountability, 260. *See also*
Professionalism
and pursuit of culture of safety,
230–284
Professionalism
addressing medical malpractice claims
risk, 272–274

addressing unprofessional conduct,
making the case for, 249
apparent pattern, 265–267
barriers to addressing behaviors
leader barriers, 248–249
team member barriers, 246–248
corrective/disciplinary action, 269–270
costs of disrespect, 251
costs of patient harm, 252
effectiveness of pyramid model, 272
egregious events, 263*t*
espresso conversation, 264–265
failure to achieve intended outcomes,
249–250
guide graduated interventions, model to
promoting professionalism pyramid,
260–261, 261*f*
high reliability and, 241–242
impact on reputation, 252
improving hand hygiene compliance,
274–277
incurred expense by risk category, 273*t*
infrastructure elements for, 254*t*
leadership commitment, 254–255
medical malpractice claims costs, 252
mission, goals, core values, and
supportive policies, 255–258
persistent pattern, 267–268
principles underlying graduated
interventions, 277–280
avoiding conflicts of interest, 279
dealing fairly in, 280
multiple opportunities to acquire,
279–280
promoting justice, 278
professionals and staff as the "second
victim," 271–272
professionals and staff as the target
of unprofessional behavior,
270–271
professionals fail to be professional,
244–246
progression of tiered interventions, 269*t*
promoting professional accountability,
infrastructure elements for,
253–254, 254*t*
resources to help address unnecessary
variation, 270
resources to help those affected, 270

Professionalism (*Cont'd.*)
  reviewing reported observations,
       processes for, 259–260
  single unprofessional incident, 261–264
  in the 21ˢᵗ century, 240–241
  surveillance tools, 258–259
  unprofessional behavior/performance
       undermines culture of safety,
       242–244
  "you are here" chart, 276*f*
Professional regulation, forms of
  group-regulation, 241
  self-regulation, 241
"Project bundle" tool, 275
Promoting Professionalism Pyramid, 261
Provost, Lloyd
  model for improvement, 3
Psychological safety, 110
  critical importance of, 126
Pyramid model, 273

Q
Quality improvement application
  annotated control chart
       example of, 46*f*
  baseline data and PDSA cycle
       example of, 42*f*–43*f*
  collect baseline data, 37–38
  common cause *vs.* special cause
       variation, 45
  component of, 47
  displaying data, run charts and control
       charts, 42–45
  establish shared goal, 31
  existing process, understanding of,
       33–35
  forming the quality improvement team,
       29–30
  generalizability in, 45–47
  hallmark of, 31
  identify barriers, 35–36
  identifying key stakeholders, 30–31
  implement on larger scale, 40
  initial test on small scale, 38–40
  key driver diagram, 36–37
       example of, 36*f*–37*f*
  metrics, 31–33
  pilot on small scale, 40
  process map, example of, 34*f*–35*f*
  rational subgroups
       example of, 44*f*
  selecting domain for improvement,
       28–29
  Specific, measurable, attainable,
       relevant, time bound (SMART)
       aim, 31
       action-oriented or achievable, 32–33
       measurable, 31
       realistic, 33
       specific, 31
       time-bound, 33
  subsequent plan-do-study-act cycles,
       40–41
       using rational subgroups in, 41–42
  targets for, 34
  using model for improvement as
       framework, 27–28, 28*f*
Quality improvement methods, 2–15, 40,
       42, 215
  change concepts in, 6–10, 7*t*–8*t*
  goal of, 28
  Lean principles, 12–14
  measures, research *vs.* process
       improvement, 5*t*
  model for, 3–12, 3*f*
  plan, do, study, act (PDSA) cycles, 10–11
  projects, 32, 228
  rapid cycle testing and implementing
       changes, 12
  science, 1
  Six Sigma, 14–15
  step in, 3–5
  testing changes, designs for, 11
  types of, 5–6
Quality improvement tools, 15–23
  case study, 20–21
  to gather information, 15–16
  for organizing information, 16–20
       affinity diagrams, 16
       cause and effect diagrams (*See*
            Fishbone diagrams; Ishikawa
            diagrams)
       failure mode and effects analysis
            (FMEA), 16–18
       key driver diagrams, 16
       Pareto charts, 18
       run charts, 18–19
       statistical process control charts, 19

PDSA cycle, 21–23
    process change, 22
    recognition, 21
    recruitment, 22
    standardization, 22
    statistical process control
        charts, 20t
    types based on type of data, 20t

R
Random variation, 19
    vs. special cause variation, 45
Rapid-cycle quality improvement
        methods, 27
Rapid response teams (RRTs),
        181, 185
Rasmussen, Jens, 63
Real-time trigger, 168
Reason, James, 110
Reason's substitution test, 117
Red blood cell (RBC), 164
Redundancies, 68
Reflux medications
    use of, 225
Reliable processes, 119
    definition of, 106–107
Root cause analyses (RCAs), 90
"80/20 rule." *See* Pareto principle
Run charts, 11, 18–19
    vs. pre- and post data
        display, 18f

S
Safe practice
    beliefs of, 66
    violations of, 63–64
Safety culture, 240
    barriers, 183
    components of, 103
    evolution stages of
        generative, 108
        proactive, 107–108
        reactive, 107
        systematic, 107
        unmindful, 107
    importance of, 240
    professionalism
        unprofessional behavior/performance
            undermines, 242–244

pursuit of
    professional accountability and,
        230–284
    surveys, 258
Safety event category impact scale, 89
Safety event reporting systems (SERS)
    implementation of, 89
Self-correction protects, 267
Shared mental model, 131, 135, 137, 142, 149
Shewhart charts. *See* Statistical process
        control charts
Simplification, 67
Situation, background, assessment,
        recommendation
        (SBAR), 111
    components of
        assessment, 112
        background, 112
        recommendation, 112
        situation, 112
Six Sigma process, 14–15
    steps in
        analyze, 15
        control, 15
        define the problem, 14
        improve, 15
        measure, 15
Sleep deprivation, 62
Socio-technical framework, 107–108
Spaghetti diagrams, 15
Specific, measurable, attainable, relevant,
        time bound (SMART) aim, 31
    action-oriented or achievable,
        32–33
    measurable, 31
    realistic, 33
    specific, 31
    time-bound, 33
Standardization, 67
Standardized infection ratios (SIRs), 277
Statistical process-control charts, 19, 45
    elements of, 20f
    for time, 22f
Stress, 62
Surveillance system, 267
Swiss-Cheese model
    of accident causation, 65
    accident causation in, 66f
    analogy, 65

T

Team member barriers, 246–248
  fear of backlash, 247
  inadequate policies, 246
  lack of awareness, 247
  misperception of downstream effects, 247
  rationalization, 247
  user-friendly reporting systems, lack of, 246–247
Teams
  behavior, 119 (*See also* Debriefing)
  component of, 114
  definition of, 105
  effective, 112–113, 126
    activities of, 113
    comprised of, 112–113
    essential behaviors for, 113
  high-performing, 114
  members, 270
Team STEPPS curriculum, 135, 147, 148
Team STEPPS™ National implementation program, 196
Teamwork, communication and, 66, 112–113, 129–152
  achieving high-functioning teams, 146–148
  emergency department
    discussion, 133–136
    learning points, 136
  learning from errors, 147*f*
  pediatrician's office, 130, 144–145
    discussion, 131–132, 145–146
    learning points, 132, 146
  pediatric intensive care unit, daily rounds, 140
    discussion, 140–142
    learning points, 142
  pediatric intensive care unit, next day, 142–143
    discussion, 143–144
    learning points, 144
  pediatric intensive care unit, patient handoff from operating room, 136–137
    discussion, 136–137, 137–139
    learning points, 139–140
  TeamSTEPPS™ framework, 148*f*
Tennessee Initiative for Perinatal Quality Care (TIPQC), 215
Test cycles, 11

Therac-25, 169
To Err is Human, 52, 157, 181, 240
Total parenteral nutrition (TPN), 51, 55
Toyota Production System (TPS), 12, 118
Training
  importance of, 269
Transfusion-feeding protocol, 225
Transfusion of prematures (TOP) trial, 213
Transparency, 107, 187, 191
  visibility and, 123–125
Triggers, 167*t*, 168
  real-time (*See* Real-time trigger)

U

Unintended variation
  types of, 19
    common cause variation (*See* Random variation)
    special cause variation (*See* Assignable variation)
Unprofessional behavior, 278
US Agency for Healthcare Research and Quality (AHRQ), 28

V

Vanderbilt University Medical Center (VUMC) leaders, 275
Ventilator-associated pneumonia (VAP), 252
Vermont Oxford Network (VON), 212–213, 228
  database, 213
  harm distribution to adverse drug events in, 217*t*
Veteran's Affairs Administration, 166
Violations
  producing conditions, 64
  of safe practice, 63
Visibility and transparency, definition of, 107

W

White spaces, 194
World Health Organization (WHO), 228
  program, 187

Y

You Are Here chart, 276, 276*f*
Your Baby's Daily Update (YBDU), 192